Diagnosis and Treatment of Male Sexual Dysfunction

Rupin Shah • Hyun Jun Park • Ashok Agarwal
Editors

Diagnosis and Treatment of Male Sexual Dysfunction

Controversies, Advances and Future Developments

Springer

Editors
Rupin Shah
Department of Urology
Lilavati Hospital & Research Centre
Mumbai, India

Ashok Agarwal
Global Andrology Forum
Moreland Hills, OH, USA

Hyun Jun Park
Department of Urology
Pusan National University Hospital, Pusan
National University School of Medicine
Busan, Korea (Republic of)

ISBN 978-3-032-12422-7 ISBN 978-3-032-12423-4 (eBook)
https://doi.org/10.1007/978-3-032-12423-4

This Springer imprint is published by the registered company Springer Nature Switzerland AG
The registered company address is: Gewerbestrasse 11, 6330 Cham, Switzerland

Foreword

The concept of male sexual dysfunction is as old as human history and was first described in ancient Egyptian and Mesopotamian texts. The Ebers Papyrus (circa 1550 BC) mentions male erectile difficulties and decreased libido, while in Mesopotamian civilization the "weakness of male power" was considered both a medical and mystical phenomenon. During the periods of Ancient Greece and Rome (fifth century BC to second century AD), the works of Hippocrates, Aristotle, and Galen began to explain male sexual functions based on physiological processes. Galen associated erectile dysfunction with "deficiency of neural stimulation or vascular obstruction" of the penis.

Modern andrology, built upon these historical foundations, reached a significant turning point in 1983 when the mechanism of erection was elucidated at the neurovascular level [1]. Since then, advances in anatomy, physiology, and pathophysiology have led to revolutionary developments in the diagnosis and treatment of male sexual dysfunction. Today, the global prevalence of erectile dysfunction ranges between 35% and 45%, rising to 52% among men over the age of forty. This corresponds to approximately 1.1 billion men affected worldwide.

This book has been prepared from a broad perspective encompassing the anatomy and physiology, epidemiology, medical, regenerative, and surgical treatments of male sexual dysfunction, as well as its psychosexual dimensions. Topics such as Peyronie's disease, anhedonia and orgasmic disorders, priapism, sexual pain in men, onco-sexology, onco-fertility, and premature ejaculation are addressed in light of current literature by experts from the Global Andrology Forum (GAF). The GAF, under the leadership of Professor Agarwal, and the academics contributing to this book should be congratulated for this excellent update.

I sincerely believe that this comprehensive work will serve as a valuable resource for clinicians and researchers in the field of sexual medicine.

Ateş Kadıoğlu, MD

FECSM Professor of Urology
Chairman of Section of Andrology
University of Istanbul
Istanbul, Turkey
10.26.2025

Reference

1. Lue TF, Zeineh SJ, Schmidt RA, Tanagho EA. Physiology of penile erection. World J Urol. 1983;1(4):194–6. https://doi.org/10.1007/BF00326801

Preface

Male sexual dysfunction (MSD) is a highly prevalent condition that affects men across all ages and backgrounds, influencing not only their sexual health but also their psychological well-being, interpersonal relationships, and overall quality of life. Because its etiology is diverse and multifactorial, patients with erectile dysfunction (ED) and related disorders present across various medical specialties, requiring clinicians to possess both breadth and depth of understanding.

In daily practice, the management of MSD is often simplified to prescribing phosphodiesterase type 5 inhibitors. However, contemporary care extends far beyond this approach. Advances in epidemiology, neurovascular and hormonal physiology, and psychosocial determinants have led to more sophisticated frameworks for evaluation and patient-centered treatment. Expanded therapeutic options, ranging from oral and injectable pharmacotherapies to device-based interventions, surgical reconstruction, and psychosexual support, are now being complemented by newer modalities such as low-intensity shockwave therapy and platelet-rich plasma injections. Although these innovations are rapidly gaining popularity, their adoption should be driven by rigorous evidence appraisal and standardized clinical protocols, which remain an urgent unmet need.

This book aims to provide clinicians with a comprehensive, up-to-date, and practical resource for the evaluation and management of male sexual dysfunction. Each chapter integrates foundational principles with current evidence, guideline recommendations, and real-world clinical considerations. A notable strength of this volume is its global multi-authorship, which brings together diverse expertise and reflects the international nature of men's health practice.

We extend our heartfelt appreciation to 24 contributors from 12 countries whose scholarship, insight, and dedication have brought this volume to fruition. Their collective expertise and unwavering commitment to advancing male reproductive health have shaped this book into an authoritative and impactful resource. We are equally grateful for the invaluable guidance of Lillie Mae Gaurano, Springer Editor for Clinical Medicine Books, and the meticulous coordination of Janaki Srinivasan,

Production Editor. Their professionalism, thoughtful oversight, and steadfast support were instrumental in ensuring the successful completion of this project.

We hope that this book serves not only as an educational reference but also as a catalyst for thoughtful, evidence-based, and empathetic care for men with sexual dysfunction.

Mumbai, India Rupin Shah
Busan, Republic of Korea Hyun Jun Park
Moreland Hills, OH, USA Ashok Agarwal

Contents

About the Editors

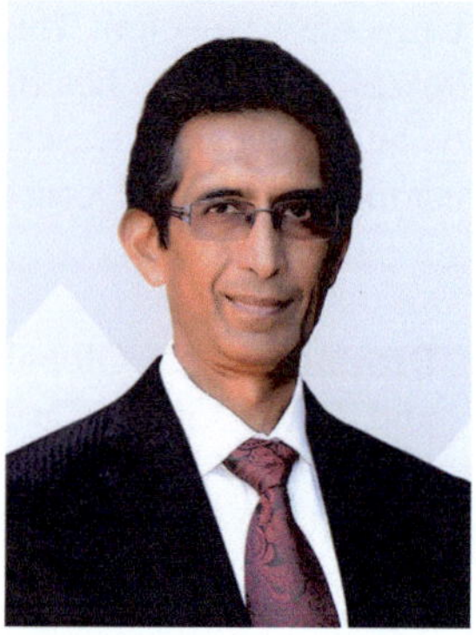

Rupin Shah is a Microsurgeon and Consultant Andrologist at the Lilavati Hospital & Research Centre, Mumbai and the Sir H N Reliance Hospital, Mumbai.

His special interest is microsurgery for male infertility, and he has pioneered reconstructive microsurgery and microsurgical sperm retrieval procedures in India.

His other major interest is the surgery for impotence, an area in which he has made numerous pioneering contributions. In 1994, he was awarded the President's video prize of the International Society of Impotence Research at the 6th World Meeting of Impotence for a new technique of microsurgical penile revascularization. He has developed the Shah penile prosthesis which is the first Indian penile prosthesis and is the most widely used penile implant in India today.

He has presented and published numerous papers and review articles. He has co-edited four books and has contributed 35 book chapters. He has held various academic positions including co-chair of the International Consultation on Sexual Medicine and is on the editorial board of "Sexual Medicine Reviews" and "Fertility and Reproduction". He is the recipient of the prestigious Dr B C Roy Award from the President of India for his role in developing Andrology in India.

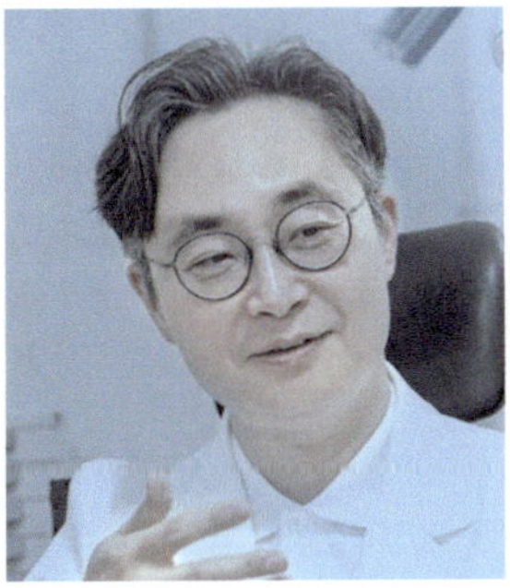

Hyun Jun Park, MD, PhD graduated from Pusan National University College of Medicine, Korea, in 1998 and first joined the Department of Urology at his alma mater in 2004 as a professor. He has been serving as an editor in chief for the *World Journal of Men's Health*. He has also been active in various academic societies, including the International Society for Sexual Medicine, Asian Society for Men's Health and Aging, Asia-Pacific Society for Sexual Medicine, Korean Association for Sexology, Korean Society for Sexual Medicine and Andrology, Korean Society for Men's Health and Aging, and Korean Society for Reproductive Medicine. Currently he is working as a Professor in the Department of Urology, Pusan National University School of Medicine and Pusan National University Hospital. The main focus of his clinical and research interests lies in sexual medicine, male infertility, and prostate diseases. He has authored or co-authored more than 180 peer-reviewed publications in international journals.

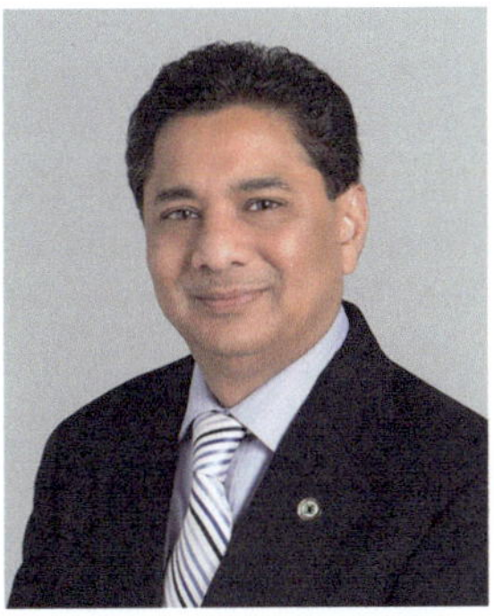

Ashok Agarwal is Director of Research at the Global Andrology Forum, Cleveland, and Professor at Case Western Reserve University. Former Head of Clinical Andrology at Cleveland Clinic (1993–2022), he is a globally recognized leader in male infertility and assisted reproduction, with over 1,030 publications, 250 book chapters, and over 50 edited textbooks. As President of the Global Andrology Foundation (2022–present), a non-profit research organization with over 900 members from 95 countries, his current focus is on promoting international collaboration through research, global surveys, and the development of evidence-based practice guidelines in male infertility and sexual medicine.

Chapter 1
Introduction to Male Sexual Dysfunction (MSD)

Balasingam Balagobi, Gokhan Calik, and Ahmed El-Sakka

Introduction

Male sexual function is a complex physiological process that is one of the most important aspects of normal physical, emotional, and psychosocial well-being. Maintaining normal sexual function depends on the involvement of multiple systems—endocrine, cardiovascular, reproductive, and nervous systems, in addition to psychiatric status [1]. Affected factors, including psychosocial ones, can impact normal sexual function.

Due to the increasing lifespan and the high incidence of MSD in the aging population, a further increase in the number of patients with MSD may be expected [1–5].

Male sexual dysfunction (MSD) refers to the impairment of normal sexual performance and may sometimes result from impaired sexual interest and pleasure [2]. Normal sexual performance includes sexual desire, penile erection, and ejaculation.

Epidemiology

MSD is common among all ages, cultures, and ethnicities. The prevalence of sexual dysfunction among males is 31% [3], and the individual types of MSD vary with age, health status, and social factors. Erectile dysfunction (ED) affects

B. Balagobi (✉)
Department of Surgery, Faculty of Medicine, University of Jaffna, Jaffna, Sri Lanka

G. Calik
Department of Urology, Faculty of Medicine, Istanbul Medipol University, Istanbul, Turkey
e-mail: gcalik@medipol.edu.tr

A. El-Sakka
Faculty of Medicine, Suez Canal University, Ismailia, Egypt

R. Shah et al. (eds.), *Diagnosis and Treatment of Male Sexual Dysfunction*,
https://doi.org/10.1007/978-3-032-12423-4_1

approximately 50% of men aged 40–70 and is correlated with conditions such as diabetes and cardiovascular disease [3]. Premature ejaculation (PE) affects 20–30% of men and is linked to psychological factors. Reduced libido, another common issue, can result from hormonal imbalances or medication use [4].

In cross-sectional, office-based studies of more than 1500 male patients, El-Sakka and collaborators demonstrated that ED is highly prevalent, and ED risk factors are also very common in the community [5, 6]. A total of 92.6% of the patients had ED, 50.8% had premature ejaculation (PE), and 7.6% had low sexual desire. Furthermore, 20% of the patients had psychogenic causes, while 80% had organic causes of ED.

Unfortunately, in many countries, there are no solid data regarding the true prevalence of MSD; however, anecdotal reports indicate a high incidence among different age groups and in patients with various comorbidities.

Social and cultural factors influence reporting and treatment-seeking behaviors. Effective management involves a holistic assessment—addressing physical, psychological, and relational aspects—and highlights the need for tailored interventions to improve quality of life.

Significance of Addressing MSD

Addressing male sexual dysfunction is important for several reasons. First, it directly impacts quality of life by influencing self-esteem, relationships, and overall well-being. Effective treatment can enhance intimate relationships and mental health, reducing anxiety and depression that are often associated with sexual performance issues.

MSD can indicate underlying health conditions such as cardiovascular disease or diabetes, which emphasizes the value of managing these conditions for overall health. Unresolved sexual problems can strain marriages or lead to relationship difficulties. Lastly, addressing sexual dysfunction promotes equality in healthcare, ensuring men receive comprehensive care for intimate health concerns. Therefore, comprehensive management of male sexual dysfunction is crucial for both individual and relational health.

Types of MSD

MSD can affect various aspects of sexual function, including desire, arousal, erection, ejaculation, and overall satisfaction. MSD is mainly divided into low libido, ED, and ejaculatory dysfunction, which includes both premature and delayed ejaculation. Other conditions that are included under MSD are Peyronie's disease, priapism, post-orgasmic illness syndrome, and anhedonic orgasm [1]. One third of males will experience one form of the above sexual dysfunctions in their lifetime. Each type may have physical, psychological, or relational causes, necessitating

tailored approaches for diagnosis and treatment. Understanding these types is crucial for addressing the complex nature of male sexual health and enhancing overall well-being.

Low Libido

It refers to a decrease or absence of sexual interest or desire for sexual activity [1]. In aging males, it is one of the most common sexual dysfunctions [4]. This defect can be due to hormonal changes as a result of normal aging, late-onset hypogonadism, neurological and vascular diseases, as well as psychiatric and relationship issues.

Erectile Dysfunction

Erectile dysfunction (ED) is defined as the persistent inability to attain or maintain a penile erection sufficient to permit satisfactory sexual function [7]. ED is commonly classified into three groups based on the etiology—organic, psychogenic, and mixed ED [8]. Organic ED results from diminished blood flow to the penis or nerve dysfunction and is usually associated with cardiovascular disease or cardiometabolic syndrome. In psychogenic ED, there is normal blood flow to the penis and nerve function; patients may achieve erection in some circumstances but not with their partner when they are trying to conceive [8]. ED is frequently associated with certain urological conditions and procedures, including lower urinary tract symptoms (LUTS)/benign prostatic hyperplasia (BPH), chronic pelvic pain syndrome, chronic prostatitis, and urethroplasty surgery for posterior urethral stricture.

Premature Ejaculation (PE)

PE is a common MSD. It is defined as ejaculation occurring without control or shortly after penetration and before the person wishes it [8]. It causes marked distress and interpersonal difficulties.

Even though intravaginal ejaculatory latency time (IELT)—the time from penetration to ejaculation—is not included in this definition, an IELT of <2 minutes and ejaculation before penetration are considered PE [9].

There are many definitions of PE. The WHO defines it as "inability to delay ejaculation sufficiently to enjoy lovemaking, which is manifested by either an occurrence of ejaculation before or very soon after the beginning of intercourse, or ejaculation that occurs in the absence of sufficient erection, making intercourse impossible" [10].

PE refers to the triad of short ejaculatory latency, lack of control over the ability to delay ejaculation, and personal distress. In patients with PE, the normal sexual response cycle is compressed with a sharp excitement phase followed by a short plateau and subsequent ejaculation.

PE is classified into primary (lifelong) and secondary (acquired) forms. Lifelong PE refers to ejaculation that occurs within 1 minute of vaginal penetration. In acquired PE, latency time may be up to 3 minutes or less [8].

Delayed Ejaculation (DE)

Delayed ejaculation (DE) is an uncommon form of MSD. DE refers to the inability to achieve ejaculation or a significant delay in ejaculation. DE is also defined as an IELT threshold beyond 20–25 minutes of sexual activity [11]. The American Psychiatric Association defines it as a marked delay, infrequency, or absence of ejaculation. One of these symptoms persists for at least 6 months and cause distress [12]. However, recent studies suggest that distress is not considered a significant factor [13].

Priapism

Priapism is defined as a penile erection lasting more than 4 hours, which is unrelated to sexual arousal [14]. It is classified into ischemic and non-ischemic subtypes based on the oxygenation of penile tissue. Ischemic priapism is the most common type; it is usually associated with pain and carries the risk of permanent loss of erectile function. Therefore, it requires rapid intervention. Non-ischemic priapism is less common and usually results from perineal trauma. It is typically not painful, and treatment is usually conservative [15]. Recurrent (stuttering) priapism is a variant of ischemic priapism, occurring during sleep and lasting less than 3–4 hours.

Peyronie's Disease

Peyronie's disease is most common after the fifth decade of life. It is an acquired connective tissue disorder of the tunica albuginea of the penis that causes fibrosis [16]. Fibrosis is thought to occur due to trauma to the erect penis during intercourse. It results in a palpable, inelastic plaque that causes penile curvature or deformity. There is an active disease phase, which is associated with severe pain. Even after the pain has resolved, erectile dysfunction is often present along with acquired penile curvature and/or shortening during erections [17].

In a study assessing the prevalence of Peyronie's disease (PD) among patients with ED, El-Sakka reported on a total of 1440 male patients with ED enrolled in this study. Of these, 7.9% had PD. Significant associations between PD and both the longer duration and increased severity of ED were detected. There were also significant associations between PD and the following sociodemographic risk factors of ED: age, obesity, smoking, duration of smoking, and number of cigarettes smoked per day. Concomitant diseases and medical comorbidities such as diabetes, dyslipidemia, psychological disorders, and the presence of at least one risk factor were significantly associated with PD in patients with ED [18].

Post-Orgasmic Illness Syndrome (POIS)

POIS is a rare disorder that causes flu-like and allergic-like symptoms. It most commonly occurs in individuals aged 21–61 years [19]. This is a chronic condition with primary onset during adolescence and secondary onset later in life. The exact pathophysiology is unknown. Symptom onset is usually within seconds, minutes, or hours after ejaculation. Symptoms can occur after masturbation, spontaneous ejaculation, or intercourse [20]. They last for 2–7 days. One or more of the following symptoms can occur: flu-like symptoms, extreme fatigue, muscle weakness, perspiration, mood disturbance or irritability, memory difficulties, concentration problems, incoherent speech, itching eyes, and nasal congestion. The three most common symptoms are fatigue, poor concentration, and irritability [19].

Anhedonic Orgasm

An orgasm involves both cognition and emotion. It requires the brain's ability to process stimuli from the pudendal nerve and the highly pleasurable contraction of sexual organs [21]. It involves the peripheral, central, and autonomic nervous systems and causes a temporary increase in heart rate, blood pressure, and respiratory rate. In anhedonic orgasm, the individual cannot feel pleasure from orgasm.

Risk Factors for MSD

Male sexual dysfunction can arise from a variety of factors, which can be categorized as physical, psychological, or lifestyle-related causes. Common risk factors include:

Aging

As men get older, sexual function can decline due to natural aging processes, associated risk factors, or medical comorbidities.

Medical Conditions

Cardiovascular disease: Conditions such as hypertension, atherosclerosis, and heart disease can affect blood flow to the penis, leading to erectile dysfunction. ED can occur due to hypertension or the use of antihypertensive medications. The prevalence of ED is twice as high compared to normotensive patients [22]. Decline in sexual function after stroke is due to vascular disorders, depression, physical disability, and adverse effects of drugs.

Depending on the severity of the stroke and the part of the brain affected, patients may experience different types of sexual dysfunction (SD). Disinhibited sexual behavior and increased libido are observed in 10% of post-stroke patients [23], although decreased desire and ED are common complaints.

Jackson et al. evaluated the link between ED and coronary artery disease (CAD) and provided a consensus report regarding evaluation and management of ED associated with CAD. They stated that ED can arise before CAD becomes symptomatic, with a time window of 3–5 years. ED and CAD share the same risk factors, and endothelial dysfunction is the common denominator. Treating ED in cardiac patients is safe, provided that their risks are properly evaluated [24].

Diabetes mellitus (DM): It is one of the common causes of MSD. High blood sugar levels can damage blood vessels and nerves, contributing to erectile dysfunction. This results in vascular insufficiency—preventing optimal blood flow to the penis; neuropathy—which prevents nerve conduction; and selective degradation of neuronal nitric oxide (NO) production. These cause failure of erection.

DM causes impotence, erectile dysfunction, ejaculatory disorders (PE or delayed ejaculation), decreased libido, and changes in semen quality.

According to various reports, 59% of diabetic men suffer from ED [25]. The prevalence of ED is three- to fivefold higher in men with DM than in non-diabetic men, affects diabetic men at an earlier age, and increases with the duration of diabetes [26].

Another study reported that, among patients with type 2 diabetes, 86.1% had various degrees of ED: mild in 7.7%, moderate in 29.4%, and severe in 49.1%. The prevalence of ED was 25% in patients younger than 50 years, increasing to 75% in those older than 50 years [27].

In another assessment study on the relation between diabetes and other sexual problems, El-Sakka and Tayeb evaluated the prevalence of Peyronie's disease (PD) in type 2 diabetic patients who were screened for ED. Of a total of 1133 male diabetic patients, 8.1% were diagnosed with PD. Penile plaque and curvature were the most common findings [28]. There were significant associations between a longer duration and poor metabolic control of diabetes and PD [28]. In the same study, they reported that type 2 DM and PD, both independently and together, negatively affect the vascular status of erection. Type 2 DM demonstrated the principal effect; however, the presence of PD has an additive impairment effect on erection and Doppler parameters [29].

Chronic kidney disease (CKD): MSD is common in patients with CKD, especially those with end-stage renal disease [2]. Disruption of the hypothalamic-pituitary-gonadal axis leads to decreased sexual function. Uremia results in ED, low sexual desire, and a reduced ejaculation rate. Some improvement is observed after renal transplant or dialysis.

Neurological disorders: Conditions such as multiple sclerosis, Parkinson's disease, and spinal cord injuries can interfere with nerve signals involved in sexual arousal and erection [2].

Hormonal imbalances: Low testosterone levels (hypogonadism) can lead to decreased libido and erectile dysfunction [30].

Surgery or trauma: Pelvic surgery, especially prostate surgery, can damage the nerves and arteries involved in erections, leading to erectile dysfunction [15]. Trauma to the pelvic area can also affect sexual function [30].

Psychological Factors

Stress: Work-related stress, financial worries, or relationship issues can affect sexual performance [31].

Anxiety: Performance anxiety or generalized anxiety disorders can interfere with sexual function [32].

Depression: Mood disorders can decrease libido and affect arousal [33].

Lifestyle Factors

Smoking: It is an independent risk factor for ED. In the short term, smoking causes alterations in cavernous smooth muscle contractile function and acute vasospasm. The long-term effects are due to increased levels of carbon monoxide and the development of atherosclerotic changes [2].

Alcohol: A small amount of alcohol intake may lead to increased libido or improvement in erectile function. However, excessive intake or chronic use of alcohol leads to hypogonadism and polyneuropathy, causing ED [2].

Drug use: Recreational drugs such as cocaine, heroin, or marijuana can interfere with sexual arousal and performance.

Obesity: Being overweight can lead to conditions such as diabetes and cardiovascular disease, which are risk factors for sexual dysfunction. Obesity is associated with a one- to threefold relative risk for ED. Among patients with ED, 79% were obese or overweight [2].

Lack of exercise: Sedentary lifestyles can contribute to obesity and cardiovascular problems, which in turn affect sexual function.

Poor diet: Diets high in saturated fats and low in fruits, vegetables, and whole grains can contribute to cardiovascular disease and diabetes, which are linked to sexual dysfunction.

Medications: Many commonly used drugs lead to MSD by decreasing libido, interfering with erectile function, or causing retrograde ejaculation. Medications used to treat conditions such as hypertension, depression, anxiety, and prostate disorders can have side effects that affect sexual function.

Drugs with sympatholytic activity inhibit ejaculation and cause retrograde ejaculation by preventing bladder neck closure. Anticholinergic drugs lead to inadequate smooth muscle relaxation within the *corpora cavernosa*, preventing the normal process of erection. Centrally acting drugs cause sedation and decreased libido. Spironolactone increases prolactin levels; as a result, it can cause impotence [2].

Cardiovascular drugs such as digoxin, beta-blockers, statins, psychotropics, histamine-2 receptor antagonists, and certain cytotoxic drugs are associated with ED [2, 30].

Relationship issues: Difficulties in a relationship, lack of communication, or unresolved conflicts can lead to stress and anxiety, which can affect sexual performance [31].

Sleep disorders: Conditions such as sleep apnea or insomnia can disrupt hormone levels and contribute to erectile dysfunction [31, 34].

Environmental factors: Long-term exposure to certain chemicals and toxins, such as pesticides and herbicides, can affect sexual function and reduce sexual desire by altering the hormonal system. Exposure to heavy metals like lead, arsenic, and cadmium can also lead to sexual dysfunction [2].

Identifying and addressing these risk factors through lifestyle changes, medical treatments, therapy, or counseling can often help improve sexual function in men experiencing dysfunction

Impact on Quality of Life

All types of MSD may affect psychosocial health and have a significant impact on the quality of life of the patient and their partner. Usually, men with SD have comorbidities such as depression, anxiety-related disorders, and transient states of altered mood. Relationship factors, including feelings of emotional disconnection from the partner during sexual activity and lack of satisfaction with the partner, are also associated with MSD. This may lead to poor self-esteem and cognitive distraction.

References

1. Nicol A, Chung E. Male sexual dysfunction: clinical diagnosis and management strategies for common sexual problems. Aust J Gen Pract. 2023;52(1–2):41–5. https://doi.org/10.31128/AJGP-09-22-6559. PMID: 36796767.
2. Chen L, Shi GR, Huang DD, Li Y, Ma CC, Shi M, Su BX, Shi GJ. Male sexual dysfunction: a review of literature on its pathological mechanisms, potential risk factors, and herbal drug intervention. Biomed Pharmacother. 2019;112:108585. https://doi.org/10.1016/j.biopha.2019.01.046. Epub 2019 Feb 21. PMID: 30798136.
3. Ramírez-Santos J, Cristóbal-Cañadas D, Parron-Carreño T, Lozano-Paniagua D, Nievas-Soriano BJ. The problem of calculating the prevalence of sexual dysfunction: a meta-analysis attending gender. Sex Med Rev. 2024;12(2):116–26. https://doi.org/10.1093/sxmrev/qead058.
4. Wylie K, Kenney G. Sexual dysfunction and the ageing male. Maturitas. 2010;65(1):23–7. https://doi.org/10.1016/j.maturitas.2009.10.018. Epub 2009 Dec 16. PMID: 20015601.
5. El-Sakka AI. Characteristics of erectile dysfunction in Saudi patients. Int J Impot Res. 2004;16:13–20.
6. El-Sakka AI. Association of risk factors and medical comorbidities with male sexual dysfunctions. J Sex Med. 2007;4(6):1691–700.
7. Ho CC, Singam P, Hong GE, Zainuddin ZM. Male sexual dysfunction in Asia. Asian J Androl. 2011;13(4):537–42. https://doi.org/10.1038/aja.2010.135. Epub 2011 Jun 6. PMID: 21643001; PMCID: PMC3739628.
8. Penzias A, Bendikson K, Butts S, Coutifaris C, Falcone T, Fossum G, Gitlin S, Gracia C, Hansen K, La Barbera A, Mersereau J. Diagnostic evaluation of sexual dysfunction in the male partner in the setting of infertility: a committee opinion. Fertil Steril. 2018;110(5):833–7. https://doi.org/10.1016/j.fertnstert.2018.07.010. PMID: 30316420.
9. Diaz VA Jr, Close JD. Male sexual dysfunction. Prim Care. 2010;37(3):473–89, vii–viii. https://doi.org/10.1016/j.pop.2010.04.002. Epub 2010 Jun 18. PMID: 20705194.
10. Bramer GR. International statistical classification of diseases and related health problems. Tenth revision. World Health Stat Q. 1988;41:32–6.
11. Abdel-Hamid IA, Ali OI. Delayed ejaculation: pathophysiology, diagnosis, and treatment. World J Mens Health. 2018;36(1):22–40. https://doi.org/10.5534/wjmh.17051. PMID: 29299903; PMCID: PMC5756804.
12. DSM V, American Psychiatric Association. Diagnostic and statistical manual of mental disorders. 5th ed. Arlington; 2013. dsm.psychiatryonline.org. Access date: 1 June 2013.
13. Rowland DL, et al. Moving toward empirically based standardization in the diagnosis of delayed ejaculation. J Sex Med. 2020;17:1896. https://pubmed.ncbi.nlm.nih.gov/32828700.
14. Melman A, Serels S. Priapism. Int J Impot Res. 2000;12(Suppl 4):S133–9. https://doi.org/10.1038/sj.ijir.3900592. PMID: 11035401.
15. EUA guidelines on sexual and reproductive health. European Association of Urology. 2024.
16. Feyisetan O. Peyronie's disease: a brief overview. Cureus. 2023;15(4):e37037. https://doi.org/10.7759/cureus.37037.
17. Gabrielsen JS. Peyronie's disease: is it genetic or not? Transl Androl Urol. 2020;9(Suppl 2):S262–8. https://doi.org/10.21037/tau.2019.10.21. PMID: 32257867; PMCID: PMC7108984.
18. El-Sakka AI. Prevalence of Peyronie's disease among patients with erectile dysfunction. Eur Urol. 2006;49(3):564–9.
19. Odusanya BO, Pearce I, Modgil V. Post orgasmic illness syndrome: a review. Int J Impot Res. 2024. https://doi.org/10.1038/s41443-024-00860-3. Epub ahead of print. PMID: 38486122.
20. Paulos MR, Avelliino GJ. Post-orgasmic illness syndrome: history and current perspectives. Fertil Steril. 2020;113(1):13–5. https://doi.org/10.1016/j.fertnstert.2019.11.021. PMID: 32033716.

21. Haney NM, Alzweri LM, Hellstrom WJG. Male orgasmic dysfunction post-radical pelvic surgery. Sex Med Rev. 2018;6(3):429–37. https://doi.org/10.1016/j.sxmr.2017.12.003. Epub 2018 Feb 12. PMID: 29396282.
22. Lou IX, Chen J, Ali K, Chen Q. Relationship between hypertension, antihypertensive drugs and sexual dysfunction in men and women: a literature review. Vasc Health Risk Manag. 2023;19:691–705. https://doi.org/10.2147/VHRM.S439334. PMID: 37941540; PMCID: PMC10629452.
23. Na Y, Htwe M, Rehman CA, Palmer T, Munshi S. Sexual dysfunction after stroke-a biopsychosocial perspective. Int J Clin Pract. 2020;74(7):e13496. https://doi.org/10.1111/ijcp.13496. Epub 2020 Mar 5. PMID: 32100415.
24. Jackson G, Montorsi P, Adams MA, Anis T, El-Sakka A, Miner M, et al. Cardiovascular aspects of sexual medicine. J Sex Med. 2010;7:1608–26.
25. Andlib N, Sajad M, Kumar R, Thakur SC. Abnormalities in sex hormones and sexual dysfunction in males with diabetes mellitus: a mechanistic insight. Acta Histochem. 2023;125(1):151974. https://doi.org/10.1016/j.acthis.2022.151974. Epub 2022 Nov 28. PMID: 36455338.
26. Defeudis G, Mazzilli R, Tenuta M, Rossini G, Zamponi V, Olana S, Faggiano A, Pozzilli P, Isidori AM, Gianfrilli D. Erectile dysfunction and diabetes: a melting pot of circumstances and treatments. Diabetes Metab Res Rev. 2022;38(2):e3494. https://doi.org/10.1002/dmrr.3494. Epub 2021 Sep 21. PMID: 34514697; PMCID: PMC9286480.
27. El-Sakka AI, Tayeb KA. Erectile dysfunction risk factors in non-insulin dependent diabetic Saudi patients. J Urol. 2003;169:1043–7.
28. El-Sakka AI, Tayeb KA. Peyronie's disease in diabetic patients being screened for erectile dysfunction. J Urol. 2005;174:1026–30.
29. El-Sakka AI, Tayeb KA. Vascular impairment of erection in patients with diabetes and Peyronie's disease: is that accumulative? J Sex Med. 2009;6:1736–42.
30. Hatzimouratidis K. Epidemiology of male sexual dysfunction. Am J Mens Health. 2007;1(2):103–25. https://doi.org/10.1177/1557988306298006.
31. Osur J. Factors associated with sexual dysfunctions in Nairobi, Kenya. J Obstet Gynaecol East Cent Afr. 2024;36. https://doi.org/10.59692/jogeca.v36i1.113.
32. Pyke RE. Sexual performance anxiety. Sex Med Rev. 2020;8(2):183–90. https://doi.org/10.1016/j.sxmr.2019.07.001.
33. Waldinger MD. Psychiatric disorders and sexual dysfunction. Handb Clin Neurol. 2015;130:469–89. https://doi.org/10.1016/B978-0-444-63247-0.00027-4. PMID: 26003261.
34. Belladelli F, Li S, Zhang CA, Del Giudice F, Basran S, Muncey W, Glover F, Seranio N, Fallara G, Montorsi F, Salonia A. The association between insomnia, insomnia medications, and erectile dysfunction. Eur Urol Focus. 2024;10:139–45. https://doi.org/10.1016/j.euf.2023.08.005.

Chapter 2
Anatomy and Physiology of Male Sexual Dysfunction

Satish P. Dipankar

Learning Objectives
- To understand the gross and microscopic anatomy of the male reproductive system.
- To understand the physiology of male sexual function and dysfunction.

Introduction

Male sexual function is a complex process involving the neurological, vascular, hormonal, and psychological systems. The key stages are as follows: *Desire (Libido)*—driven primarily by testosterone and emotional factors; *Erection*—triggered by nerve signals that relax the penile smooth muscle, allowing blood flow into the penis; *Ejaculation*—a reflexive process regulated by sympathetic nerves and involving rhythmic muscle contractions; *Detumescence*—the return to a flaccid state as blood drains from the penis.

Male sexual dysfunction (MSD) encompasses conditions such as erectile dysfunction (ED), premature ejaculation (PE), and low libido. These issues, which are more common than often realized, can significantly affect a man's quality of life, mood, and relationships. Understanding the anatomy and physiology of the male reproductive system, including its role in hormone production, is crucial for accurately diagnosing and treating these conditions. The system includes both external and internal organs. The external organs are the scrotum, testes, and penis. The internal organs are the epididymis, vas deferens, seminal vesicles, prostate gland, bulbourethral glands, and urethra.

S. P. Dipankar (✉)
Department of Physiology, All India Institute of Medical Sciences,
Mangalagiri, Andhra Pradesh, India

R. Shah et al. (eds.), *Diagnosis and Treatment of Male Sexual Dysfunction*,
https://doi.org/10.1007/978-3-032-12423-4_2

External Reproductive Organs

Scrotum

The scrotum is a thick, fibromuscular, cutaneous pouch located below the penis that contains the external spermatic fascia, two testes, the epididymis, and the vas deferens (Figs. 2.1 and 2.2).

The layers of the scrotum, from the outside to the inside; are as follows:

Outer layer It consists of various tissues, including skin, smooth muscle, connective tissue, and serous membrane. The skin is the outermost layer and contains sweat glands and hair follicles.

Dartos muscle It is a smooth muscle located beneath the scrotal skin. When the dartos muscle contracts, the scrotal skin wrinkles and tightens, helping to regulate the temperature of the testes.

Cremaster muscle It is a paired structure made up of thin layers of both striated and smooth muscle. The muscle's name comes from the Greek word "suspender." In reality, it has two parts: a lateral and a medial cremaster muscle. The cremaster is an involuntary muscle responsible for the cremasteric reflex [1].

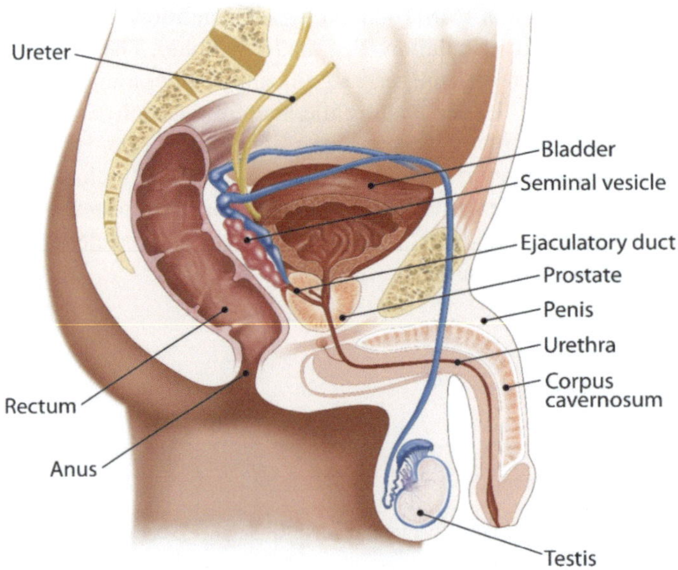

Fig. 2.1 Male reproductive system (sagittal view)

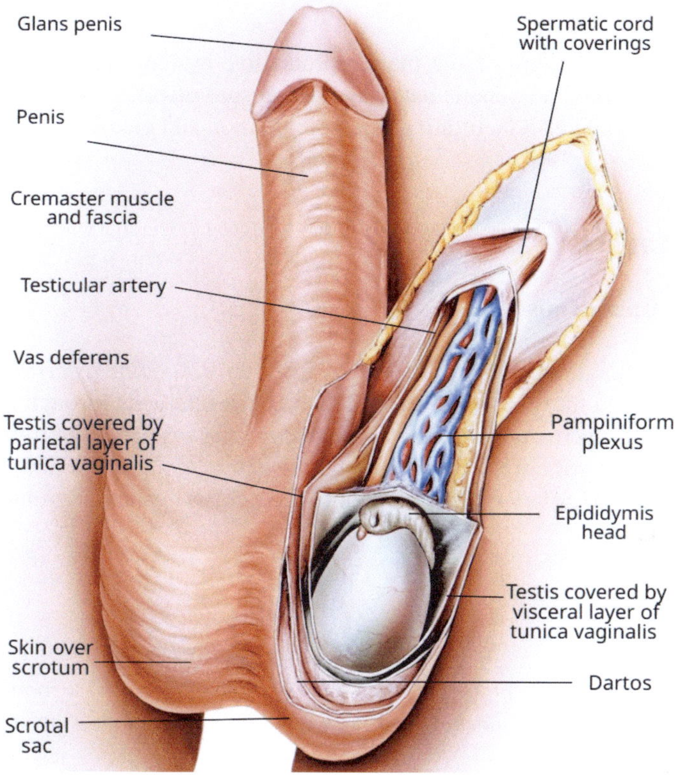

Fig. 2.2 Scrotum and testis

Tunica dartos This layer of connective tissue encircles the dartos muscle, providing structural support to the scrotum.

Scrotal septum A connective tissue septum separates the scrotum into two compartments, each holding one testis.

The testes are located within the scrotum, a skin-covered, heavily pigmented, and muscular sac that is positioned behind the penis and hangs outside the abdominopelvic cavity. This extra-abdominal location plays a vital role in regulating temperature for spermatogenesis. For optimal sperm production in the seminiferous tubules, the temperature needs to be about 2–4 °C lower than the body's core temperature. The scrotal environment maintains this temperature difference through a combination of vascular, muscular, and skin adaptations, helping to preserve the structure and function of germ cell development.

Blood Supply of the Male Reproductive System

The vascular architecture of the male reproductive system comprises a complex interplay of arterial and venous pathways that ensure effective delivery of oxygen and nutrients, while also facilitating thermoregulation and erectile physiology.

Arterial Supply

Testes and Epididymis

The primary blood supply to the testes is from the *testicular arteries*, which are direct branches of the abdominal aorta. These arteries descend through the inguinal canal within the spermatic cord. This course also involves the *cremasteric artery* (a branch of the inferior epigastric artery) and the *artery to the vas deferens* (a branch of the inferior vesical artery), which supply the epididymis and surrounding structures as well [2].

Scrotum

The scrotal wall receives blood from the *external pudendal arteries* (branches of the femoral artery) and the *internal pudendal arteries* (branches of the internal iliac artery) [3].

Penis

The *internal pudendal artery* is the principal arterial supply to the penis. It branches into:

- *Dorsal arteries of the penis*: Supply the skin and fascia.
- *Deep arteries of the penis (cavernosal arteries)*: Important for penile erection, supplying the corpora cavernosa.
- *Artery of the bulb of the penis*: Supplies the corpus spongiosum and bulbourethral glands [4].

Accessory Glands

The prostate gland is supplied by the inferior vesical, internal pudendal, and middle rectal arteries. The blood supply to the seminal vesicles and vas deferens comes from branches of the inferior vesical artery, with additional contributions from the dedicated artery to the vas deferens [5].

Venous Drainage

Testes and Epididymis

The venous drainage of the testes is highly specialized. The pampiniform plexus—a network of small veins surrounding the testicular artery in the spermatic cord—plays a crucial role in this process. This plexus functions as a counter-current heat exchanger, cooling arterial blood to help maintain the ideal temperature for spermatogenesis. The veins of the pampiniform plexus eventually merge to form a single testicular vein on each side.

The right testicular vein typically drains directly into the inferior vena cava (IVC).

The left testicular vein drains at a right angle into the left renal vein [6].

Scrotum

Venous drainage of the scrotal wall is via the external pudendal veins, which connect to the great saphenous vein [7].

Penis

The superficial and deep dorsal veins of the penis drain into the internal pudendal veins and the prostatic venous plexus [7].

Accessory Glands

The prostatic venous plexus drains the prostate gland into the internal iliac veins [8].

Testes

The testes are a pair of oval-shaped glands suspended in the scrotum, a pouch that keeps them at a lower temperature, which is essential for sperm production. Each testis, typically measuring 4–5 cm in length, is protected by multiple layers. The outer layer is the *tunica vaginalis*, a double-layered membrane that reduces friction between the testes and the surrounding tissue. Beneath it is the *tunica albuginea*, a tough, fibrous capsule. This capsule thickens at the back to form the mediastinum testis, which sends partitions inward, dividing the testis into 250–300 lobules (Fig. 2.3).

Layers and Coverings

Tunica vaginalis An outer, serous sac derived from the peritoneum, with a parietal layer lining the scrotum and a visceral layer covering the testis itself. This sac contains a small amount of fluid to reduce friction [9].

Tunica albuginea A tough, fibrous capsule of dense, irregular connective tissue that surrounds the testis directly. It extends inward to form septa, which divide the testis into about 250–300 lobules.

Tunica vasculosa The innermost layer, which is a network of blood vessels that lines the lobules [10].

Internal Structures

Seminiferous tubules Coiled tubules within the lobules where spermatogenesis occurs. These tubules are lined with Sertoli cells and developing sperm cells.

Rete testis A network of channels that collect sperm from the seminiferous tubules.

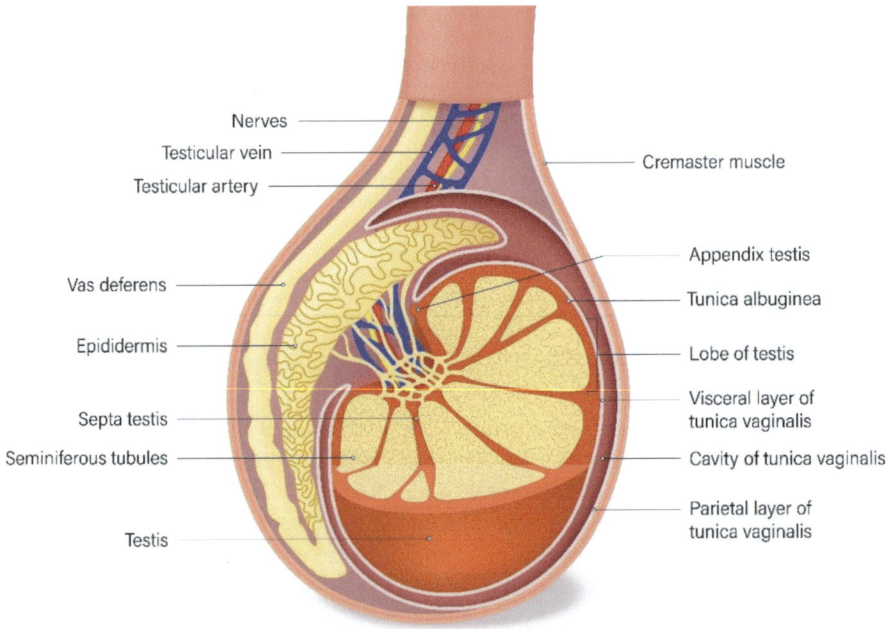

Fig. 2.3 Testis histology

Efferent ductules Small ducts that transport sperm from the rete testis to the epididymis.

Interstitial cells of Leydig Cells located in the connective tissue between the seminiferous tubules. They produce and secrete testosterone and other androgens [11].

Spermatogenesis

Spermatogenesis is the process of male gamete (sperm) development. This intricate and continuous process occurs in the seminiferous tubules of the testes and begins during puberty, continuing throughout a man's life. The entire process takes approximately 64–74 days in humans.

The stages of spermatogenesis are divided into three main stages: spermatocytogenesis, meiosis, and spermiogenesis [12].

Spermatocytogenesis This is the initial phase involving mitotic division. Diploid stem cells called spermatogonia (2n), located at the base of the seminiferous tubules, divide to produce more spermatogonia and a new population of diploid cells called primary spermatocytes (2n). This step ensures a continuous supply of cells for sperm production [13].

Meiosis The primary spermatocytes (2n) then undergo two rounds of meiotic division.

- Meiosis I: Each primary spermatocyte divides into two haploid cells, known as secondary spermatocytes (n). This is a crucial step because it reduces the chromosome number by half.
- Meiosis II: Each secondary spermatocyte divides again, this time into two haploid cells called spermatids (n). As a result, one primary spermatocyte ultimately produces four spermatids [13].

Spermiogenesis This is the final stage, in which the immature, rounded spermatids undergo a remarkable transformation into mature, elongated spermatozoa (sperm). During this process, the cells discard most of their cytoplasm, develop a head containing the condensed nucleus, and form a long, motile tail (flagellum). The Golgi apparatus forms the acrosome, a cap-like structure that covers the head and contains enzymes essential for fertilizing an egg. The mature sperm are then released into the lumen of the seminiferous tubule [13].

Regulation The hypothalamus releases *gonadotropin-releasing hormone* (GnRH). GnRH stimulates the anterior pituitary to secrete *follicle-stimulating hormone* (FSH) and *luteinizing hormone* (LH). FSH targets Sertoli cells, promoting spermatogenesis and the release of *androgen-binding protein* (ABP). LH acts on the interstitial cells of Leydig, stimulating *testosterone* production [14].

Androgen Production (Steroidogenesis)

The testes primarily produce testosterone, a crucial androgen.

Functions of Testosterone

- *Primary sex characteristics*: Development of male reproductive organs (testes, prostate, seminal vesicles) during fetal development and puberty.
- *Secondary sex characteristics*: Appearance of facial and body hair, deepening of the *voice, increased muscle mass, and bone density.*
- *Spermatogenesis*: Essential for the maturation of sperm cells.
- *Libido*: Increases sex drive.
- *Negative feedback loop*: High levels of testosterone and inhibin (a hormone released by Sertoli cells) inhibit the release of GnRH, LH, and FSH, regulating hormone levels [15].

Testicular thermoregulation plays a pivotal role in maintaining male fertility, and its disruption can have several clinically significant consequences for male infertility [16].

Sertoli Cells

These are large, column-shaped cells located in the seminiferous tubules of the testes. Acting as "nurse" cells, they provide physical support and nutrition to the developing sperm cells (spermatogonia, spermatocytes, and spermatids). Sertoli cells are crucial for male fertility and are characterized by their large, irregularly shaped nuclei. They form tight junctions with each other to create the blood-testis barrier (BTB), which protects the developing sperm from the immune system. The BTB divides the seminiferous tubule into two compartments:

- *Basal compartment*: This is where spermatogonia and early primary spermatocytes reside.
- *Adluminal compartment*: This is where later stages of spermatogenesis (meiotic and post-meiotic germ cells) take place [12].

The BTB protects developing sperm cells from the male's immune system. Since sperm cells are haploid and genetically different from the rest of the body, they could be recognized as foreign antigens and attacked by immune cells. The barrier also controls the passage of substances from the blood into the seminiferous tubules, maintaining a stable and protected microenvironment for spermatogenesis [17]. Sertoli cells are essential for the hormonal regulation of spermatogenesis [18]. They secrete androgen-binding protein (ABP), which binds to testosterone and helps concentrate it within the seminiferous tubules. High local concentrations of testosterone are vital for stimulating and maintaining spermatogenesis [19]. Sertoli cells also produce the hormone *inhibin*, which acts on the anterior pituitary gland to inhibit the release of FSH. This establishes a negative feedback loop that regulates the rate of spermatogenesis [20]. Additionally, Sertoli cells secrete *activin*, which can stimulate FSH secretion. The balance between inhibin and activin helps finely tune hormonal control [21]. During fetal development, Sertoli cells release *anti-Müllerian hormone* (AMH), which causes the regression of the Müllerian ducts (the primordia of the female reproductive tract), a crucial step in male sexual differentiation [22]. As sperm cells mature, they shed excess cytoplasm, and Sertoli cells act as phagocytes, engulfing and degrading this residual cytoplasm—an essential process for the final maturation of sperm. They also phagocytose degenerating germ cells [23]. Sertoli cells produce testicular fluid, which is vital for transporting non-motile sperm from the seminiferous tubules to the rete testis and epididymis. Therefore, Sertoli cells are indispensable to spermatogenesis, functioning as the "nurses" that support and nourish developing sperm, the "gatekeepers" that safeguard the protected environment through the blood-testis barrier, and the "regulators" that release hormones to oversee the entire process [24].

Germ Cells

These are a special category of cells that are responsible for producing gametes, which are necessary for sexual reproduction and for passing on genetic information to the next generation. They are distinct from somatic cells, which comprise all the other cells that make up the body's tissues and organs [25].

Primordial Germ Cells (PGCs) The first germ cells to be set aside during early embryonic development are called primordial germ cells (PGCs) [26]. PGCs originate very early in the embryo's development, outside the developing gonads. They then undertake a long journey, migrating through the embryo's tissues to colonize the developing gonads (the testes in males and ovaries in females). Once they arrive, they differentiate into the specific germ cells for that sex: spermatogonia in males and oogonia in females [27].

Sperm Sperm are smaller than most body cells, and 100–300 million are produced daily. Sperm have a head, mid-piece, and tail, with the head containing a compact nucleus and an acrosome.

Sperm Transport Sperm must travel from the seminiferous tubules through the epididymis and out of the body during ejaculation [28].

Epididymis

The epididymis is a vital part of the male reproductive system, found in most male vertebrates. It is a long, coiled tube located on the back of each testicle within the scrotum. It has the following parts:

- *Head (caput)*: The broad, superior end of the epididymis, where sperm from the testes first enter. At this point, the sperm are immature and nonmotile. The head is also responsible for absorbing excess fluid, which concentrates the sperm.
- *Body (corpus)*: The central part of the epididymis, where sperm begin to gain motility.
- *Tail (cauda)*: The most distal part of the epididymis, located at the bottom of the testicle. This is the primary site for storing mature sperm. The tail connects directly to the vas deferens, the tube that carries sperm away from the epididymis during ejaculation [29].

The primary functions of the epididymis are:

- *Sperm maturation*: As sperm travel through the epididymis, a process that can take several days, they undergo significant changes. They mature and acquire the ability to swim (motility) and fertilize an egg.
- *Sperm storage*: The tail of the epididymis serves as a storage reservoir for mature sperm, holding them until ejaculation. Sperm mature in the epididymis, taking about 12 days to traverse its length. More mature sperm are stored in the tail of the epididymis until they are ejaculated.
- *Sperm transport*: The smooth muscle contractions of the epididymis propel sperm from the testes toward the vas deferens.

Vas Deferens

The ductus deferens, also known as the vas deferens, is a muscular tube that follows a distinct path, carrying sperm from the epididymis to the urethra. It ascends from each testis within the spermatic cord, passes through the inguinal canal, and enters the pelvic cavity. After looping over the bladder, it joins the seminal vesicle duct to form the ejaculatory duct. During sexual arousal, muscular contractions of its walls push sperm forward, where they mix with seminal fluids to create semen.

Seminal Vesicles

These are a pair of accessory glands—also known as vesicular glands—located in the male reproductive system. Situated behind the bladder, they produce a significant portion of the seminal fluid that contributes to semen. Each seminal vesicle is a coiled tube that connects with the vas deferens to form the ejaculatory duct, which passes through the prostate gland and opens into the urethra.

Their primary function is to secrete a fluid that makes up 60–70% of the semen's volume. This fluid is alkaline to neutralize the acidic environment of the urethra and vagina, which is crucial for sperm survival. The fluid consists of nutrients—including fructose, citric acid, prostaglandins, and fibrinogen. Components of seminal fluid include fructose, prostaglandins, and clotting factors. Fructose is not produced anywhere else in the body except in the seminal vesicles. It provides a forensic test in rape cases. Nutrients help support sperm until fertilization occurs; prostaglandins may also assist by softening the mucus of the cervix and by causing reverse contractions of parts of the female reproductive tract, such as the fallopian tubes, to ensure that sperm are less likely to be expelled [30].

During ejaculation, sympathetic nerves of the autonomic nervous system stimulate the seminal vesicles to contract. This contraction expels their fluid, which then mixes with sperm and prostatic secretions [31].

Prostate Gland

The prostate gland is a small, walnut-sized exocrine gland that is located in the pelvis, below the bladder, and above the urogenital diaphragm. It has an average weight of about 11 g, usually ranging between 7 and 16 g. The urethra, which carries urine from the bladder and semen from the reproductive ducts, passes directly through the prostate [32]. Anatomically, the prostate is divided into several lobes and zones. An elastic, fibromuscular capsule surrounds it and contains glandular and connective tissue [44].

Prostatic fluid, characterized by its slightly alkaline, milky, or white appearance, constitutes 20–30% of the total semen volume. Its alkalinity helps neutralize the acidity of the vaginal tract, prolonging the lifespan of sperm. The prostatic fluid is expelled in the first part of the ejaculate, together with most of the sperm. This expulsion is a result of the intricate action of smooth muscle tissue within the prostate, highlighting the complexity of the reproductive process. In comparison with the few spermatozoa expelled together with mainly seminal vesicular fluid, those in prostatic fluid have better motility, more prolonged survival, and better protection of genetic material. With prostatic infection, the pH of prostatic fluid increases markedly [33]. The key components of prostatic fluid include citric acid, prostate-specific antigen (PSA), seminal plasmin, acid phosphatase, zinc, and others.

During ejaculation, the smooth muscle of the prostate contracts under sympathetic nervous system control, pushing prostatic fluid into the urethra. There, it mixes with sperm from the testes and fluid from the seminal vesicles to form semen. The combined fluids create an optimal environment for sperm survival and motility, aiding successful fertilization [34].

Bulbourethral Glands

Known as Cowper's glands, they are a pair of small, pea-sized exocrine glands located below the prostate, with one on each side of the membranous urethra within the urogenital diaphragm of the pelvic floor. Each gland has a duct approximately 2.5 cm long, which passes through the penile bulb and opens into the proximal part of the penile urethra. The glands consist of lobules containing numerous acini lined with columnar epithelium. They are surrounded by smooth muscle fibers, which assist in expelling their secretions [35]. The glands produce a clear, viscous fluid called pre-ejaculate fluid, also known as Cowper's fluid. This fluid is released into the urethra before semen is ejaculated. It serves as a lubricant for the urethra, helping to prepare it for the passage of semen. This is especially important for facilitating the movement of sperm and semen through the urethra. The bulbourethral fluid is alkaline, and its secretion helps neutralize any residual acidity from urine in the male urethra.

The fluid helps flush out any remaining urine, debris, or bacteria from the urethra, creating a cleaner and more favorable environment for semen to pass through [36].

Penis

The penis is an external male sex organ through which males urinate and ejaculate semen (Fig. 2.4). Parts of the penis include the root, shaft, glans, epithelium, skin over the shaft, and the foreskin covering the glans. In its flaccid state, the penis is smaller, and the foreskin covers the glans. During an erection, the penis can be straight or curved, pointing upward, downward, or straight. The average erect human penis measures 13.12 cm (5.17 inches) in length, with a circumference of 11.66 cm (4.59 inches). The size of the flaccid penis does not predict erectile length as men age [15]. Nonsexual erections occur during REM sleep (the stage during which dreaming occurs).

Penile Anatomy

The penis is divided into three parts: the root, shaft, and glans [37].

Root Also called the radix penis, which is the most proximal or internal part of the penis. It is not visible externally and is located within the perineum, the area between the anus and the scrotum. Key structures of the root include the erectile tissues, or crura, which are two diverging proximal projections of the corpora cavernosa attached to the ischiopubic arch. The root of the penis plays a vital role in both erection and urination.

The erectile tissues fill with blood during sexual arousal, aiding in erection. The muscles connected to the root help sustain the erection and assist in expelling urine and semen from the urethra [38].

Shaft Also referred to as the body of the penis; it is the elongated part that extends from the root. It contains the urethra, through which both urine and semen pass. The shaft is composed of two cylindrical masses of erectile tissue and one urethra.

The two erectile tissues are as follows:

(i) *Corpora cavernosa*: Two large cylinders of erectile tissue running along the dorsal side of the penile shaft. Each corpus cavernosum begins at the root, where it attaches to the crus of the penis, and extends through the shaft, ending near the glans. Cavernosal arteries run along the center of each corpus cavernosum. Each corpus cavernosum is surrounded by the tunica albuginea, a dense, fibroelastic connective tissue. The tunica albuginea has an inner circular layer and an outer longitudinal layer, forming an incomplete septum between the two corpora. The corpora cavernosa are filled with interconnected vascular spaces (sinusoids) lined by endothelium, separated by fibrous septae rich in smooth muscle. During erection, these spaces fill with blood, compressing venous outflow and resulting in penile rigidity. The deep fascia of the penis, known as Buck's fascia, is a strong layer that encloses the erectile tissues and is continuous with the fascia covering the crura and bulb muscles. The tunica albuginea is a dense, fibroelastic layer that forms separate capsules around the corpora cavernosa, helping to maintain their shape during an erection. Ligaments include the suspensory ligament, which connects the erectile bodies to the pubic symphysis, and the fundiform ligament, which descends from the linea alba and encircles the root of the penis, providing support. The corpora cavernosa mainly ensure penile rigidity during an erection (Fig. 2.5).

(ii) *Corpus spongiosum*: The corpus spongiosum is a single column of erectile tissue that runs along the ventral (underside) of the penis, between the two corpora cavernosa. It begins proximally as the bulb of the penis, located in the superficial perineal pouch. Distally, it expands to form the glans penis, which caps the corpora cavernosa. The urethra runs through the middle of the corpus spongiosum. It encloses the spongy (penile) urethra and extends from the perineum to the tip of the penis. The tunica albuginea also surrounds it, although this layer is thinner than that surrounding the corpora cavernosa. The corpus spongiosum contains the spongy (penile) urethra and extends distally to form the glans penis. Its primary role is to prevent the urethra from collapsing during an erection, keeping a clear channel for ejaculation and urination [39].

The proximal part forms the bulb of the penis, while the distal expansion forms the glans.

Glans The rounded end of the penis. It is a highly sensitive structure, rich in nerve endings. This sensitivity is a key aspect of its function. It is covered by the prepuce, or foreskin, in uncircumcised males. The *corona* is the raised rim or ridge at the base

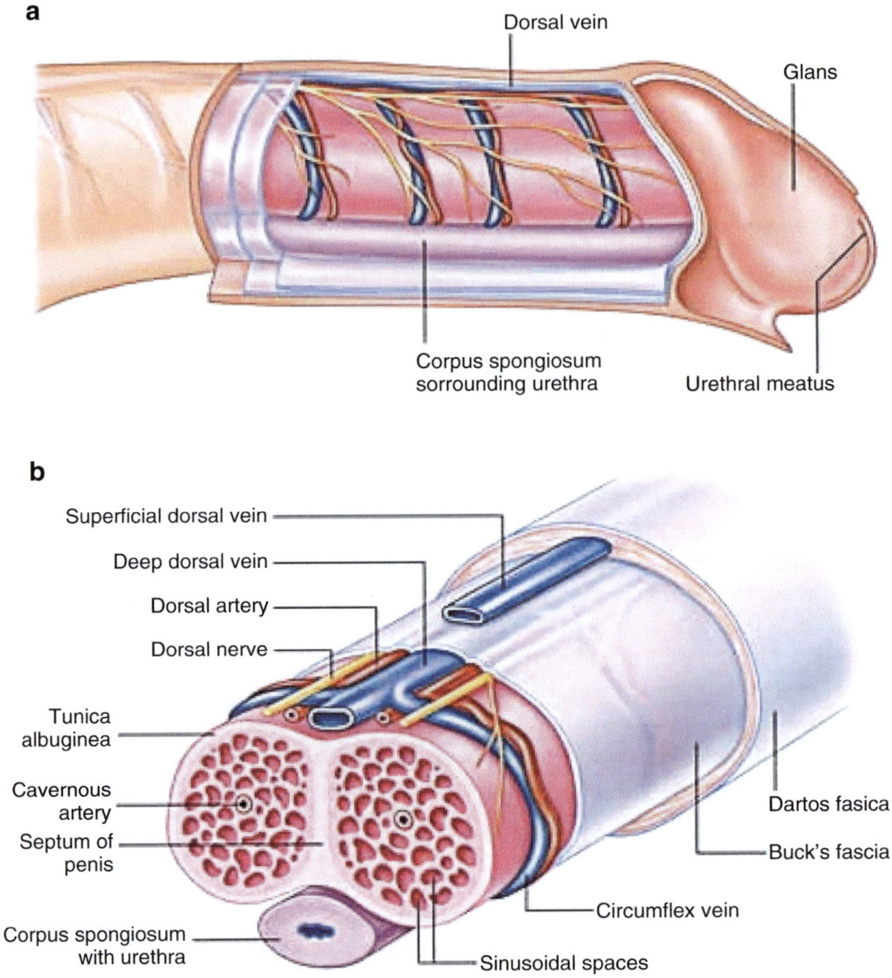

Fig. 2.4 Penis and its erectile tissues

of the glans, where it meets the penile shaft. The *meatus*, located at the very tip of the glans, is the opening for both urine and semen. It is also known as the external urethral orifice, serving as the exit point for these fluids. The *frenulum* is a small, sensitive band of tissue located on the underside of the glans, connecting it to the shaft. It plays a significant role in sexual pleasure, enhancing the understanding of male genital anatomy.

Blood Supply

The penis receives a complex dual blood supply system, consisting of arterial inflow and venous outflow mechanisms, with the venous system playing a critical role in erectile function through specialized structures, including intertrabecular veins and the subtunica venous plexus [40].

Arterial blood supply The *internal pudendal artery* provides the main arterial blood supply to the penis, originating as a branch of the *internal iliac artery* and becoming the *common penile artery* distally. The common penile artery divides into three distinct branches:

- *Cavernous arteries*: Supply the corpora cavernosa and branch into *helicine arteries* throughout each corporal body.
- Dorsal arteries: Supply blood to the glans penis during engorgement.
- *Bulbourethral arteries*: Supply the corpus spongiosum and penile bulb.

The helicine arteries are *resistance vessels* that supply the trabecular tissue and sinusoids of the erectile chambers. In the flaccid state, these arteries are tortuous and

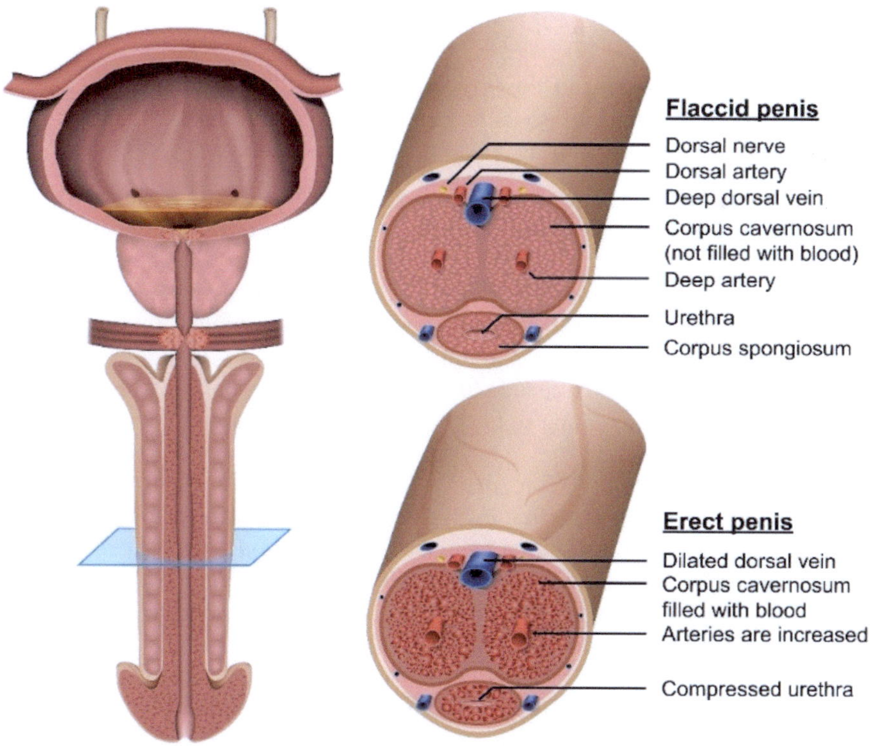

Fig. 2.5 Blood supply of the penis and its erectile tissues

constricted, but during erection, they straighten and dilate to allow blood to fill the corpora cavernosa (Fig. 2.5) [40].

Venous drainage system It operates through a sophisticated network that begins with blood from the peripheral sinusoids traveling through the trabecular network. Blood flows centrifugally from central to peripheral sinusoids in the flaccid state, but during erection, blood rapidly flows to both central and peripheral sinusoids.

The venous system consists of three main groups. *Superficial veins* primarily drain the penile skin and communicate with the deep dorsal veins. *Intermediate veins* include the deep dorsal vein, which drains cavernous tissue. *Deep veins* include the prostatic and crural venous plexuses [41].

Sub-tunica venous plexus It is a critical component of the venous outflow system, located between the tunica albuginea and the peripheral sinusoids. This plexus serves as an intermediate drainage pathway, where blood from the *trabecular network* collects before exiting via *emissary veins.*

Emissary veins and venous outflow Emissary veins serve as the final common pathway for venous drainage, situated between the inner circular and outer longitudinal layers of the tunica albuginea. These veins either drain via the *internal pudendal veins* or communicate with veins that converge on the *deep dorsal vein* and drain via the *periprostatic plexus* [40].

Role in regulating blood outflow by veno-occlusive mechanism The *intertrabecular veins* and *subtunica venous plexus* are essential for this mechanism, which maintains penile erection. During erection, several coordinated events occur:

- *Compression of the subtunical venous plexus*: The expanding sinusoids compress the subtunical venous plexus against the tunica albuginea, reducing venous outflow.
- *Emissary vein occlusion*: Stretching of the tunica albuginea compresses the emissary veins between the sinusoids and the inelastic tunica albuginea, further decreasing venous outflow to a minimum.
- *Pressure dynamics*: The trapped blood raises intracavernous pressure to approximately 100 mmHg, creating rigidity while maintaining blood flow [40].

Physiological regulation The regulation of blood outflow occurs through smooth muscle relaxation and contraction cycles. During sexual stimulation, nitric oxide-induced smooth muscle relaxation causes *arterial dilation*, which increases blood inflow. *Sinusoidal expansion* traps incoming blood. *Venous compression* by the subtunical venous plexuses reduces outflow. *Stretching* of the tunica occludes the emissary veins and minimizes venous drainage [41].

Detumescence process It involves the gradual restoration of venous outflow through the following three phases:

- *Initial phase*: Transient pressure increase as smooth muscles contracts against an occluded venous system.
- *Second phase*: Slow pressure decrease with gradual reopening of venous channels.
- *Final phase*: Rapid pressure decrease with fully restored venous outflow capacity [40].

The *subtunica venous plexus and intertrabecular veins are fundamental to erectile function*, serving as the primary regulators of venous outflow through their compression and decompression during the erectile cycle. This mechanism ensures adequate blood retention for maintaining an erection while allowing controlled drainage during detumescence [40, 41].

Nerve Supply of the Penis

The penis, a marvel of biological engineering, is delicately balanced under the dual control of the autonomic and somatic nervous systems (Fig. 2.6). Each system, with its unique roles, is crucial for the complex function of the penis. The autonomic system, responsible for involuntary functions like blood flow and glandular secretions, works in harmony with the somatic system, which provides sensory input and voluntary motor control.

Autonomic innervation The autonomic nervous system, a key regulator of involuntary functions such as blood flow and gland secretions, controls the automatic processes of penile function (Table 2.1).

Parasympathetic nervous system (PSNS) Responsible for erection (tumescence). Nerve fibers originate from the S2–S4 segments of the sacral spinal cord, forming the pelvic splanchnic nerves. These nerves converge to form the cavernous nerves, which extend to the corpora cavernosa (the primary erectile tissues) of the penis [42]. Upon sexual arousal, these nerves release neurotransmitters, most notably nitric oxide (NO). Nitric oxide causes the smooth muscles within the penile arteries (helicine arteries) and the corpora cavernosa to relax. This relaxation allows a significant increase in blood flow into the erectile tissues, causing them to expand and become rigid. The expanding corpora cavernosa then compresses the veins against the rigid tunica albuginea, trapping the blood and maintaining the erection [43].

Sympathetic nervous system (SNS) It plays a pivotal role in maintaining the flaccid state of the penis, a key aspect of sexual function. Nerve fibers originate from the T11 to L2 segments of the thoracolumbar spinal cord and travel through the hypogastric and pelvic plexuses to reach the penis [44]. In the flaccid state, the sympathetic system maintains a tonic contraction of the penile smooth muscles and arteries, limiting blood flow. During sexual climax, the sympathetic system triggers the emission phase of ejaculation, causing the smooth muscles of the epididymis, vas deferens, seminal vesicles, and prostate to contract, propelling semen into the urethra. Simultaneously, the parasympathetic system, primarily via the pelvic splanchnic nerves, is responsible for the rhythmic contractions of the bulbospongiosus and ischiocavernosus muscles, which are initiated by the somatic nervous system during sexual arousal and orgasm. The expulsion phase, a somatic reflex, follows this. After ejaculation, the sympathetic system reasserts its constricting effect on the penile arteries, leading to the outflow of blood and detumescence (the end of the erection) [45].

Somatic innervation It provides sensory input and voluntary motor control.

Pudendal nerve Provides both sensory and motor innervation to the penis. This large nerve originates from the S2 to S4 segments of the spinal cord. Its main branch is the dorsal nerve of the penis [46].

Sensory role The dorsal nerve of the penis is the primary source of sensory input from the skin of the penile shaft and the highly sensitive glans penis. This sensory information travels back to the central nervous system, contributing to the reflex arcs that control erection and ejaculation.

Motor role The pudendal nerve provides motor innervation to the bulbospongiosus and ischiocavernosus muscles at the base of the penis. The rhythmic contractions of these muscles, initiated by the somatic nervous system during orgasm, are responsible for the forceful expulsion of semen during the final phase of ejaculation [47].

Mechanism of penile erection Penile erections happen because of vasocongestion, where tissues become engorged with blood due to more arterial blood entering the penis than leaving through the veins. During sexual arousal, nitric oxide (NO) is released from nerve endings near blood vessels in the corpora cavernosa and spongiosum. The release of NO activates a signalling pathway that relaxes the smooth muscles around the penile arteries, causing them to dilate. This dilation allows more blood to flow into the penis and prompts the endothelial cells in the arterial walls to release more NO, maintaining vasodilation. The cavernosal arteries dilate, allowing more blood to enter the corpora cavernosa. This increased blood causes the sinusoids to fill and swell, leading to penile tumescence (swelling) and rigidity. As the corpora cavernosa expand, they compress the thin-walled penile venules, preventing blood from draining out. The combined effect of increased blood inflow and restricted outflow results in an erection of the penis [48].

Clinical significance Conditions affecting the cavernosal arteries, such as atherosclerosis, can restrict blood flow and cause erectile dysfunction (ED) [49].

Besides aging, ED is linked to diabetes, vascular issues, mental health conditions, prostate problems, certain medications such as antidepressants, and testicular problems that cause low testosterone levels. These physical and emotional factors can disrupt the vasodilation process and lead to difficulty achieving an erection [50].

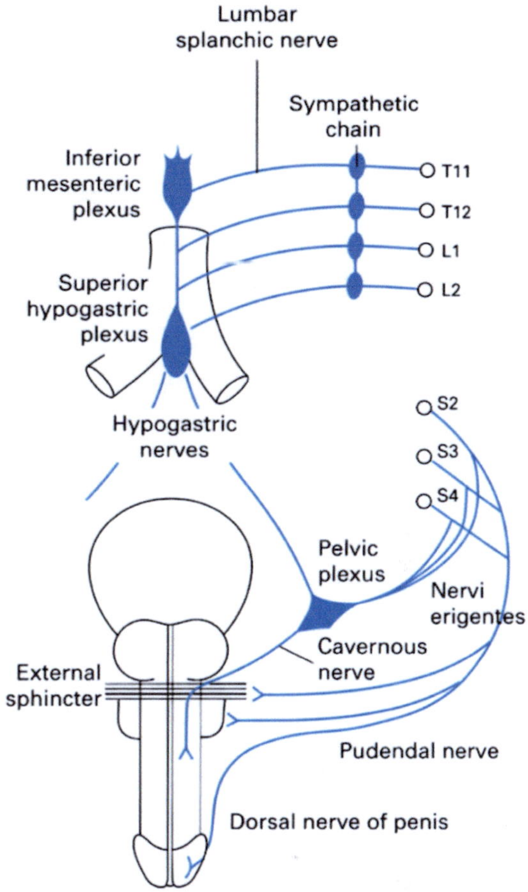

Fig. 2.6 Nerve supply of the penis

Table 2.1 Neural regulation of erection

Nerve system	Origin	Role	Nerves involved
Parasympathetic	Sacral spinal cord segments (S2–S4)	*Erection*: Facilitates tumescence by releasing nitric oxide, which relaxes the smooth muscles of the penile arteries and corpora cavernosa. This allows increased blood flow into the penis and traps it for rigidity (veno-occlusion)	*Pelvic splanchnic nerves*, *Cavernous nerves* (also contain sympathetic fibers)
Sympathetic	Thoracolumbar spinal cord segments (T11–L2)	*Detumescence and flaccidity*: Mediates the return to the flaccid state by releasing norepinephrine, which causes contraction of the smooth muscles in the penile arteries and corpora cavernosa. This restricts blood inflow and increases venous outflow. It also plays a role in ejaculation	*Hypogastric nerves*, Cavernous nerves (also contain parasympathetic fibers)
Somatic	Sacral spinal cord segments (S2–S4)	*Sensation and rigidity*: Provides sensory innervation to the penis, including the glans. Its motor function controls the contraction of the ischiocavernosus and bulbospongiosus muscles, which help to increase and maintain penile rigidity during the "rigid erection" phase	*Pudendal nerve*, *Dorsal nerve of penis* (a branch of the pudendal nerve)

References

1. Mellick LB, Mowery ML, Al-Dhahir MA. Cremasteric Reflex. In: StatPearls [Internet]. Treasure Island (FL): StatPearls Publishing; 2025 Jan–. Updated 2023 Apr 19.PMID: 30020720. Available from: https://www.ncbi.nlm.nih.gov/books/NBK513348/
2. Jones O. The testes and epididymis [Internet]. TeachMeAnatomy; 2023 [cited 2025 Dec 11]. Available from: https://teachmeanatomy.info/pelvis/the-male-reproductive-system/testes-epididymis/.
3. Garcia RA, Sajjad H. Anatomy, Abdomen and Pelvis, Scrotum. 2023 Jul 24. In: StatPearls [Internet]. Treasure Island (FL): StatPearls Publishing; 2025 Jan–. PMID: 31751083. Available from: https://www.ncbi.nlm.nih.gov/books/NBK549893/.
4. Halls JE, Patel DV, Walkden M, Patel U. Priapism: pathophysiology and the role of the radiologist. Br J Radiol. 2012;85 Spec No 1(Spec Iss 1):S79–85.
5. Zaunbrecher N, Arbor TC, Samra NS. Anatomy, abdomen and pelvis: internal iliac arteries. In: StatPearls [Internet]. Treasure Island (FL): StatPearls Publishing; 2025 Jan–. Updated 2023 Jan 17 [cited 2025 Dec 11]. Available from: https://www.ncbi.nlm.nih.gov/books/NBK537311/.
6. Gupta R, Gupta A, Aggarwal N. Variations of gonadal veins: embryological prospective and clinical significance. J Clin Diagn Res. 2015;9(2):AC08–10.
7. Moscovici J, Galinier P, Hammoudi S, Lefebvre D, Juricic M, Vaysse P. Contribution to the study of the venous vasculature of the penis. Surg Radiol Anat. 1999;21(3):193–9.
8. Singh O, Bolla SR. Anatomy, abdomen and pelvis, prostate. Treasure Island: StatPearls; 2023.
9. Garriga V, Serrano A, Marin A, Medrano S, Roson N, Pruna X. US of the tunica vaginalis testis: anatomic relationships and pathologic conditions. RadioGraphics. 2009;29(7):2017–32.

10. Anand Kumar MS. Basics of human andrology. Singapore: Springer Singapore; 2017.
11. Norio Inaba YN. Testis: anatomy, physiology & pathology (human reproductive system – anatomy, roles and disorders). New York: Nova Science; 2012.
12. O'Donnell L, Stanton P, de Kretser DM. Endocrinology of the Male Reproductive System and Spermatogenesis. [Updated 2017 Jan 11]. In: Feingold KR, Ahmed SF, Anawalt B, et al., editors. Endotext [Internet]. South Dartmouth (MA): MDText.com,Inc.;2000. PMID: 25905260. Available from: https://www.ncbi.nlm.nih.gov/books/NBK279031/.
13. Suede SH, Malik A, Sapra A. Histology, Spermatogenesis. 2023 Mar 6. In: StatPearls [Internet]. Treasure Island (FL): StatPearls Publishing; 2025 Jan–. PMID: 31985935. Available from: https://www.ncbi.nlm.nih.gov/books/NBK553142/.
14. Oduwole OO, Peltoketo H, Huhtaniemi IT. Role of follicle-stimulating hormone in spermatogenesis. Front Endocrinol (Lausanne). 2018;9:763.
15. Gunton. Testes. Endocrine Society of Australia; 2023.
16. Hamada A, Esteves SC, Agarwal A. Varicocele and male infertility. Cham: Springer International Publishing; 2016.
17. Jiang XH, Bukhari I, Zheng W, Yin S, Wang Z, Cooke H, et al. Blood-testis barrier and spermatogenesis: lessons from genetically-modified mice. Asian J Androl. 2014;16(4):572.
18. Abel MH, Baker PJ, Charlton HM, Monteiro A, Verhoeven G, De Gendt K, et al. Spermatogenesis and Sertoli cell activity in mice lacking Sertoli cell receptors for follicle-stimulating hormone and androgen. Endocrinology. 2008;149(7):3279–85.
19. Walker WH. Testosterone signaling and the regulation of spermatogenesis. Spermatogenesis. 2011;1(2):116–20.
20. Shah W, Khan R, Shah B, Khan A, Dil S, Liu W, et al. The molecular mechanism of sex hormones on Sertoli cell development and proliferation. Front Endocrinol (Lausanne). 2021;12:648141.
21. Hedger MP, Winnall WR. Regulation of activin and inhibin in the adult testis and the evidence for functional roles in spermatogenesis and immunoregulation. Mol Cell Endocrinol. 2012;359(1–2):30–42.
22. Josso N, Rey RA, Picard JY. Anti-Müllerian hormone: a valuable addition to the toolbox of the pediatric endocrinologist. Int J Endocrinol. 2013;2013:1–12.
23. Wang H, Wang H, Xiong W, Chen Y, Ma Q, Ma J, et al. Evaluation on the phagocytosis of apoptotic spermatogenic cells by Sertoli cells in vitro through detecting lipid droplet formation by Oil Red O staining. Reproduction. 2006;132(3):485–92.
24. Griswold MD. The central role of Sertoli cells in spermatogenesis. Semin Cell Dev Biol. 1998;9(4):411–6.
25. Suzuki A, Kurihara Y, Saga Y. Mechanism of mammalian germ cell development: toward assisted new reproductive technologies. Reprod Med Biol. 2012;11(2):73–7.
26. Clark AT, Gkountela S, Chen D, Liu W, Sosa E, Sukhwani M, et al. Primate primordial germ cells acquire transplantation potential by carnegie stage 23. Stem Cell Rep. 2017;9(1):329–41.
27. Nikolic A, Volarevic V, Armstrong L, Lako M, Stojkovic M. Primordial germ cells: current knowledge and perspectives. Stem Cells Int. 2016;2016(1):1741072.
28. Teves ME, Roldan ERS. Sperm bauplan and function and underlying processes of sperm formation and selection. Physiol Rev. 2022;102(1):7–60.
29. James ER, Carrell DT, Aston KI, Jenkins TG, Yeste M, Salas-Huetos A. The role of the epididymis and the contribution of epididymosomes to mammalian reproduction. Int J Mol Sci. 2020;21(15):5377.
30. John Hall MH. Function of the seminal vesicles. In: Guyton and Hall textbook of medical physiology. 14th ed. Philadelphia: Elsevier; 2020.
31. Hsieh J, Kuo Y, Chang H, Liu S, Chen J, Tsai VFS. The role of sympathetic and parasympathetic nerve systems on the smooth muscle of rat seminal vesicles – experimental results and speculation for physiological implication on ejaculation. Andrology. 2014;2(1):59–64.
32. Leissner KH, Tisell LE. The weight of the human prostate. Scand J Urol Nephrol. 1979;13(2):137–42.

33. Zaichick S, Zaichick V, Nosenko S, Moskvina I. Mass fractions of 52 trace elements and zinc/trace element content ratios in intact human prostates investigated by inductively coupled plasma mass spectrometry. Biol Trace Elem Res. 2012;149(2):171–83.
34. Banerjee PP, Banerjee S, Brown TR, Zirkin BR. Androgen action in prostate function and disease. Am J Clin Exp Urol. 2018;6(2):62–77.
35. Standring S. Gray's anatomy: the anatomical basis of clinical practice. 42nd ed. London: Elsevier; 205AD.
36. Zukerman Z, Weiss DB, Orvieto R. Does preejaculatory penile secretion originating from Cowper's gland contain sperm? J Assist Reprod Genet. 2003;20(4):157–9.
37. Schmidt MH, Schmidt HS. Sleep-related erections: neural mechanisms and clinical significance. Curr Neurol Neurosci Rep. 2004;4(2):170–8.
38. Hsu G, Hsieh C, Wen H, Hsu W, Wu C, Fong T, et al. Anatomy of the human penis: the relationship of the architecture between skeletal and smooth muscles. J Androl. 2004;25(3):426–31.
39. Dwyer ME, Salgado CJ, Lightner DJ. Normal penile, scrotal, and perineal anatomy with reconstructive considerations. Semin Plast Surg. 2011;25(3):179–88.
40. Dean RC, Lue TF. Physiology of penile erection and pathophysiology of erectile dysfunction. Urol Clin N Am. 2005;32(4):379–95.
41. Sangiorgi G, Cereda A, Benedetto D, Bonanni M, Chiricolo G, Cota L, et al. Anatomy, pathophysiology, molecular mechanisms, and clinical management of erectile dysfunction in patients affected by coronary artery disease: a review. Biomedicine. 2021;9(4):432.
42. Tubbs RS, Shoja MM, Loukas M. Abdominal pre- and para-aortic and inferior hypogastric plexuses. In: Nerves and nerve injuries. Elsevier; 2015. p. 647–58.
43. Akorede BA, Hassan SA, Akhigbe RE. Penile erection and cardiovascular function: effects and pathophysiology. Aging Male. 2024;27(1):2336627.
44. Andersson KE, Hedlund P, Alm P. Sympathetic pathways and adrenergic innervation of the penis. Int J Impot Res. 2000;12(Suppl 1):S5–12.
45. Prieto D. Physiological regulation of penile arteries and veins. Int J Impot Res. 2008;20(1):17–29.
46. Kinter KJ, Newton BW. Anatomy, Abdomen and Pelvis, Pudendal Nerve. 2023 Feb 10. In: StatPearls [Internet]. Treasure Island (FL): StatPearls Publishing; 2025 Jan–. PMID: 32134612. Available from: https://www.ncbi.nlm.nih.gov/books/NBK554736/.
47. Weech D, Ameer MA, Ashurst JV. Anatomy, Abdomen and Pelvis, Penis Dorsal Nerve. [Updated 2023 Aug 8]. In: StatPearls [Internet]. Treasure Island (FL): StatPearls Publishing; 2025 Jan-. PMID: 30247841. Available from: https://www.ncbi.nlm.nih.gov/books/NBK525966/.
48. Hsieh C, Wang C, Hsu G, Chen S, Ling P, Wang T, et al. Penile veins play a pivotal role in erection: the haemodynamic evidence. Int J Androl. 2005;28(2):88–92.
49. Mulcahy JJ. Male sexual function: a guide to clinical management. Totowa: Humana Press; 2001.
50. Richard Sadovsky KC. How a primary care clinician approaches erectile dysfunction. In: Breaugh MJ, editor. Male sexual function: a guide to clinical management. Totowa: Humana Press; 2001.

Chapter 3
Erectile Dysfunction: Epidemiology and Diagnosis

Luca Boeri, Tuncay Toprak, and Selahittin Çayan

Introduction

Erectile dysfunction (ED) is defined as the consistent inability to attain or maintain an erection sufficient to perform satisfactory sexual intercourse [30]. ED is a common male problem at all ages and exerts a great impact on the quality of life of sufferers and their partners. Epidemiological studies have shown that more than 150 million men worldwide have ED in different extents [20]. Due to racial and regional differences as well as different definitions of ED, there is a large gap in the existing epidemiological data on ED. In the United States, the incidence of ED is 25.9 cases per 1000 people, and it increases with age, with more than 70% of men over 70 years old affected by ED. However, despite being a common and important disorder, due to psychological and referral reasons, the prevalence of ED is still not standardized worldwide.

The occurrence of ED is associated with many comorbidities and risk factors, such as aging, smoking, obesity, decreased androgen levels, cardiovascular and metabolic disorders, depression, prostate surgery, and penile trauma [30]. Moreover, previous longitudinal studies have demonstrated a strong connection between ED and the future risk of developing cardiovascular events [24]. For this reason, it is of utmost importance that men with ED undergo a detailed diagnostic workup, not only for the appropriate management of the disease itself but also for preventive purposes in terms of general health status. Besides medical and sexual history and

L. Boeri (✉)
Fondazione IRCCS Ca' Granda Ospedale Maggiore Policlinico, Milan, Italy

T. Toprak
University of Health Sciences, Hamidiye Faculty of Medicine, FSM Health Practice & Research Center, Deparment of Urology, Istanbul, Turkey

S. Çayan
Faculty of Medicine, Department of Urology, Mersin University, Mersin, Turkey

R. Shah et al. (eds.), *Diagnosis and Treatment of Male Sexual Dysfunction*,
https://doi.org/10.1007/978-3-032-12423-4_3

physical examination, which are the cornerstones of the ED diagnostic pathway, various diagnostic tools are available to further investigate men with erectile difficulties, but a definitive consensus about their use is still lacking.

The purpose of this chapter is to explore the controversies, advances, and future developments in the epidemiology and diagnosis of erectile dysfunction.

ED Prevalence

Several epidemiological studies have investigated the prevalence of ED in different countries and populations.

ED has a high prevalence and incidence worldwide [12]. One of the most famous epidemiological studies, the Massachusetts Male Aging Study (MMAS) reported an overall prevalence of 52% for ED in men aged 40–70 years in the Boston area [14]. More specifically, minimal, moderate, and complete ED was reported by 17.2%, 25.2%, and 9.6% of participants, respectively. Similarly, in the Cologne study of men aged 30–80 years, the prevalence of ED was 19.2%, with a steep age-related increase from 2.3% to 53.4% [4]. The long-term data from the MMAS study reported an incidence rate of ED (new cases per 1000 men annually) of 26 [15] and a Dutch study reported a rate of 19.2 (mean follow-up of 4.2 years) [31]. More recently, Capogrosso et al., in a cross-sectional, real-life study among 439 men seeking first medical help for new-onset ED, found that one in four patients was younger than 40 years, with almost 50% of the young men complaining of severe ED [6]. Mark et al., by using data from the 2021 *National Survey of Sexual Wellbeing* of 1822 cisgender men ranging in age from 18 to 87 years (mean age of 47.5 years) in the United States, found an ED prevalence of 24.2% [19]. ED prevalence and severity were associated with aging; moreover, most individuals who met the criteria for ED had not sought medical care related to this concern. This study further confirmed the psychological stigma that is still associated with ED in men.

Differences among these studies can be explained by differences in methodology, ages, and socioeconomic and cultural status of the populations studied.

Risk Factors Associated with ED

As previously reported, age is one of the most recognized risk factors for ED. Several studies have demonstrated that ED prevalence and severity increase with aging [4, 19], but this condition is also common in young men (e.g., men younger than 40 years). A psychogenic cause of ED is likely in young men, but its severity is reported to be similar to that of older men. For example, Pozzi et al., in a cross-sectional study with 2009 consecutive patients presenting for ED, found that one out of nine participants had a psychogenetic form of the disease [25], and men with psychogenic ED had a similar severity of ED compared to those with organic causes.

Therefore, this form of ED, which is typical of young men, should not be underestimated given the high repercussions in terms of severity on the patient's quality of life.

Other common risk factors for ED are diabetes mellitus (DM), dyslipidemia, hypertension, cardiovascular disorders, obesity/increased waist circumference, metabolic syndrome, hyperhomocysteinemia, lack of exercise, and smoking, with a demonstrated association between ED and the quantity and duration of smoking [30]. Erectile dysfunction is also one of the symptoms of hypogonadism [1], sleep disorders, and obstructive sleep apnea. Several pharmacotherapeutic agents have a negative impact on erectile function, including thiazide diuretics and β-blockers(except nebivolol), antidepressant/antipsychotic medications as well as treatments for benign prostatic hyperplasia (such as 5α-reductase inhibitors) [30].

As previously reported, men with DM are at a significantly higher risk for ED than those without DM. Moreover, ED has an earlier onset and higher severity in men with DM compared to euglycemic ones [7]. This interplay is related to the many risk factors that ED and DM have in common. As hyperglycemia is associated with increased oxidative stress, and the hyperproduction of reactive oxygen species (ROS), in DM a cascade of events occurs: reduced NO, increased prothrombotic factors such as tissue factor and plasminogen activator inhibitor-1, an increase in endothelin-1, with subsequent thrombosis and vasoconstriction, as well as an increase in nuclear factor kappa B and activation protein 1 with subsequent inflammation, culminating in ED [10].

In line with this, Corona et al. reported a 19.4%, 15.4%, 10.4%, and 21.6% prevalence of mild, mild-to-moderate, moderate, and severe ED in men with DM, respectively [7]. The severity of ED is highly dependent on the type and duration of DM, type of treatment, and comorbidities [16]. A study conducted by Fedele et al. on a large population of men with DM showed a 26% and 37% prevalence of ED among those with type 1 DM (T1DM) and type 2 DM (T2DM), respectively [13]. Similarly, a recent meta-analysis showed that the overall prevalence rate of ED in patients with DM was 52.5% (95% confidence interval [CI], 48.8–56.2), with prevalence rates of 37.5% and 66.3% in those with T1DM and T2DM, respectively [18]. Accordingly, patients with DM had an approximately 3.5-fold higher prevalence of ED than those without DM.

Not only is DM associated with ED, but also its mild form called prediabetes. Prediabetes is a common clinical condition characterized by mild hyperglycemia, which has been considered a relevant risk factor for the further development of DM and CVDs. In a cross-sectional study with 372 men with new-onset ED, Boeri et al. found that 23% of participants had glucose values suggestive of unrecognized prediabetes status [2]. Men with ED and prediabetes had lower testosterone values, higher rates of comorbidities, and more severe ED than those with normal glucose values. Moreover, men with ED and prediabetes showed lower rates of response to PDE5i than normoglycemic men [3], thus further corroborating the importance of endothelial dysfunction and nitric oxide activity in men with ED and DM.

The increasing incidence and adverse consequences of CVDs have driven research efforts to identify risk factors and, in particular, to recognize modifiable factors and possible strategies to prevent or reverse their occurrence. Research in several fields has identified numerous lifestyle, clinical, biochemical, and instrumental parameters that can predict major adverse cardiovascular events (MACE) in general or in specific populations. Over the last few decades, several studies have recognized that ED is a frequent risk factor for MACE [9]. The sharing of risk factors between CVDs and ED explains the epidemiologic relationship between these conditions. ED is found in more than 50% of men with a history of CVD [21] and, on the other hand, one out of eight men with ED reports previous CVD [8]. This suggests that ED is a symptom that occurs frequently before a MACE. Accordingly, a recent meta-analysis of observational longitudinal studies has shown a 59% and 34% increased relative risk of ischemic heart disease and stroke, respectively, in men with ED [36]. The entire process has been proposed by Montorsi et al. in their well-known "artery size hypothesis." This hypothesis argues that ED and CVD are different manifestations of systemic arterial damage and, due to the smaller diameter of penile arteries, ED occurs earlier than heart disease, stroke, or peripheral artery disease (PAD) with an equal extent of artery damage [22]. Accordingly, it is estimated that ED precedes the first CV event by 3 years on average. For this reason, ED should be considered an alarm bell. Men with ED should be carefully assessed for CV risk factors to prevent future MACE. In men with ED, who should be considered at high CV risk until proven otherwise, it is important to take into account not only traditional risk factors but also unconventional ones. The assessment of family history of cardiometabolic events, alcohol abuse, fatherhood, partner's sexual interest, and the severity of the impairment in erection during intercourse or masturbation should be considered [24]. In addition, alterations in metabolic parameters have demonstrated their predictive value, including impaired fasting glucose, slightly increased triglycerides, and obesity without metabolic complications. Decreased penile blood flow upon intracavernosal injection of vasodilating agents has been associated with increased CV risk. Recognizing these risk factors may help in identifying, among subjects with ED, those who warrant stricter lifestyle or pharmacological interventions to minimize their CV risk. Taking care of a patient with ED is an opportunity to implement a strict correction of modifiable risk factors [35].

Epidemiological studies have demonstrated consistent evidence for an association between BPH and sexual dysfunction, regardless of age, other comorbidities, and lifestyle factors [32]. The *Multinational Survey on the Aging Male* study, performed in the United States, France, Germany, Italy, Netherlands, Spain, and the United Kingdom, systematically investigated the relationship between LUTS and sexual dysfunction in >12,000 men aged 50–80 years. In 83% of men who were reported to be sexually active, the overall prevalence of LUTS was 90%, with an overall 49% prevalence of ED and a reported complete absence of erections in 10% of patients [28]. Lower urinary tract symptoms/benign prostatic hyperplasia and erectile dysfunction share similar pathophysiological pathways (NO–cGMP signaling, increased sympathetic nervous system activity, atherosclerosis); moreover, they also have common risk factors, such as metabolic syndrome, obesity, and hypertension [5]. It is therefore not surprising that both conditions can coexist, particularly in aging men, and a common therapeutic approach is recommended.

It is well known that treatment with 5-alpha-reductase inhibitors might affect sexual function, while surgical treatment of BPH has minimal or no effect on ED [30].

Lastly, sexual problems are highly prevalent among patients with psychiatric disorders. They may be caused by the psychopathology of the psychiatric disorder, but also by its pharmacotherapy [34]. Both positive symptoms (e.g., psychosis, hallucinations), as well as negative symptoms (e.g., anhedonia) of schizophrenia, may negatively interfere with interpersonal and sexual relationships. Atypical antipsychotics have fewer sexual side effects than classic antipsychotics. Mood disorders may affect libido, sexual arousal, orgasm, and erectile function. Except for bupropion, agomelatine, mirtazapine, vortioxetine, amineptine, and moclobemide, all antidepressants cause sexual side effects [34]. Selective serotonin reuptake inhibitors (SSRIs) may particularly delay ejaculation and female orgasm, but also can cause decreased libido and erectile difficulties. SSRI-induced sexual side effects are dose-dependent and reversible. Some personality characteristics are a risk factor for sexual dysfunction. Also, patients with eating disorders may suffer from sexual difficulties [34].

Diagnosis of ED

The complexity of the erectile process and the fact that the factors causing erectile dysfunction are often not unique can make the diagnostic process difficult. Additionally, in clinical practice, inadequate reimbursement, limited budgets, and the availability of commonly used oral pharmacotherapy for many patients, have led to a direct conclusion rather than a diagnostic process. However, it is extremely important not to abandon adequate diagnosis. This ensures safety, especially for the patient himself, and satisfies his basic need for a rational justification of his symptoms. It is important to document pathological vascular findings, especially when considering the possible diseases underlying erectile dysfunction. Therefore, the diagnostic workup is more important than the current practice.

Validated Questionnaires to Assess ED

Many questionnaires have been developed to diagnose ED and evaluate treatment progress. These include the International Index of Erectile Function (IIEF), which measures the domains of erectile function, sexual desire, sexual intercourse, orgasm, and satisfaction, and the abbreviated versions IIEF erectile function domain (IIEF-EF) and Sexual Health Inventory for Men (SHIM). Erectile Hardness Score

(EHS) measures penis hardness [27]. Although not validated in different languages for different countries, they are all internationally accepted.

Taking Clinical and Sexual History

The patient's history and physical examination provide important clues in elucidating the etiology of ED. For many patients, talking about sexual disorders can be embarrassing. In this respect, the examination environment must be comfortable and the doctor must provide an environment where the patient feels safe. It may be of great practical importance for further diagnosis and a better understanding of the problem. For this reason, patient examination should take place with due sincerity and within a sufficient period of time, without being affected by external factors. In addition to age and taking a history, risk factors such as hypertension, obesity, diabetes, dyslipidemia, and cardiovascular diseases should be considered first [30]. Up to 70% of patients with diabetes, hypertension, and dyslipidemia develop ED. In a large study, Rosen et al. found that the incidence of these comorbidities was twice as high in patients with ED compared with those without, and that approximately 65% of all ED patients had at least one of these risk factors [29]. Up to 25% of all patients with ED have diabetes, and up to 17% have previously unknown impaired glucose tolerance [2]. ED may be an early symptom and clinical predictor of cardiovascular events. On average, ED occurs approximately 25 months before coronary artery disease and myocardial infarction occur [36]. Patients with ED have a 33% increased mortality compared with patients without ED. Cardiovascular disease exclusion is therefore reasonable in patients with ED.

Additionally, nicotine use, an important modifiable risk factor for ED, should also be assessed. The patient's alcohol and recreational drug use should also be evaluated. It is also important to inquire about neurological systemic diseases such as epilepsy or multiple sclerosis. Previous surgeries in the pelvic region, such as urological tumor surgery, sigmoid and rectal resections, and reconstructive procedures of the abdominal aorta and iliac vessels, should also be considered. Reconstructive urethral surgeries can also negatively affect erectile function. A history of pelvic trauma is also important.

Another issue that should be assessed in erectile dysfunction is the medications used by the patient. Especially antihypertensives, drugs that affect lipid metabolism, and diuretics can cause erectile dysfunction (Table 3.1). It is important to determine the social and psychological status of the patient in the general medical history. It is important to determine the type of sexual disorder and distinguish between libido disorders, ejaculation disorders, and erectile dysfunction. Unlike primary ED, which occurs from adolescence onwards, secondary ED is characterized by its onset occurring temporarily following normal erectile function. To understand the underlying cause, how ED started, erection quality, masturbation, and frequency of sexual intercourse should be evaluated. There is an age-related decrease in the frequency of sexual intercourse. It is important to question how the patient evaluated his

Table 3.1 Medications most commonly associated with ED

Antihypertensives (i.e., thiazide diuretics, beta-blockers)
Antidepressants (e.g., selective serotonin reuptake inhibitors, tricyclics)
Antipsychotics
Antiandrogens (GnRH analogues and antagonists; 5-ARIs)
Recreational drugs (e.g., heroin, cocaine, marijuana, methadone, synthetic drugs, anabolic steroids, excessive alcohol intake)

GnRH gonadotropin-releasing hormone, *5-ARIs* 5α-reductase inhibitors

situation before the onset of ED. The cause of situation- or partner-related ED is predominantly psychogenic. Similarly, ED that occurs only during sexual intercourse and not at any time or during masturbation should be attributed predominantly to functional problems.

Psychosexual developmental defects and conflict situations with the partner may require the partner to be included in the psychosexual evaluation. Sexual deviations require evaluation by a psychiatrist. A diagnosis of psychogenic or idiopathic ED is made after other diagnoses have been excluded.

Physical Examination

During the physical examination, secondary sexual characteristics and external genital organs should be examined. Abnormalities in beard and hair distribution, body fat pattern, and general structure, as well as loss of libido, fatigue, sweating, and sleep disorders, raise suspicion of hypogonadism. Since severe androgen deficiency is often associated with testicular atrophy, it is particularly important to evaluate the testicle for size and consistency. Blood pressure, the patient's body weight, and BMI should also be determined. Measurement of abdominal circumference should be performed separately as it may indicate metabolic syndrome. Penile plaques, suggestive of induratio penis plastica, should be assessed since they might cause ED [30].

Hormonal Status and Metabolic Assessment

The role of androgens in sexual function is complex, and their importance in erection is still a matter of debate. While full erection is observed in infants and castrated individuals, low serum testosterone levels lead to sexual dysfunctions such as ED, decreased nocturnal erections, and loss of libido. Additionally, administering testosterone to patients with severe hypogonadism results in improvements in erectile function, increased nocturnal erections, and improved libido. However, when serum testosterone levels are normal, testosterone is not superior to placebo. A significant testosterone deficiency (<12 nmol/L) is associated with androgen deficiency symptoms and can be detected in up to 19% of ED patients [17]. Androgen deficiency leads to apoptosis in cavernous smooth muscle, a decrease in NO-containing nerve fibers, and disruption of signal transmission at the cellular level. Moreover, hypogonadism is associated with a low response to PDE5i. Therefore, serum testosterone levels need to be monitored in every man with ED who may have hypogonadism based on risk factors. It would be appropriate to take a blood sample for testosterone between 7:00 and 11:00 in the morning due to circadian rhythms. In case of low values, a second test should be requested along with LH measurement to evaluate the pituitary-gonadal axis. Additional useful investigations are prolactin, estradiol, and, in patients with borderline total testosterone values (8–12 nmol/L), SHBG, and albumin to calculate the free testosterone. Hyperprolactinemia can negatively affect erectile function, and treatment of hyperprolactinemia results in the improvement of erectile function. Hypothyroidism or hyperthyroidism can also negatively affect erectile function [30].

Further laboratory investigations include examining fasting blood sugar and HbA1c, as well as lipid profiles. In addition, PSA can also be checked in men who need screening for prostate cancer.

Organic Versus Psychogenic ED: How to Distinguish

Considering that ED, as a sexual dysfunction, creates psychosocial effects on the patient and their partners, the distinction between organic and non-organic ED has been debated for a long time.

Psychogenic, neurogenic, vascular, myogenic, or hormonal disorders may independently cause ED or may also act in combination. There is a strong focus on organic causes due to diagnostic methods that allow examination of functions important for erection. However, especially in long-term ED, psychological effects or psychogenic factors are almost always observed.

Psychogenic inputs, such as mental or sensory stimuli, can be triggers for the erectile urge. On the other hand, opposing stimuli, such as fear or past traumatic events, negatively affect erection. The causes of primary disorders usually arise from the family environment and upbringing, while secondary disorders usually occur acutely and develop partly depending on the partner or the situation. These conditions can often be accompanied by other sexual disorders. Of prognostic importance is whether ED is characterized predominantly by a loss of libido or an inability to maintain initial arousal due to fear of failure or other disorders. Libido disorders may have developed as a result of organic causes. Anxiety disorders, depression, and problems with partners can cause psychogenic ED. The prevalence of sexual performance-related anxiety varies between 9% and 25% and can lead to the development of psychogenic ED [23].

As a whole, psychogenic ED, accounting for approximately 10% of cases [25], is more common in young individuals, if the condition starts suddenly, if it is associated with a personal and traumatic event, if it is present with a specific partner and if morning erections and masturbation are fully present.

Vascular Reasons for Erectile Dysfunction

For an adequate erection, in addition to arterial perfusion, the cavernous occlusion mechanism must also be intact. Therefore, states of arterial inflow and venous outflow can be distinguished. Approximately 50%–80% of organically caused ED results from arterial circulatory disorders. In addition to arteriosclerotic changes, pudendal vascular injury or iatrogenic causes should be distinguished. Clinically, arterial disorders are characterized by difficulty or delay in initiating erection, the symptomatology develops slowly and usually does not depend on the partner or the situation.

Advanced Tests to Diagnose ED: Current Status and Controversies

Nocturnal Penile Tumescence and Rigidity Test

In healthy men, four to five erectile phases occur physiologically at night during the REM phases of sleep, lasting approximately 20–30 min. Considering that psychological factors do not affect nocturnal erections, the measurement of nocturnal erections serves as a reference method for distinguishing organic from psychogenic erectile dysfunction [26]. Because studies in the sleep laboratory are personnel dependent and time-consuming, various measures of nocturnal erection have been developed. From this perspective, simple logic-based measurements such as a snap measuring tape provide information about the increase in erectile tumescence and allow a qualitative assessment. When recording nocturnal erections with the help of RigiScan®, changes in tumescence at the base and tip of the penis are recorded continuously and can be correlated with the corresponding hardness. However, the specificity and sensitivity of the method are much lower than previously thought [37], because rigidity and tumescence measurements record the quality of nocturnal erections, not the quality of sleep. Due to low specificity and sensitivity and the high cost, the method is not suitable for routine use. The test is especially important in forensic cases and the evaluation of postoperative or post-traumatic ED, especially in isolated lesions of the autonomic innervation (cavernous nerve).

Intracavernous Injection Test

In the diagnostic evaluation of ED, detecting vascular ED by injection into the corpus cavernosum remains important today, and its diagnostic value increases when combined with color-coded duplex sonography of the profunda penile arteries. In this procedure, delivery of a vasoactive substance into the left or right corpus cavernosum causes a largely physiological erection. In this way, blood flow, functional integrity of smooth muscles in the corpus cavernosum, and cavernous closure mechanism are tested, and vascular disorders are evaluated without the need for nerve stimulation. Injection of the vasoactive substance at a low dosage (for example, 5–10 μg of prostaglandin E1 or equivalent dose of bimix or tri-mix) into one of the corpus cavernosa is performed laterally with a 31 G insulin needle. A standardized dose for this examination has never been defined. If a low dose is used the risk of priapism is lower but there may be incomplete corporal smooth muscle relaxation, resulting in a false diagnosis of a vascular problem. Conversely, with a high dose, the risk of priapism is higher but the correct vascularity of the penis is studied.

There is no need for compression of the base of the penis. The test result is evaluated approximately 15–20 min after cavernosal injection for swelling and hardness and is classified as follows:

- E0 = No reaction
- E1 = Low tumescence, no rigidity
- E2 = Medium tumescence, low rigidity
- E3 = Full tumescence, low rigidity
- E4 = Full tumescence, medium rigidity
- E5 = Full tumescence, full rigidity

In cases E0–E3, the test is interpreted as negative, and patients are classified as "non-responders". A negative test is associated with cavernous or venous insufficiency in >90% of cases. If an erection occurs at a level of E4–E5, the test result is considered positive. Before the injection, an informed consent form should be obtained from the patient regarding priapism. When evaluating the test, the quality of the erection, as well as the onset and duration of the erection, should be taken into consideration. The course and result of the test in this way allow important conclusions to be drawn about the etiology of ED.

If, as a result of the test, there is a rapid and sustained erection at low doses and nonspecific findings on Doppler sonography, then arterial or venous/cavernous insufficiency, that is, the vascular etiology of ED, is largely excluded.

If the erection develops slowly and reaches a sufficient level only after 15–30 min, it is usually a sign of a significant arterial perfusion disorder. This situation can be confirmed with Doppler sonography.

A positive test result largely excludes venous or cavernous insufficiency, while a negative test is associated with a 90% chance of venous/cavernous insufficiency.

Unstable angina pectoris, severe cardiovascular insufficiency, and significant liver dysfunction constitute contraindications for intracavernous injection testing.

Side effects include pain, hematoma, prolonged erections (>3 h), priapism (>4 h), and infections.

Dynamic Duplex Ultrasound of the Penis

Doppler sonography of the penis remains an integral part of the diagnosis of organic causes of ED. As a noninvasive and inexpensive method, it detects arterial penile circulation disturbances. Stimulation of the corpus cavernosum with the help of vasoactive substances makes it possible to examine the arteria profunda penis that feeds the corpus cavernosum. Ultrasound is usually performed 5–10 min after vasoactive substance injection, with tumescence still increasing. Examination before the onset of a rigid erection allows a more reliable assessment of the dilatation capacity of the examined vessel, since physiologically arterial perfusion decreases sharply after the beginning of phase III of the erection.

Evaluation of Doppler sonography is based on the absolute height of the pulse curve. A widened pulse curve, with a low peak rate and amplitude, is a sign of reduced arterial perfusion.

According to the intracavernous injection test result, the normal value is considered to be a strong pulse of the vessel, a diameter of the profunda penile vessel reaching 1 mm, and dilatation after intracavernous injection being >75% compared to the beginning. Maximum flow velocities of >30 cm/s are expected to be achieved, and achievement of these levels largely excludes a serious arterial perfusion defect. It is important to include both flow velocity and diameter increase in the assessment of vascular structure, as increased flow velocities can be measured, especially in the area of vascular stenosis. Therefore, maximum flow rate as the sole evaluation criterion may lead to bias. Additional evaluation of curve shape and determination of systolic rise rate allows for improved significance. End-diastolic flow velocities >3 cm/s may indicate inadequate relaxation of the corpus cavernosum muscles or the presence of cavernous insufficiency with increased venous drainage. Moreover, the determination of the resistance index (RI) is an accepted parameter to evaluate venous integrity, and is based on end-diastolic flow. An RI < 0.8 with normal systolic flow velocity and incomplete erectile response is indicative of veno-occlusive insufficiency [33]. However, it should be mentioned that a false positive diagnosis of veno-occlusive insufficiency can occur due to inadequate relaxation of the corporal smooth muscles.

According to the intracavernous injection test, the normal values of the systolic and end-diastolic flow rates of the profunda penile artery and the resistance index are as follows.

1. Maximum systolic flow velocity >30 cm/s
2. End diastolic velocity <4–5 cm/s
3. Resistance index >0.8

Neurological Tests

While questioning the patient's medical history, sensory or motor lesions that are indicative of a neurological disorder should be identified. Attention should be paid to neurological diseases that are generally clinically known or easily detected. Usually, ED is not the primary manifestation in such diseases. The bulbocavernosus reflex, which records the conduction pathways between the penis and the sacral erection center, can be measured clinically and electrophysiologically. An electrical stimulus is applied to the penile shaft via ring electrodes and the reflex response is obtained via two needle electrodes in the bulbocavernosus muscles. Simultaneous recording of cortical evoked potentials is performed via needle electrodes attached to relevant reference points on the scalp. The integrity of the bulbocavernous reflex provides information about the integrity of the short conduction pathways between the sacral erectile center and the penis. Standardization of these procedures has made it possible to examine at least the somatosensory aspect of penile innervation and thus detect some forms of neurogenic ED. However, bulbocavernous reflex measurement is controversial in the evaluation of ED today. Another part of the efferents is the parasympathetic nervous system, and after passing through the lower hypogastric plexus, this system moves towards the corpus cavernosum as the cavernous nerve and inhibits the tonic activity of the smooth muscles of the corpus cavernosum. It is not possible to directly detect autonomic nerve lesions below the pelvic floor level. Indirect symptoms of autonomic innervation dysfunction include weakened urine flow and signs of bladder dysfunction detectable on urodynamics. Direct recording of the electrical activity of smooth muscle cells in the corpus cavernosum is technically possible today, but interpretation is difficult. Despite the reproducibility, the application of this method should still be considered experimental.

Penile Angiography

Angiography of the penile vessels was considered the gold standard in the evaluation of vascular disorders for many years. However, it is an invasive and complex diagnostic method for penile perfusion. Doppler sonography correlates more than 90% with selective angiography results. Angiography with noninvasive duplex sonography, which is advantageous in terms of time, cost, and personnel, is now only indicated in problems requiring expert opinion in forensic situations or in patients with primary ED and suspected congenital vascular dysplasia before any vascular surgical intervention. MRI-guided angiography of the penis allows visualization of the internal iliac artery and vein. However, sufficient resolution of the penile vessels cannot be achieved in this way, so its use is not accepted compared to traditional penile angiography.

Psychosocial Intervention and Therapy

Psychosocial interventions include different modalities (e.g., sexual skills training, marital therapy, psychosexual education), and cognitive and behavioural therapy (CBT—group or couple format). Cognitive and behaviour therapy is aimed at altering dysfunctional cognitive and behavioral patterns influencing ED, and increasing adjustment during the course of the disorder. The CBT approach combined with medical treatment for ED has received empirical support and is considered an optimal procedure [11]. ED patients with suspected psychogenic etiology or with concomitant psychological disorders should be referred to a sex therapist.

Conclusion

The diagnosis of ED in men is important to reveal a condition often hidden due to shame and with a great negative impact on a couple's quality of life. Moreover, given the fact that ED is a risk factor for future cardiovascular events, the correct identification of the disease is crucial also for the patient's general health. An accurate medical and sexual history should always be performed along with a general and genital physical examination to identify potential treatable risk factors for ED. Hormonal and gluco-metabolic laboratory examinations are essential in the diagnostic workup of men with ED. Nowadays there are still no clear indications for NPT or CDDU tests, but the majority of experts indicate these assessments when vascular disorders are suspected. Finally, if sexual history and diagnostic tools suggest a psychogenic disease, a psychologist expert in sexual disorders should be involved in the diagnostic and therapeutic workup.

References

1. Boeri L, Capogrosso P, Ventimiglia E, Cazzaniga W, Pederzoli F, Moretti D, Dehò F, Montanari E, Montorsi F, Salonia A. Does calculated free testosterone overcome total testosterone in protecting from sexual symptom impairment? Findings of a cross-sectional study. J Sex Med. 2017;14:1549–57.
2. Boeri L, Capogrosso P, Pederzoli F, Ventimiglia E, Frego N, Chierigo F, Montanari E, Montorsi F, Salonia A. Unrecognized prediabetes is highly prevalent in men with erectile dysfunction—results from a cross-sectional study. J Sex Med. 2018;15:1117–24.
3. Boeri L, Capogrosso P, Ventimiglia E, Pozzi E, Chierigo F, Belladelli F, Zuabi R, Schifano N, Abbate C, Dehò F, et al. Undiagnosed prediabetes status is associated with a reduced effectiveness of phosphodiesterase type 5 inhibitors in men with erectile dysfunction. Int J Impot Res. 2020;32:393–400.
4. Braun M, Wassmer G, Klotz T, Reifenrath B, Mathers M, Engelmann U. Epidemiology of erectile dysfunction: results of the "Cologne Male Survey". Int J Impot Res. 2000;12:305–11.

5. Calogero AE, Burgio G, Condorelli RA, Cannarella R, La Vignera S. Lower urinary tract symptoms/benign prostatic hyperplasia and erectile dysfunction: from physiology to clinical aspects. Aging Male. 2018;21:261–71.
6. Capogrosso P, Colicchia M, Ventimiglia E, Castagna G, Clementi MC, Suardi N, Castiglione F, Briganti A, Cantiello F, Damiano R, et al. One patient out of four with newly diagnosed erectile dysfunction is a young man—worrisome picture from the everyday clinical practice. J Sex Med. 2013;10:1833–41.
7. Corona G, Giorda CB, Cucinotta D, Guida P, Nada E, Gruppo di studio SUBITO-DE. Sexual dysfunction at the onset of type 2 diabetes: the interplay of depression, hormonal and cardiovascular factors. J Sex Med. 2014;11:2065–73.
8. Corona G, Rastrelli G, Maseroli E, Fralassi N, Sforza A, Forti G, Mannucci E, Maggi M. Low testosterone syndrome protects subjects with high cardiovascular risk burden from major adverse cardiovascular events. Andrology. 2014;2:741–7.
9. Corona G, Rastrelli G, Isidori AM, Pivonello R, Bettocchi C, Reisman Y, Sforza A, Maggi M. Erectile dysfunction and cardiovascular risk: a review of current findings. Expert Rev Cardiovasc Ther. 2020;18:155–64.
10. Defeudis G, Gianfrilli D, Di Emidio C, Pofi R, Tuccinardi D, Palermo A, Lenzi A, Pozzilli P. Erectile dysfunction and its management in patients with diabetes mellitus. Rev Endocr Metab Disord. 2015;16:213.
11. Dewitte M, Bettocchi C, Carvalho J, Corona G, Flink I, Limoncin E, Pascoal P, Reisman Y, Van Lankveld J. A psychosocial approach to erectile dysfunction: position statements from the European Society of Sexual Medicine (ESSM). Sex Med. 2021;9:100434.
12. Eardley I. The incidence, prevalence, and natural history of erectile dysfunction. Sex Med Rev. 2013;1:3–16.
13. Fedele D, Coscelli C, Santeusanio F, Bortolotti A, Chatenoud L, Colli E, Landoni M, Parazzini F. Erectile dysfunction in diabetic subjects in Italy. Gruppo Italiano Studio Deficit Erettile nei Diabetici. Diabetes Care. 1998;21:1973–7.
14. Feldman HA, Goldstein I, Hatzichristou DG, Krane RJ, McKinlay JB. Impotence and its medical and psychosocial correlates: results of the Massachusetts Male Aging Study. J Urol. 1994;151:54–61.
15. Johannes CB, Araujo AB, Feldman HA, Derby CA, Kleinman KP, McKinlay JB. Incidence of erectile dysfunction in men 40 to 69 years old: longitudinal results from the Massachusetts male aging study. J Urol. 2000;163:460–3.
16. Kamenov ZA. A comprehensive review of erectile dysfunction in men with diabetes. Exp Clin Endocrinol Diabetes. 2015;123:141–58.
17. Kanakis GA, Nordkap L, Bang AK, Calogero AE, Bártfai G, Corona G, Forti G, Toppari J, Goulis DG, Jørgensen N. EAA clinical practice guidelines-gynecomastia evaluation and management. Andrology. 2019;7:778.
18. Kouidrat Y, Pizzol D, Cosco T, Thompson T, Carnaghi M, Bertoldo A, Solmi M, Stubbs B, Veronese N. High prevalence of erectile dysfunction in diabetes: a systematic review and meta-analysis of 145 studies. Diabet Med J Br Diabet Assoc. 2017;34:1185–92.
19. Mark KP, Arenella K, Girard A, Herbenick D, Fu J, Coleman E. Erectile dysfunction prevalence in the United States: report from the 2021 National Survey of Sexual Wellbeing. J Sex Med. 2024;21:296–303.
20. McCabe MP, Sharlip ID, Lewis R, Atalla E, Balon R, Fisher AD, Laumann E, Lee SW, Segraves RT. Incidence and prevalence of sexual dysfunction in women and men: a consensus statement from the Fourth International Consultation on Sexual Medicine 2015. J Sex Med. 2016;13:144–52.
21. Montorsi F, Briganti A, Salonia A, Rigatti P, Margonato A, Macchi A, Galli S, Ravagnani PM, Montorsi P. Erectile dysfunction prevalence, time of onset and association with risk factors in 300 consecutive patients with acute chest pain and angiographically documented coronary artery disease. Eur Urol. 2003;44:360–4. discussion 364–5.

22. Montorsi P, Montorsi F, Schulman CC. Is erectile dysfunction the "tip of the iceberg" of a systemic vascular disorder? Eur Urol. 2003;44:352–4.
23. Nguyen HMT, Gabrielson AT, Hellstrom WJG. Erectile dysfunction in young men—a review of the prevalence and risk factors. Sex Med Rev. 2017;5:508–20.
24. Pozzi E, Capogrosso P, Boeri L, Belladelli F, Baudo A, Schifano N, Abbate C, Dehò F, Montorsi F, Salonia A. Longitudinal risk of developing cardiovascular diseases in patients with erectile dysfunction—which patients deserve more attention? J Sex Med. 2020;17:1489–94.
25. Pozzi E, Fallara G, Capogrosso P, Boeri L, Belladelli F, Corsini C, Costa A, Candela L, Cignoli D, Cazzaniga W, et al. Primary organic versus primary psychogenic erectile dysfunction: findings from a real-life cross-sectional study. Andrology. 2022;10:1302–9.
26. Qin F, Gao L, Qian S, Fu F, Yang Y, Yuan J. Advantages and limitations of sleep-related erection and rigidity monitoring: a review. Int J Impot Res. 2018;30:192–201.
27. Rosen RC, Riley A, Wagner G, Osterloh IH, Kirkpatrick J, Mishra A. The international index of erectile function (IIEF): a multidimensional scale for assessment of erectile dysfunction. Urology. 1997;49:822–30.
28. Rosen R, Altwein J, Boyle P, Kirby RS, Lukacs B, Meuleman E, O'Leary MP, Puppo P, Robertson C, Giuliano F. Lower urinary tract symptoms and male sexual dysfunction: the multinational survey of the aging male (MSAM-7). Eur Urol. 2003;44:637–49.
29. Rosen RC, Fisher WA, Eardley I, Niederberger C, Nadel A, Sand M, Men's Attitudes to Life Events and Sexuality (MALES) Study. The multinational Men's Attitudes to Life Events and Sexuality (MALES) study: I. Prevalence of erectile dysfunction and related health concerns in the general population. Curr Med Res Opin. 2004;20:607–17.
30. Salonia A, Bettocchi C, Boeri L, Capogrosso P, Carvalho J, Cilesiz NC, Cocci A, Corona G, Dimitropoulos K, Gül M, et al. European Association of Urology guidelines on sexual and reproductive Health-2021 update: male sexual dysfunction. Eur Urol. 2021;80:333–57.
31. Schouten BWV, Bosch JLHR, Bernsen RMD, Blanker MH, Thomas S, Bohnen AM. Incidence rates of erectile dysfunction in the Dutch general population. Effects of definition, clinical relevance and duration of follow-up in the Krimpen study. Int J Impot Res. 2005;17:58–62.
32. Seftel AD, de la Rosette J, Birt J, Porter V, Zarotsky V, Viktrup L. Coexisting lower urinary tract symptoms and erectile dysfunction: a systematic review of epidemiological data. Int J Clin Pract. 2013;67:32–45.
33. Sikka SC, Hellstrom WJG, Brock G, Morales AM. Standardization of vascular assessment of erectile dysfunction: standard operating procedures for duplex ultrasound. J Sex Med. 2013;10:120–9.
34. Waldinger MD. Psychiatric disorders and sexual dysfunction. Handb Clin Neurol. 2015;130:469–89.
35. Yannas D, Frizza F, Vignozzi L, Corona G, Maggi M, Rastrelli G. Erectile dysfunction is a hallmark of cardiovascular disease: unavoidable matter of fact or opportunity to improve men's health? J Clin Med. 2021;10:2221.
36. Zhao B, Hong Z, Wei Y, Yu D, Xu J, Zhang W. Erectile dysfunction predicts cardiovascular events as an independent risk factor: a systematic review and meta-analysis. J Sex Med. 2019;16:1005–17.
37. Zou Z, Lin H, Zhang Y, Wang R. The role of nocturnal penile tumescence and rigidity (NPTR) monitoring in the diagnosis of psychogenic erectile dysfunction: a review. Sex Med Rev. 2019;7:442–54.

Chapter 4
Advances in the Treatment of Erectile Dysfunction

Naveen Kumar, Murat Gül, and Amarnath Rambhatla

Introduction

Erectile dysfunction (ED) is the inability to achieve or maintain rigidity of the penis suitable for satisfactory sexual intercourse [1].

Its prevalence rises with increasing age and is also associated with many comorbidities such as cardiovascular diseases, diabetes mellitus, hypertension, obesity, sedentary lifestyle, and lower urinary tract symptoms [2]. These diseases mainly affect the penile arteries, nerves, smooth muscle, cavernosal endothelium, as well as hormone levels. Some patients have psychogenic ED, while most others have predominantly organic causes. All these factors ultimately lead to failure in relaxation of the cavernosal smooth muscle. Relaxation of the cavernosal smooth muscle leads to inflow of blood into the corporal bodies through the cavernosal arteries and helicine arterioles. This results in an increase in penile tumescence, which facilitates compression of venules by the tunica albuginea and a decrease in venous drainage of the penis, leading to full rigidity of the penis during an erection [3].

The true prevalence of ED is difficult to determine due to hesitation on the patient's part to seek help as well as reluctance by physicians to enquire about sexual health. However, studies have reported the prevalence of ED to be 30–50 million men in the United States and at least 150 million men globally [4]. The prevalence

N. Kumar (✉)
Department of Urology, All India Institute of Medical Sciences, Patna, India

M. Gül
Department of Urology, Selcuk University School of Medicine, Konya, Turkey

A. Rambhatla
Vattikuti Urology Institute, Henry Ford Health, Detroit, MI, USA
e-mail: arambha1@hfhs.org

R. Shah et al. (eds.), *Diagnosis and Treatment of Male Sexual Dysfunction*,
https://doi.org/10.1007/978-3-032-12423-4_4

increases from 40% of men in their 40s to 70% of men in their 70s. It is estimated that approximately 325 million men will be suffering from ED by 2025 [5].

Initial treatment for ED consists of counseling patients regarding a healthy lifestyle, eating a balanced diet, and cessation of smoking, alcohol, and drug consumption. Oral phosphodiesterase-5 (PDE5) inhibitors like sildenafil and tadalafil are the first-line treatment for ED. They reduce the degradation of cyclic guanosine monophosphate (cGMP) by inhibiting the PDE5 enzyme, which helps relax cavernosal smooth muscle. Many patients respond to these medications; however, some patients with more advanced ED require intraurethral prostaglandin E1 pellets, intracavernosal injections (ICIs) of vasoactive medications, or vacuum erection devices. Penile prosthetic implants are utilized as a last resort when all of the above measures fail or are unacceptable to patients.

Over the last decade, there have been several advancements in the treatment of ED. This chapter aims to present these recent advances, including novel oral and topical pharmacological therapies, non-pharmacological treatments such as regenerative therapies, and improvements in implanted devices and surgical techniques.

Novel Pharmacological Therapies

Oral Agents

Dopamine receptor agonists have been found to have erectogenic effects in animal studies, and preclinical studies have shown increased dopamine activity in the medial preoptic area (MPOA), the paraventricular nucleus (PVN), and the nucleus accumbens, mediated by D2 dopaminergic receptors. During an erection in men, D2 receptor agonists activate the nitric oxide (NO) synthase enzyme in oxytocinergic neurons, leading to oxytocin release under stimulation of NO in the spinal cord and extrahypothalamic brain areas, leading to an erection [6, 7].

A mixed dopamine receptor agonist, apomorphine, was first introduced in 2000 for the treatment of ED. However, its popularity decreased after PDE5 inhibitors came into the market due to low efficacy and multiple side effects. This investigation has led to the search for a molecule with selective action on the D2 receptor and its subtypes, which may lead to fewer side effects. The D4 receptor, a subtype of the D2 receptor family, has been suggested as a potential target for erectogenic effects with reduced collateral emetic effects. Only preclinical studies have confirmed the role of D4 receptor agonists in ED, and the search for a suitable molecule is still underway [8].

Adrenocorticotropic hormone (ACTH), melanocyte-stimulating hormone (MSH), and endorphins are derived from a common precursor molecule, proopiomelanocortin, and they induce penile erection by acting on the melanocortin (MC) receptor subtypes, mainly MC3 and MC4 receptors present in the hypothalamus, midbrain, and brainstem. Many MC receptor agonists have been developed with selective action on various receptor subtypes. The nonselective MC receptor agonist melanotan and its carboxylate derivative bremelanotide have been found to induce penile erection when used for unrelated reasons. As only MC3 and MC4 receptors are present in the hypothalamus, it is postulated that MC3 and MC4 receptor agonists may be promising agents for ED, and some of these agents have been clinically tried for effect against ED, but due to serious collateral side effects such as priapism, these agents need to be tested further [9].

Soluble guanylate cyclase (sGC) stimulators and activators are a novel therapeutic class for treating erectile dysfunction independent of nitric oxide (NO) levels. In patients who do not respond adequately to PDE5 inhibitors, sGC is an enzyme in the erection pathway activated by NO, leading to the conversion of guanosine triphosphate (GTP) into cyclic guanosine monophosphate (cGMP) [10]. In ED, impaired NO signaling leads to reduced cGMP levels by insufficient activation of sGC. YC-1 was the first compound in the class developed in the 1990s. sGC stimulators, such as YC-1, BAY 41-2272, BAY 63-2521 (Riociguat), BAY 41-8543, and BAY 60-4552, increase the enzyme's sensitivity to NO, elevating cGMP levels even at low NO levels. sGC activators, such as BAY 58-2667 (Cinaciguat), BAY 60-2770, and HMR-1766, directly activate sGC independently of NO, providing an alternative promising pathway for cGMP synthesis, as they can activate sGC in conditions when the iron in the heme group is oxidized (sGC-Fe^{3+}) or in the absence of the heme group. Heme (Fe^{3+}) oxidation can make sGC insensitive to endogenous NO, inhibiting the activation of the sGC-cGMP-PKG pathway [11]. To summarize, their dual mechanism of action, both enhancing and substituting for NO, offers a novel approach to manage ED, potentially overcoming the limitations of PDE5 inhibitors, particularly in conditions where NO bioavailability is severely compromised, such as in diabetes or cardiovascular diseases and offering hope for patients with more advanced forms of ED.

RhoA/Rho kinase is a critical enzyme involved in cavernous smooth muscle contraction. Rho kinase inhibitors reduce smooth muscle contraction, leading to relaxation of cavernosal smooth muscle, vasodilation, and an increased accumulation of blood in the corpora cavernosa, thereby enhancing erectile function [12]. Inhibitors of this enzyme include Y-27632 and HA-1077 (Fasudil), which induce relaxation of cavernosal tissues in vitro and induce penile erection in vivo in male rats [13]. SAR407899 and azaindole-1 in this class have also been found to induce penile erection in diabetic rabbits and rats [14]. However, the RhoA/Rho kinase system is present in all vascular tissues, and thus their inhibition leads to profound systemic hypotension [15]. Due to the potential for systemic side effects, none of the drugs in this class are currently being tried in the treatment of ED.

Topical Agents

Topical therapies for ED represent a promising alternative to oral medications, especially for men who experience adverse effects or limited efficacy. They offer localized treatment, minimizing systemic side effects and provide a convenient alternative, not requiring intracavernosal or intraurethral administration. Alprostadil, a prostaglandin E1 analogue, is the leading substance used for topical therapy. Combined with a soft enhancer of percutaneous absorption (SEPA), it is marketed under the brand name Topiglan [16]. Alprostadil induces vasodilation by increasing cyclic adenosine monophosphate (cAMP) levels, leading to enhanced blood flow to the penile tissues, facilitating an erection. The efficacy of topical alprostadil has been supported by various clinical trials, showing significant improvement in erectile function compared to placebo [17, 18]. Additionally, the application of these agents directly to the skin of the penis ensures rapid onset of action, often within 5–30 min, making them a suitable option for spontaneous sexual activity.

Other topical formulations under investigation include nitric oxide donors, such as some PDE5 inhibitors, and combination therapies that aim to potentiate the local effects of each component [19]. Moreover, the development of novel delivery systems, such as nanobioliposomal and proniosomal formulations, aims to improve the permeability and stability of these agents, ensuring consistent and effective dosing [20, 21]. These formulations are still at an experimental stage and have not been studied clinically.

Testosterone replacement therapy has been used concomitantly to treat ED and hypogonadism. A study showed the efficacy of 6-month application of 1% testosterone gel in patients with hypogonadism and ED [22]. The TADTEST study confirmed the benefit of the addition of 1% testosterone hydrogel to PDE5 inhibitors in men with ED and baseline testosterone levels ≤3 ng/mL [23]. However, testosterone replacement therapy should only be prescribed after a thorough endocrine evaluation of hypogonadism with biochemical confirmation in a patient who is symptomatic.

Eroxon is a novel topical treatment for ED available without prescription in the United Kingdom and Europe and approved by the *Food and Drug Administration (FDA)* in United States, based on two unpublished phase 3 trials evaluating its efficacy, with FM57 being the initial trial and then FM71 conducting a head-to-head comparison with 5 mg tadalafil and showing significant improvement in erectile function compared to baseline as well as achieving significant improvement in erectile function at 24 weeks. It has a unique formulation of 35% ethanol, propylene glycol, and glycerine, which stimulates the nerve terminals on the glans, leading to increased blood flow and an erection with onset within 10 min, much earlier than oral tadalafil, with a favorable safety profile.

Despite their advantages, limitations of topical therapy include local irritation or allergic reactions experienced by some patients and variable penetration efficiency of the active compound due to differences in penile tissue characteristics. Their continued development and refinement may hold the potential to offer a targeted and effective patient-centered approach.

Regenerative Therapies

Non-pharmacological therapies are being investigated for their potential to regenerate erectile function. These can be employed when pharmacological therapies are ineffective and/or when a patient is not a candidate for vacuum erection devices or penile prosthesis implants, or the patient wishes to try and regain natural erections. The goal of regenerative therapies is to restore or regenerate cavernosal smooth muscle cells, endothelial cells, and nerves. There is a wide array of pathologies that can potentially be treated with regenerative therapies such as patients with refractory ED secondary to other pathologies (i.e., diabetes, hypertension), damage to pelvic and cavernous nerves during prostatectomy or radiotherapy, and trauma to the pelvic cavernous nerves or the genital vascular supply. By reversing the underlying causes of dysfunction, these treatments seek to develop a dependable and long-lasting solution for ED and restore physiological processes rather than only treat the symptoms. These include low-intensity shockwave therapy, injection of platelet-rich plasma (PRP) or stem cell-based therapies, and gene therapies aimed at the restoration of cavernous endothelial cells and nerves.

Low-Intensity Shockwave Therapy (LiSWT)

LiSWT has emerged as a promising non-invasive treatment for erectile dysfunction (ED), particularly for men who do not want to take or do not respond to traditional treatments such as phosphodiesterase type 5 inhibitors (PDE5i). LiSWT aims to address the underlying vascular deficiencies through the application of low-intensity acoustic energy (<0.2 mJ/mm^2) waves to the penile tissue, which induces mechanical stress that triggers a cascade of biological responses at the cellular level, including neovascularization, tissue regeneration (including nerve regeneration), and reduction of inflammation—which is crucial for achieving and maintaining erections [24]. This therapy is generally well-tolerated, with minimal transient side effects, including mild pain or discomfort at the treatment site, erythema, and bruising. LiSWT does not lead to any systemic side effects, such as hypotension or headache, which are associated with PDE5 inhibitors [25].

Vardi et al. in 2010 conducted one of the first pilot studies evaluating the efficacy of LiSWT in ED [26]. They applied LiSWT to the corpus and pillars of the penis of 20 men with vasculogenic ED who had previously responded to PDE5 inhibitors. There was improvement in erection length, stiffness, and penile endothelial function—along with significant improvement in International Index of Erectile Function (IIEF) score and Erection Hardness Score (EHS). A meta-analysis by Lu et al. in 2017 analyzed 14 studies including seven randomized controlled trials involving 833 patients [27]. The study found that LiSWT significantly improved erectile function, as measured by the International Index of Erectile Function (IIEF) and EHS, with better efficacy in patients with mild to moderate ED, regardless of variation in treatment protocols. However, the outcome was related to energy flux density, number of shock waves per treatment, and duration of LiSWT. A global survey of doctors treating ED reported LiSWT to be the most commonly employed regenerative therapy—despite imprecise guidelines [28]. In patients with severe vasculogenic ED, LiSWT was recently tried in combination with daily low-dose tadalafil, resulting in significant improvement in erection at 3 months in the combination group [29]. An umbrella review of five systematic reviews and meta-analyses in 2024 concluded that LiSWT may significantly enhance IIEF and EHS scores compared to placebo in patients with mild-to-moderate vasculogenic ED, despite variation in shock wave generating devices, treatment duration, setting parameters, and patient characteristics. Lower energy density (0.09 mJ/mm^2), greater number of pulses, and shorter treatments (<6 weeks) led to higher efficacy [30]. However, insufficient clinical evidence with heterogeneous study designs and variability in treatment protocols has led to FDA not yet approving its application in ED. The variability in treatment protocols—including differences in the number of sessions, energy levels, and treatment intervals—also mandates further research to optimize therapeutic outcomes.

Platelet-Rich Plasma (PRP)

PRP therapy remains an experimental but promising option for men seeking alternative treatments for ED. It is derived from the patient's own blood and contains an increased proportion of platelets, which are rich in growth factors such as platelet-derived growth factor (PDGF), vascular endothelial growth factor (VEGF), and transforming growth factor-beta (TGF-β) which can promote tissue repair and regeneration. PRP injections are believed to stimulate the repair of damaged penile tissues, angiogenesis, and increased collagen deposition, leading to stronger and longer-lasting erections. Additionally, PRP may promote the regeneration of nerve tissues, which can improve erectile function. The evidence supporting PRP therapy for ED is still in the preliminary stages, with small-scale studies and case reports showing encouraging results. Intracavernosal administration of PRP has been shown to improve erectile function in animal models with neurogenic ED [31]. In a study on human participants, four ED patients treated with PRP showed improved erectile function [32]. A randomized, placebo-controlled trial confirmed PRP as a safe and effective short-term treatment for the management of mild to moderate ED [33]. A meta-analysis analyzing seven non-randomised studies and three randomised studies showed significant improvement in IIEF scores after 1, 3, and 6 months of PRP treatment compared to baseline, and also a significant increase in IIEF scores compared to placebo [34]. EHS, reported in two studies, was not significantly different after PRP treatment compared to baseline. Nonetheless, there was heterogeneity in optimal dosing, injection route, and frequency of PRP administration, as well as in the study design and included population.

One of the key advantages of PRP therapy is its minimal invasiveness and low risk of adverse effects, due to the use of autologous material, thus reducing the risk of allergic reactions or infections. However, further large-scale, randomized controlled trials are needed to establish standardized protocols, long-term efficacy, and safety profiles. Although PRP has not been approved by the FDA for the treatment of ED and is considered experimental, it currently remains an option at some centers, especially in cases where other treatments have failed.

Stem Cells

Stem cells are undifferentiated cells of various origins, often derived from adipose tissue, bone marrow, or placental tissue. They are transplanted by the intracavernosal route, and these cells can differentiate into various cell types and have the ability to repair and regenerate smooth muscle cells, endothelial cells, and nerve fibers, which are crucial for the erectile response. Stem cells secrete paracrine factors, including cytokines and growth factors, which promote tissue repair and angiogenesis.

Preclinical studies in rodent models of ED have shown promising results. Mainly diabetic, vascular, nerve injuries, and aging models have been studied, and their efficacy in erectile dysfunction has been seen both in vitro and in vivo [35, 36]. A meta-analysis by Hou et al. showed the effect of adipose tissue-derived mesenchymal stem cells (AT-MSCs) in repairing cavernous tissue of rats [37]. AT-MSCs modified growth factors such as nerve growth factor, VEGF, hepatocyte growth factor, and neurotrophic factors like brain-derived neurotrophic factor, had better efficacy in improving erectile function compared to AT-MSCs alone.

Very few clinical studies with small patient populations receiving stem cell therapy have been reported, which have shown improvements in erectile function, as measured by the IIEF and EHS scores, with minimal side effects [38]. Most of them were phase I/II clinical studies, evaluating the safety and tolerability of stem cell therapy in patients with ED. These studies did not report any significant harmful effects resulting from stem cell administration. The intracavernous stem cell injection clinical trial (INSTIN) was a phase 1/2 pilot clinical trial evaluating the efficacy of intracavernosal injection of autologous bone marrow stem cells in patients with post-radical prostatectomy erectile dysfunction. In stage I, 12 patients were treated and there was no safety-related issue, with considerable improvement in erectile function at 1 year, which declined slightly over long-term follow-up of 62.1 months. In stage 2, six additional patients were given ICI of bone marrow stem cells, with a significant increase in IIEF scores at 6 months without any side effects [39, 40]. A study by Haahr et al. showed that ICI of autologous AT-MSCs improved erectile function in men with post-radical prostatectomy erectile dysfunction [41].

Even with these encouraging outcomes, stem cell therapy for ED remains in the experimental phase and is not commonly accepted [42]. There are still a number of obstacles to overcome, such as improving distribution strategies, choosing the best source of stem cells, and ensuring long-term efficacy and safety. Additionally, the cultivation and maintenance of cells requires a lot of time and resources, and the risk of an immunological reaction is significant. Millions of cells need to be infused to overcome the low engraftment rate in vivo; however, this approach bears the risk of tumor growth in the future [43]. Mesenchymal stem cell secretomes are increasingly being utilized due to the advantages of utilizing cytokines and trophic factors secreted from cells while eliminating the potential for tumor formation. There is a minimal immune reaction to secretome therapy, and it can be preserved after production as a readily available solution [44]. Developing a treatment approach that takes into account the complex interactions of paracrine components after damage is one of the major challenges facing stem cell secretome research [45]. A better understanding of the molecular mechanisms governing secretome composition and expression is necessary to get over this drawback and make this a practical treatment option. Furthermore, it might be possible to alter the secretome secretion profile by stem cell preconditioning or genetic manipulation.

Recent studies have evaluated a combined treatment approach, with stem cells modified or supplemented with angiogenic and/or neurotrophic genes and proteins, such as those present in PRP. The aim is to facilitate stem cell adherence in damaged penile tissues and improve therapeutic efficacy, depending on the animal model used or when bioengineered with particular substances (i.e., hydrogels) [46, 47]. Rats treated with comodified AT-MSCs with Smad7 and VEGF gene showed greater improvements in their erectile function [48]. However, the results of this approach have yet to be determined vis-à-vis the complexities involved in modifying stem cells.

Gene Therapy

Gene therapy seeks to alter the function of preexisting cell populations. Although there was initial interest, progress in the field has been hindered due to safety concerns arising from deaths associated with gene therapy in the late 1990s and early 2000s. Contrary to methods used for treating cancer and inflammatory diseases, genetic therapy for ED focuses on achieving low cell disruption and minimal impact on the body as a whole rather than aiming for strong overall effectiveness. Gene therapy can be delivered using vectors or without them [49]. The vector serves as the carrier for the gene, and these vectors are typically viral in nature. The most effective method for transferring genes, specifically to the penis, is still uncertain; however, the nonharmful characteristics of ED and the specific smooth muscle targets in the area make it possible to transfer DNA without the use of plasmids [50].

The primary gene therapy candidate for treating erectile dysfunction (ED) is the Maxi-K gene, which encodes calcium-sensitive potassium channels that regulate intracellular calcium levels [51]. The initial human trial of gene transfer through Maxi-K channels was published in 2006. A small cohort of men was administered a single dose of Maxi-K (human) into the corpora and were observed for a duration of

24 weeks. A total of three men received treatment at each of three different dosages: 500, 1000, and 5000 mg. Additionally, two men were treated with a dosage of 7500 mg. The treated men did not experience any negative events, and there was no presence of plasmids (indicating leftover genetic material) found in their semen. There was a noticeable increase in erectile function as measured by IIEF scores at the 5000 and 7500 mg dosages, which remained consistent after 24 weeks. Although this treatment modality appears to be safe and potentially effective, no further studies have been published on it [52].

The exploration of gene therapy for the activation of alternative molecular signaling pathways has involved the examination of nitric oxide synthase (NOS), which is recognized to be relevant to erectile function in males. Following the administration of an adenoviral vector carrying the endothelial NOS (eNOS) gene via injection into the body, older rats exhibited elevated levels of eNOS and cGMP, and a greater intracorporal pressure when compared to rats that received only the vehicle [53]. In another study, adenoviral vectors carrying the eNOS gene were introduced into MSCs before being injected intracavernosally in aged rats [54]. The animals that received treatment showed higher levels of eNOS protein, NOS activity, and cGMP. Gene therapy using viral vectors targeting neuronal nitric oxide synthase (nNOS) and inducible NOS (iNOS) has the potential to enhance erectile function in animal models [55]. Penile nNOS was introduced into rats aged 5 and 24 months through transfection. The intracorporal pressure in aged rats was elevated compared to the control group after transfecting penile nNOS through electroporation [56].

Various growth factors, including vascular endothelial growth factor (VEGF), neurotrophin-3, glial cell-derived neurotrophic factor (GDNF), and brain-derived neurotrophic factor, have been suggested to improve erectile function. Bennett and colleagues investigated [57] the transmission of neurotrophin-3 mediated by herpes simplex virus (HSV) in a rat model of diabetes. The administration of HSV-NT3 was compared to the administration of the β-galactosidase (Lac-z) gene, which was inserted into HSV and served as a control. The researchers observed a marked increase in the number of neurons stained with NOS and higher levels of intracorporal pressure in the neurotrophin-3 group compared to the Lac-z group.

GDNF belongs to the transforming growth factor-β family and plays a role in preserving autonomic axons [58]. The neurons located in the penis rely on GDNF for their survival and regeneration. Kato and colleagues conducted two studies [59, 60] that investigated the use of HSV to deliver GDNF and neurturin (NTN) in an animal model of cavernous nerve injury. At 2 and 4 weeks following the injection of HSV-GDNF and HSV-NTN near the injury site, intracorporal pressure and histology were assessed. At the 4-week mark, the intracorporal pressure showed a significant improvement in groups treated with GDNF and NTN, reaching approximately twice the level of the control group. This improvement was observed when comparing these groups to the group treated with HSV transfected with green fluorescent protein and LacZ. The HSV-NTN groups exhibited significantly elevated levels of fluorogold-positive neurons in the major pelvic ganglion compared to the control groups.

Choe and colleagues [61] investigated the role of Sonic Hedgehog (SHH), a well-established regulator of penile smooth muscle. The laboratory developed a nanofiber hydrogel that can be injected into the cavernosa to provide extended-release following cavernous nerve injury in an animal model. Rats were administered injections of Sonic Hedgehog (SHH) at a concentration of 6.25 mg per rat ($n = 1$) or 2 mg per rat ($n = 5$). The administration of SHH inhibited apoptosis and maintained smooth muscle integrity by 48% when delivered to both the cavernous nerve and cavernosa. Furthermore, the combined delivery of SHH to these areas resulted in the preservation of smooth muscle at 100%.

Botulinum NeuroToxin (BoNT)

Botulinum neurotoxin (BoNT), which is synthesized by bacterial strains belonging to the Clostridia family, is classified into seven distinct serotypes (A, B, C, D, E, F, and G). Among these serotypes, serotype A (BoNT-A) is the most potent and commonly employed for therapeutic applications. When the BoNT affects the cholinergic synapse at the neuromuscular junction in humans, it inhibits the release of acetylcholine from the neurons before the synapse. Consequently, there is a deficiency in the stimulation of acetylcholine receptors after the synapse, leading to temporary muscle weakness. The temporal and reversible characteristics of BoNT are believed to result from a combination of factors, including the reconstitution of the SNARE protein complex, the formation of new nerve terminals and synaptic connections, and the gradual recovery of the original nerve terminals [62].

A hypothesis regarding the mechanism by which BoNT-A may treat ED is based on its effectiveness in treating priapism. For patients experiencing priapism, a condition characterized by prolonged and painful erections, a method of treatment involves the direct injection of adrenergic agonists into the corpora cavernosa. This stimulates the contraction of smooth muscle, leading to the cessation of the erection process [63]. In contrast, the intracavernosal injection (ICI) of BoNT-A hinders the release of norepinephrine from sympathetic neurons. This results in reduced activation of alpha-adrenergic receptors, potentially leading to enhanced relaxation of smooth muscle and improved erectile function [64]. However, BoNT-A also inhibits the release of acetylcholine from parasympathetic cholinergic neurons, leading to a reduction in the production of subendothelial nitric oxide. The ultimate outcome is that the expansion of cavernosal smooth muscle relies exclusively on the discharge of neuronal nitric oxide from nonadrenergic noncholinergic neurons. An objection to this theory is that BoNT-A has demonstrated efficacy in enhancing erectile function in men who do not respond to tri-mix [64]. Phentolamine, a component of tri-mix medication, functions as an alpha-adrenergic antagonist, operating through the same mechanism as previously described. Due to BoNT-A's ability to treat patients that tri-mix cannot, it is probable that there are additional unidentified mechanisms by which it exerts its effects. Ghanem et al. conducted intracavernous injections of saline, 1 unit of BoNT-A, and 2 units of BoNT-A in a group of 30 rats. After 4 weeks, penile tissue was collected for analysis. The treatment groups exhibited a statistically significant increase in the average resting sinusoidal diameter of the penile tissue, as compared to the control group [64].

De Young et al. conducted a separate study on rats ($n = 10$) and found a greater average resting sinusoidal diameter. However, these results did not have enough statistical evidence to be considered significant [65].

Clinical trials by Giuliano et al. demonstrated that sympathetic hyperactivity plays a significant role in ED, and as a result, BoNT injections can be beneficial for its treatment [66–69]. Supporting these clinical trials, two recent randomized controlled trials showed promising results that ICI of BonT-A is safe and effective for the treatment of ED [70, 71].

Overall, the use of BoNT-A as a potential treatment for vasculogenic ED shows promise. Furthermore, in order to delve deeper into the actual therapeutic effectiveness and clinical safety of BoNT-A in treating ED, it is necessary to carry out more double-blinded randomized controlled trials in addition to the results obtained from the pilot studies mentioned earlier. Optimally, future studies should possess substantial statistical power by utilizing larger samples derived from diverse patient populations across multiple clinical centers.

Surgical Therapy

In the present age of consumerism, patients are increasingly seeking products of superior quality. As a result of the ongoing investment by prosthesis companies in research and design development, newer-generation prostheses that are more innovative and superior have been created. Over time, advancements in penile prostheses, including features like kink-resistant tubing, rear-tip extenders, lockout valve, tactile pump, polypropylene cylinder coating, and antibiotic-impregnated devices, have enhanced the mechanical reliability and durability of these devices. Although there have been significant scientific advancements and positive long-term results for both function and patient satisfaction, a minority of patients still express dissatisfaction with the procedure and the use of penile prostheses. While many of these dissatisfactions with the surgical procedure may stem from technical issues like intraoperative complications or unsatisfactory surgical outcomes, factors such as inadequate preoperative informed consent and suboptimal patient selection can also contribute to a heightened risk of patient dissatisfaction. Additional factors contributing to patient dissatisfaction after penile prosthesis surgery include a decrease in perceived length, absence of engorgement in the glans, perception of unnaturalness by the partner, or a general sense of sexual dissatisfaction experienced by the patient and/or partner [72].

Infection is the most significant complication that can arise from penile prosthesis implantation surgery. Historically, the incidence of infection for initial penile implants has been documented to range from 1% to 3%, while the rate can reach up to 10% for implants that require revision or replacement [73]. The presence of a biofilm on the surface of the prosthetic is essential for the occurrence of postoperative infection. Biofilms pose a significant challenge, as they make their microbial colonies impervious to antibiotic treatment. Antibiotic coatings are widely recognized as a highly efficient innovation that prevents the establishment of microbial colonies [74]. The manufacturer has the option to precoat the implant with this coating, or the surgeon can bind it to the hydrophilic implant by immersing it in an antibiotic solution before inserting it. The implementation of this intervention has resulted in the current infection rate of 1%–3%, which is comparatively lower among surgeons who perform a large number of procedures [73].

An intriguing advancement in the treatment of prosthesis infection caused by biofilms is the utilization of ultrasound-targeted microbubble destruction (UTMD) as an intervention. The effectiveness of this groundbreaking intervention has been demonstrated in laboratory settings, and animal models for the control of *Staphylococcus epidermidis* biofilms. The combined use of UTMD, and vancomycin therapy has shown a synergistic effect in the treatment [75]. Human β-defensin 3, a peptide, has demonstrated effectiveness in eradicating *Staphylococcal* biofilms, especially when used in combination with UTMD [60]. While most research on this subject has concentrated on titanium orthopedic prostheses, UTMD may have potential in treating infections related to penile prostheses—and should be further investigated [76].

In addition, the field of material science continuously advances, with the continual development and introduction of novel substances frequently. Within this framework, modern penile prosthetics depend on specific material configurations—specifically, expansile and contractile metal alloys—to replicate the physiological rigid erection, enabling successful penetrative sexual intercourse. Researchers have also investigated the use of heat-sensitive polymers that can alter their shape and stiffness for the development of penile implants. For instance, a specific type of prosthesis created by Le and colleagues [77] utilizes a heat-activated nickel-titanium-based shape memory alloy. This alloy can transition from a relaxed to an erect state simply by applying a heating pad and from an erect to a relaxed state by using an ice pack. This specific prosthesis has the capability to generate the necessary mechanical forces to achieve a firm erection that is adequate for successful penetration during sexual intercourse. Furthermore, the efficacy of this prosthesis is comparable to that of conventional penile implants that rely on hydraulic mechanisms [77]. In addition, the research team has recently developed a contactless prosthesis that utilizes magnetic induction to attain a predetermined form [62]. The novel prosthesis was surgically inserted into an animal model and multiple cadavers while they were in a relaxed state. The prosthesis was then activated within 45 s using an external magnetic device. The researchers observed that the implant allowed for a firm erection that was essential for penetration, and it also demonstrated the ability to withstand significant buckling forces [78]. While still in its early stages of development, this device has the potential to offer a significant advantage in terms of durability and ease of operation by eliminating the need for pumps and hydraulic tubing.

A novel penile implant device (Zephyr FTM) was developed in Switzerland specifically for phalloplasty patients. It is available in both malleable and inflatable forms, both of which can produce a physiological erection that is suitable for penetrative sexual intercourse in this specific group of patients [79].

One area of focus is automating penile prosthesis for remote patient control [80]. A potential "touchless" IPP has been described in preclinical tests that eliminates the need for manual pumping, and is controlled by an external remote device that sends fluid from the reservoir to the cylinders, as well as an implantable battery comparable to a sacral neuromodulation device [81]. There exist several patents for this technology, which may be available soon [82]. A vibrating penile implant to boost partner happiness has been studied; however, the lifespan of a battery-powered device may be reduced [83].

In general, penile implants have been utilized for many years as essential elements of ED treatment, and they continue to be the most reliable option for patients who do not respond to medical therapy. Various advancements and innovations have been introduced alongside current technological improvements, resulting in improved device durability, increased patient satisfaction, and reduced post-operative complications. Future researchers should view advancements in materials science, innovations in prosthesis design, and improvements in surgical techniques as a promising opportunity to create an optimal implant.

Conclusion

Overall, the field of treating ED is progressing quickly due to a better comprehension of the underlying causes of the condition and the creation of new and innovative treatments. Although there has been notable advancement, continuous research and clinical trials are crucial to further enhance these treatments and ensure they cater to the varied requirements of patients. The future holds potential for more efficient, tailored, and user-friendly solutions in the management of erectile dysfunction, thanks to ongoing advancements.

References

1. Muneer A, Kalsi J, Nazareth I, Arya M. Erectile dysfunction. BMJ. 2014;348:g129. https://doi.org/10.1136/bmj.g129. PMID: 24468580.
2. Shamloul R, Ghanem H. Erectile dysfunction. Lancet. 2013;381(9861):153–65. https://doi.org/10.1016/S0140-6736(12)60520-0. Epub 2012 Oct 5. PMID: 23040455.
3. Andersson KE. Mechanisms of penile erection and basis for pharmacological treatment of erectile dysfunction. Pharmacol Rev. 2011;63(4):811–59. https://doi.org/10.1124/pr.111.004515. Epub 2011 Aug 31. PMID: 21880989.
4. McKinlay JB. The worldwide prevalence and epidemiology of erectile dysfunction. Int J Impot Res. 2000;12(Suppl 4):S6–S11. https://doi.org/10.1038/sj.ijir.3900567. PMID: 11035380.

5. Ayta IA, McKinlay JB, Krane RJ. The likely worldwide increase in erectile dysfunction between 1995 and 2025 and some possible policy consequences. BJU Int. 1999;84(1):50–6. https://doi.org/10.1046/j.1464-410x.1999.00142.x. PMID: 10444124.
6. Melis MR, Sanna F, Argiolas A. Dopamine, erectile function and male sexual behavior from the past to the present: a review. Brain Sci. 2022;12(7):826. https://doi.org/10.3390/brainsci12070826.
7. Melis MR, Succu S, Mascia MS, Cortis L, Argiolas A. Extra-cellular dopamine increases in the paraventricular nucleus of male rats during sexual activity. Eur J Neurosci. 2003;17:1266–72. https://doi.org/10.1046/j.1460-9568.2003.02558.x.
8. Argiolas A, Argiolas FM, Argiolas G, Melis MR. Erectile dysfunction: treatments, advances and new therapeutic strategies. Brain Sci. 2023;13(5):802. https://doi.org/10.3390/brainsci13050802. PMID: 37239274; PMCID: PMC10216368.
9. Mallory CW, Lopategui DM, Cordon BH. Melanotan tanning injection: a rare cause of priapism. Sex Med. 2021;9(1):100298. https://doi.org/10.1016/j.esxm.2020.100298. Epub 2021 Jan 15. PMID: 33460908; PMCID: PMC7930850.
10. Pereira DA, Silveira THR, Calmasini FB, Silva FH. Soluble guanylate cyclase stimulators and activators: new horizons in the treatment of priapism associated with sickle cell disease. Front Pharmacol. 2024;15:1357176. https://doi.org/10.3389/fphar.2024.1357176.
11. Sandner P, Zimmer DP, Milne GT, Follmann M, Hobbs A, Stasch JP. Soluble guanylate cyclase stimulators and activators. Handb Exp Pharmacol. 2021;264:355–94. https://doi.org/10.1007/164_2018_197. Erratum in: Handb Exp Pharmacol 2021;264:425. PMID: 30689085.
12. Zewdie KA, Ayza MA, Tesfaye BA, Wondafrash DZ, Berhe DF. A systematic review on rho-kinase as a potential therapeutic target for the treatment of erectile dysfunction. Res Rep Urol. 2020;12:261–72.
13. Bivalacqua TJ, Champion HC, Usta MF, Cellek S, Chitaley K, Webb RC, Lewis RL, Mills TM, Hellstrom WJ, Kadowitz PJ. RhoA/Rho-kinase suppresses endothelial nitric oxide synthase in the penis: a mechanism for diabetes-associated erectile dysfunction. Proc Natl Acad Sci U S A. 2004;101(24):9121–6. https://doi.org/10.1073/pnas.0400520101. Epub 2004 Jun 7. PMID: 15184671; PMCID: PMC428483.
14. Lasker GF, Pankey EA, Allain AV, Murthy SN, Stasch JP, Kadowitz PJ. The selective rho-kinase inhibitor azaindole-1 has long-lasting erectile activity in the rat. Urology. 2013;81(2):465.e7–14. https://doi.org/10.1016/j.urology.2012.10.039. PMID: 23374844; PMCID: PMC3564057.
15. Löhn M, Plettenburg O, Ivashchenko Y, Kannt A, Hofmeister A, Kadereit D, Schaefer M, Linz W, Kohlmann M, Herbert JM, et al. Pharmacological characterization of SAR407899, a novel rho-kinase inhibitor. Hypertension. 2009;54:676–83.
16. Hamzehnejadi M, Tavakoli MR, Homayouni F, Jahani Z, Rezaei M, Langarizadeh MA, Forootanfar H. Prostaglandins as a topical therapy for erectile dysfunction: a comprehensive review. Sex Med Rev. 2022;10(4):764–81. https://doi.org/10.1016/j.sxmr.2022.06.004. PMID: 37051966.
17. Schanz S, Hauck EW, Schmelz HU, Weidner W, Fierlbeck G. Topical treatment of erectile dysfunction with prostaglandin E_1 ethyl ester. J Dtsch Dermatol Ges. 2009;7(12):1055–9. https://doi.org/10.1111/j.1610-0387.2009.07101.x. PMID: 19469786. English, German.
18. Padma-Nathan H, Yeager JL. An integrated analysis of alprostadil topical cream for the treatment of erectile dysfunction in 1732 patients. Urology. 2006;68(2):386–91. https://doi.org/10.1016/j.urology.2006.02.027. PMID: 16904458
19. Yonessi N, Saeedi M, Mohammadalipour Malekshah A. A double-blind placebo-controlled evaluation of the effect of topical sildenafil on erectile dysfunction. J Mazandaran Univ Med Sci. 2005;15(49):9–15.
20. Mohamed SA, Rofaeil RR, Salem H, Elrehany M, Asiri YI, Al Fatease A, Abdelkader H. Proniosomal gel-loaded phosphodiesterase inhibitors (sildenafil, Vardenafil, and Tadalafil): prospects for topical penile therapy of Tadalafil for treatment of erectile dysfunc-

tion. Gels. 2023;9(8):597. https://doi.org/10.3390/gels9080597. PMID: 37623052; PMCID: PMC10453270.

21. Abdelalim LR, Abdallah OY, Elnaggar YSR. High efficacy, rapid onset nanobiolosomes of sildenafil as a topical therapy for erectile dysfunction in aged rats. Int J Pharm. 2020;591:119978. https://doi.org/10.1016/j.ijpharm.2020.119978. Epub 2020 Oct 22. PMID: 33122159.
22. Corona G, Petrone L, Fisher AD, Mansani R, Bandini E, Boddi V, Lotti F, Forti G, Maggi M. Six-month administration of 1% testosterone gel is able to restore erectile function in hypogonadal patients with erectile dysfunction. Arch Ital Urol Androl. 2008;80(3):103–8. PMID: 19009866.
23. Buvat J, Montorsi F, Maggi M, Porst H, Kaipia A, Colson MH, Cuzin B, Moncada I, Martin-Morales A, Yassin A, Meuleman E, Eardley I, Dean JD, Shabsigh R. Hypogonadal men nonresponders to the PDE5 inhibitor tadalafil benefit from normalization of testosterone levels with a 1% hydroalcoholic testosterone gel in the treatment of erectile dysfunction (TADTEST study). J Sex Med. 2011;8(1):284–93. https://doi.org/10.1111/j.1743-6109.2010.01956.x. PMID: 20704642.
24. Dong L, Chang D, Zhang X, Li J, Yang F, Tan K, Yang Y, Yong S, Yu X. Effect of low-intensity extracorporeal shock wave on the treatment of erectile dysfunction: a systematic review and meta-analysis. Am J Mens Health. 2019;13(2):1557988319846749. https://doi.org/10.1177/1557988319846749. PMID: 31027441; PMCID: PMC6487775.
25. Brunckhorst O, Wells L, Teeling F, Muir G, Muneer A, Ahmed K. A systematic review of the long-term efficacy of low-intensity shockwave therapy for vasculogenic erectile dysfunction. Int Urol Nephrol. 2019;51(5):773–81. https://doi.org/10.1007/s11255-019-02127-z. Epub 2019 Mar 22. PMID: 30903393; PMCID: PMC6499893.
26. Vardi Y, Appel B, Jacob G, Massarwi O, Gruenwald I. Can low-intensity extracorporeal shockwave therapy improve erectile function? A 6-month follow-up pilot study in patients with organic erectile dysfunction. Eur Urol. 2010;58:243–8.
27. Lu Z, Lin G, Reed-Maldonado A, Wang C, Lee YC, Lue TF. Low-intensity extracorporeal shock wave treatment improves erectile function: a systematic review and meta-analysis. Eur Urol. 2017;71(2):223–33. https://doi.org/10.1016/j.eururo.2016.05.050. Epub 2016 June 16. PMID: 27321373.
28. Al Hashimi M, Pinggera GM, Mostafa T, Rambhatla A, Hamoda T, Shah R, et al. Regenerative therapy in erectile dysfunction: a survey on current global practice trends and GAF expert recommendations. World J Mens Health. 2025;43:359–75. https://doi.org/10.5534/wjmh.240086. Epub ahead of print. PMID: 39028131.
29. Kalyvianakis D, Mykoniatis I, Pyrgidis N, Kapoteli P, Zilotis F, Hatzichristou D. The effect of combination treatment with low-intensity shockwave therapy and daily tadalafil on severe erectile dysfunction: a double-blind, randomized, sham-controlled clinical trial. J Sex Med. 2024;21(6):533–8. https://doi.org/10.1093/jsxmed/qdae038. PMID: 38600694.
30. Medrano-Sánchez EM, Peña-Cantonero B, Candón-Ballester P, Blanco-Díaz M, Díaz-Mohedo E. Effectiveness of low-intensity extracorporeal shock wave therapy in erectile dysfunction: an analysis of sexual function and penile hardness at erection: an umbrella review. J Pers Med. 2024;14(2):177. https://doi.org/10.3390/jpm14020177. PMID: 38392610; PMCID: PMC10890328.
31. Wu YN, Wu CC, Sheu MT, Chen KC, Ho HO, Chiang HS. Optimization of platelet-rich plasma and its effects on the recovery of erectile function after bilateral cavernous nerve injury in a rat model. J Tissue Eng Regen Med. 2016;10(10):E294–304. https://doi.org/10.1002/term.1806. Epub 2013 Aug 16. PMID: 23950105.
32. Matz EL, Pearlman AM, Terlecki RP. Safety and feasibility of platelet-rich fibrin matrix injections for treatment of common urologic conditions. Investig Clin Urol. 2018;59(1):61–5. https://doi.org/10.4111/icu.2018.59.1.61. Epub 2017 Dec 21. PMID: 29333517; PMCID: PMC5754585.
33. Poulios E, Mykoniatis I, Pyrgidis N, Zilotis F, Kapoteli P, Kotsiris D, Kalyvianakis D, Hatzichristou D. Platelet-rich plasma (PRP) improves erectile function: a double-blind,

randomized, placebo-controlled clinical trial. J Sex Med. 2021;18(5):926–35. https://doi.org/10.1016/j.jsxm.2021.03.008. Epub 2021 Apr 24. PMID: 33906807.
34. Huang H, Qin J, Wen Z, Liu Y, Chen C, Wang C, Li H, Yang X. Efficacy and safety of platelet-rich plasma (PRP) in erectile dysfunction (ED): a systematic review and meta-analysis. Transl Androl Urol. 2024;13(6):970–82. https://doi.org/10.21037/tau-24-30. Epub 2024 May 29. PMID: 38983474; PMCID: PMC11228668.
35. Gur S, Abdel-Mageed AB, Sikka SC, Hellstrom WJ. Advances in stem cell therapy for erectile dysfunction. Expert Opin Biol Ther. 2018;18:1137–50.
36. Feng H, Liu Q, Deng Z, Li H, Zhang H, Song J, Liu X, Liu J, Wen B, Wang T. Human umbilical cord mesenchymal stem cells ameliorate erectile dysfunction in rats with diabetes mellitus through the attenuation of ferroptosis. Stem Cell Res Ther. 2022;13(1):450. https://doi.org/10.1186/s13287-022-03147-w. PMID: 36064453; PMCID: PMC9444126.
37. Hou QL, Ge MY, Zhang CD, Tian DD, Wang LK, Tian HZ, et al. Adipose tissue-derived stem cell therapy for erectile dysfunction in rats: a systematic review and meta-analysis. Int Urol Nephrol. 2017;49:1127–37.
38. Castiglione F, Cakir OO, Satchi M, Fallara G, Pang KH, European Society for Sexual Medicine Scientific Collaboration and Partnership. The current role and implications of stem cell therapy in erectile dysfunction: a transformation from caterpillar to butterfly is required. Eur Urol Focus. 2023;9:28–31.
39. Yiou R, Hamidou L, Birebent B, Bitari D, Le Corvoisier P, Contremoulins I, et al. Intracavernous injections of bone marrow mononucleated cells for postradical prostatectomy erectile dysfunction: final results of the INSTIN clinical trial. Eur Urol Focus. 2017;3:643–5.
40. Yiou R, Hamidou L, Birebent B, Bitari D, Lecorvoisier P, Contremoulins I, et al. Safety of intracavernous bone marrow-mononuclear cells for postradical prostatectomy erectile dysfunction: an open dose-escalation pilot study. Eur Urol. 2016;69:988–91.
41. Haahr MK, Jensen CH, Toyserkani NM, Andersen DC, Damkier P, Sørensen JA, et al. Safety and potential effect of a single intracavernous injection of autologous adipose-derived regenerative cells in patients with erectile dysfunction following radical prostatectomy: an open-label phase I clinical trial. EBioMedicine. 2016;5:204–10.
42. Margiana R, Pilehvar Y, Amalia FL, Lestari SW, Supardi S, I'tishom R. Mesenchymal stem cell secretome: a promising therapeutic strategy for erectile dysfunction? Asian J Urol. 2024;11(3):391–405. https://doi.org/10.1016/j.ajur.2024.02.003. Epub 2024 Feb 9. PMID: 39139521; PMCID: PMC11318444.
43. Matz EL, Thakker PU, Gu X, Terlecki RP, Dou L, Walker SJ, Lue T, Lin G, Atala A, Yoo JJ, Zhang Y, Jackson JD. Administration of secretome from human placental stem cell-conditioned media improves recovery of erectile function in the pelvic neurovascular injury model. J Tissue Eng Regen Med. 2020;14(10):1394–402. https://doi.org/10.1002/term.3105. Epub 2020 July 31. PMID: 32652851.
44. Matz E, Dou L, Zhang Y, Terlecki R, Atala A, Jackson J. 322 stem cell conditioned media profiles and potential uses in erectile dysfunction. J Sex Med. 2018;15:S254–5. https://doi.org/10.1016/j.jsxm.2018.04.285.
45. Mirotsou M, Jayawardena TM, Schmeckpeper J, Gnecchi M, Dzau VJ. Paracrine mechanisms of stem cell reparative and regenerative actions in the heart. J Mol Cell Cardiol. 2011;50:280–9.
46. Liu G, Sun X, Bian J, Wu R, Guan X, Ouyang B, Huang Y, Xiao H, Luo D, Atala A, Zhang Y, Deng C. Correction of diabetic erectile dysfunction with adipose derived stem cells modified with the vascular endothelial growth factor gene in a rodent diabetic model. PLoS One. 2013;8(8):e72790. https://doi.org/10.1371/journal.pone.0072790. PMID: 24023647; PMCID: PMC3758339.
47. Shao J, Nie P, Yang W, Guo R, Ding D, Liang R, Wei B, Wei H. An EPO-loaded multifunctional hydrogel synergizing with adipose-derived stem cells restores neurogenic erectile function via enhancing nerve regeneration and penile rehabilitation. Bioeng Transl Med. 2022;7(3):e10319. https://doi.org/10.1002/btm2.10319. PMID: 36176612; PMCID: PMC9471998.

48. He L, Yu T, Xiao Y, Huang Y, Guan Y, Zhao F, et al. Co-overexpression of VEGF and Smad7 improved the therapeutic effects of adipose-derived stem cells on neurogenic erectile dysfunction in the rat model. Andrologia. 2022;54:e14538. https://doi.org/10.1111/and.14538.
49. Melman A, Davies KP. Gene therapy in the management of erectile dysfunction (ED): past, present, and future. Sci World J. 2009;9:846–54.
50. Melman A, Rojas L, Christ G. Gene transfer for erectile dysfunction: will this novel therapy be accepted by urologists? Curr Opin Urol. 2009;19(6):595–600.
51. Christ G, Spray D, Brinkt P. Characterization of K currents in cultured human corporal smooth muscle cells. J Androl. 1993;14(5):319–28.
52. Melman A, Bar-Chama N, McCullough A, et al. hMaxi-K gene transfer in males with erectile dysfunction: results of the first human trial. Hum Gene Ther. 2006;17(12):1165–76.
53. Champion HC, Bivalacqua TJ, D'Souza FM, et al. Gene transfer of endothelial nitric oxide synthase to the lung of the mouse in vivo. Circ Res. 1999;84(12):1422–32.
54. Bivalacqua TJ, Deng W, Kendirci M, et al. Mesenchymal stem cells alone or ex vivo gene modified with endothelial nitric oxide synthase reverse age-associated erectile dysfunction. Am J Physiol Heart Circ Physiol. 2007;292(3):1278–90.
55. Garban H, Marquez D, Magee T, et al. Cloning of rat and human inducible penile nitric oxide synthase. Application for gene therapy of erectile dysfunction Biol Reprod. 1997;56(4):954–63.
56. Magee TR, Ferrini M, Garban HJ, et al. Gene therapy of erectile dysfunction in the rat with penile neuronal nitric oxide synthase. Biol Reprod. 2002;67(3):1033–41.
57. Bennett N, Kim J, Wolfe D, et al. Improvement in erectile dysfunction after neurotrophic factor gene therapy in diabetic rats. J Urol. 2005;173(5):1820–4.
58. Markus A, Patel TD, Snider WD. Neurotrophic factors and axonal growth. Curr Opin Neurobiol. 2002;3:523–31.
59. Kato R, Wolfe D, Coyle CH, et al. Herpes simplex virus vector-mediated delivery of neurturin rescues erectile dysfunction of cavernous nerve injury. Gene Ther. 2009;16(1):26–33.
60. Kato R, Wolfe D, Coyle CH, et al. Herpes simplex virus vector-mediated delivery of glial cell line-derived neurotrophic factor rescues erectile dysfunction following cavernous nerve injury. Gene Ther. 2007;14(18):1344–52.
61. Choe S, Kalmanek E, Bond C, et al. Optimization of sonic hedgehog delivery to the penis from self-assembling nanofiber hydrogels to preserve penile morphology after cavernous nerve injury. Nanomedicine. 2019;20:102033. https://doi.org/10.1016/j.nano.2019.102033.
62. Simpson LL. Molecular pharmacology of botulinum toxin and tetanus toxin. Annu Rev Pharmacol Toxicol. 1986;26:427–53.
63. Reddy AG, Alzweri LM, Gabrielson AT, et al. Role of penile prosthesis in priapism: a review. World J Men's Health. 2018;36:4–14.
64. Ghanem H, Raheem AA, AbdelRahman IFS, et al. Botulinum neurotoxin and its potential role in the treatment of erectile dysfunction. Sex Med Rev. 2018;6:135–42.
65. De Young L, Campbell J, Radomski S, et al. 142 intracavernosal injection of botulinum toxin to improve erectile function in older rats. J Sex Med. 2017;14(Supplement 1):S40–1.
66. Giuliano F, Denys P, Joussain C. Safety and effectiveness of repeated botulinum toxin A intracavernosal injections in men with erectile dysfunction unresponsive to approved pharmacological treatments: real-world observational data. Toxins. 2023;15:382.
67. Giuliano F, Denys P, Joussain C. Effectiveness and safety of Intracavernosal IncobotulinumtoxinA (Xeomin®) 100 U as an add-on therapy to standard pharmacological treatment for difficult-to-treat erectile dysfunction: a case series. Toxins. 2022;14:286.
68. Giuliano F, Joussain C, Denys P. Long term effectiveness and safety of intracavernosal botulinum toxin A as an add-on therapy to phosphosdiesterase type 5 inhibitors or prostaglandin E1 injections for erectile dysfunction. J Sex Med. 2022;19:83–9.
69. Giuliano F, Joussain C, Denys P, Laurin M, Behr-Roussel D, Assaly R. Intracavernosal onabotulinumtoxin A exerts a synergistic pro-erectile effect when combined with sildenafil in spontaneously hypertensive rats. J Sex Med. 2022;19:899–906.

70. Abdelrahman IFS, Raheem AA, Elkhiat Y, Aburahma AA, Abdel-Raheem T, Ghanem H. Safety and efficacy of botulinum neurotoxin in the treatment of erectile dysfunction refractory to phosphodiesterase inhibitors: results of a randomized controlled trial. Andrology. 2022;10(2):254–61. https://doi.org/10.1111/andr.13104. Epub 2021 Oct 7. PMID: 34618409.
71. El-Shaer W, Ghanem H, Diab T, Abo-Taleb A, Kandeel W. Intra-cavernous injection of BOTOX® (50 and 100 units) for treatment of vasculogenic erectile dysfunction: randomized controlled trial. Andrology. 2021;9(4):1166–75. https://doi.org/10.1111/andr.13010. Epub 2021 Apr 20. PMID: 33784020.
72. Pastuszak AW, Lentz AC, Farooq A, et al. Technological improvements in three-piece inflatable penile prosthesis design over the past 40 years. J Sex Med. 2015;12(Suppl 7):415–21.
73. Darouiche RO, Bella AJ, Boone TB, et al. North American consensus document on infection of penile prostheses. Urology. 2013;82(4):937–42.
74. Lindsey JP, Lue TF, Shindel AW. The future of penile prostheses for the treatment of erectile dysfunction. Transl Androl Urol. 2020;9(Suppl 2):S244–51.
75. Hu J, Zhang N, Li L, et al. The synergistic bactericidal effect of vancomycin on UTMD treated biofilm involves damage to bacterial cells and enhancement of metabolic activities. Sci Rep. 2018;8(1):192.
76. Li S, Zhu C, Fang S, et al. Ultrasound microbubbles enhance human β-defensin 3 against biofilms. J Surg Res. 2015;199(2):458–69.
77. Le B, McVary K, McKenna K, Colombo A. A novel thermal-activated shape memory penile prosthesis: comparative mechanical testing. Urology. 2017;99:136–41.
78. Le BV, McVary KT, McKenna K, Colombo A. Use of magnetic induction to activate a "touchless" shape memory alloy implantable penile prosthesis. J Sex Med. 2019;16(4):596–601.
79. Pigot GLS, Sigurjónsson H, Ronkes B, Al-Tamimi M, van der Sluis WB. Surgical experience and outcomes of implantation of the ZSI 100 FtM malleable penile implant in transgender men after phalloplasty. J Sex Med. 2020;17(1):152–8.
80. Robles-Torres JI, Gómez-Guerra L, Ramos-Cuevas D, Sánchez-Uresti A, Gutiérrez-González A. PD40-04 semiautomatic inflatable electronic penile implant prototype. J Urol. 2018;199:e804–5.
81. Barnard JT, Cakir OO, Ralph D, Yafi FA. Technological advances in penile implant surgery. J Sex Med. 2021;18(7):1158–66. https://doi.org/10.1016/j.jsxm.2021.04.011. Epub 2021 June 25. PMID: 34183291.
82. https://patents.google.com/patent/US20170079760A1/en.
83. Cheriyan A. Prosthetics in urology: current status and future directions. Indian J Urol. 2023;39(1):12–20. https://doi.org/10.4103/iju.iju_90_22. Epub 2022 Dec 29. PMID: 36824106; PMCID: PMC9942223.

Chapter 5
Surgical Treatment of Erectile Dysfunction

Sidney Glina and Osama Shaeer

History

There are several historical reports of surgical procedures for the treatment of impotence in ancient civilizations. However, the earliest reports documented in medical literature include ligation of the dorsal vein of the penis, reported as early as 1897 [1], and the transplantation of testicular tissue, whether from humans or animals, to the abdominal wall, dating to the early 1900s [2, 3]. This was followed by the combination of shortening the bulbocavernosus, plicating the ischiocavernosus, and ligation of the deep dorsal vein in 1935 [4].

In 1936, the first attempt to create an erection with the implantation of rib cartilage into the penis was reported [5]. The use of synthetic implants was first reported in 1952 with the implantation of an acrylic splint (extracorpora cavernosa) [6]. Then, in 1960, Beheri of Egypt performed the first intracavernosal penile prosthesis implantation, dilating the corpora with Hegar dilators, and implanting a polyurethane stent [7]; the author published a report on successful treatment of 700 patients in 1966 [8].

In the 1970s, with the advent of medical-grade silicone, the present-day penile implants started evolving. In 1973, Scott et al. described the first three-piece inflatable penile implant, with two cylinders in the penis, a pump, and a reservoir, connected by tubing [9]. Small and Carrion [10] described the first malleable implant, in the form of two rods constructed out of a silicon-sponge interior and silicon exterior. The progress in penile implants set off from there, continuously evolving and developing.

S. Glina (✉)
Urology Division of the Centro Universitário FMABC, São Paulo, Brazil
e-mail: sidney.glina@fmabc.net

O. Shaeer
Faculty of Medicine, Cairo University, Giza, Egypt

R. Shah et al. (eds.), *Diagnosis and Treatment of Male Sexual Dysfunction*,
https://doi.org/10.1007/978-3-032-12423-4_5

Penile Prosthesis Implantation

Penile prosthesis implantation (PPI) is the surgical procedure whereby a penile prosthesis is implanted into the corpora cavernosa of the penis, aiming at restoring rigidity. PPI became the gold standard for treating organic erectile dysfunction refractory to other forms of treatment, with high success, and satisfaction rates.

Patient Selection and Counseling

The recommendations from the *International Consultation on Sexual Medicine* state that penile prosthesis implantation should be considered the optimal treatment in motivated men with organic erectile dysfunction (ED) after failure or rejection of other treatment options. The patient should be informed of any alternative treatment options [11]. Such treatment options include—and are not limited to—phosphodiesterase-5 inhibitors, hormonal modulation in candidate cases, intracavernosal injections, and vacuum erection devices, under the umbrella of controlling risk factors, such as diabetes or smoking.

In addition to awareness of alternative treatment modalities, patients should be counseled for appropriate expectations, and increased risks associated with comorbidities, such as diabetes, and smoking, prior implantation, and scarred corporal bodies.

Patients should be informed of possible complications, such as infection and its consequences, tissue injury, and mechanical failure [11]. Patients with possible reasons for a lower success rate or lower satisfaction should be counseled preoperatively. Shortening of the penis following radical prostatectomy or due to an overhanging suprapubic fat pad should be discussed. Penile length is preferably documented before surgery in the flaccid-stretched state. Patients should be informed about adjuvant techniques that may help enhance length. Peyronie's patients should be informed that the deformity may require correction with adjuvant techniques, ranging from modeling to excision, and grafting. The possible effect on sensitivity of the penis with mobilization of the neurovascular bundle should be discussed. So are the added operative time, and its effect on infection rates. Implant types should be discussed with the patient at length. Recommendations based on medical factors, lifestyle factors, and financial aspects should be made. Ideally, the partner should also be informed of possible outcomes, positive or negative. Unrealistic expectations can result in postoperative dissatisfaction. These factors should generally be documented in the consent prior to surgery [11].

Psychological evaluation prior to PPI is not routine; nevertheless, operating on a patient with an undiagnosed or missed psychiatric condition may pose difficulties in the postoperative period, particularly if complications arise [12].

In a survey of preoperative counseling attitudes of penile implant surgeons, 87% assessed patients' grip strength to ensure their ability to operate the scrotal pump.

96.5% discussed patients' expectations before surgery. 42.6% asked patients about sexual orientation, and 63.5% commonly asked about partner sexual function. Only 49.6% obtained a psychiatric history, but 68.7% evaluated the impact of sexual function on patient self-esteem [13]. However, Dos Reis et al. [12] reported that a preoperative evaluation protocol combining standardized and validated tools showed that more than one-quarter of patients with a medical indication for penile prosthesis implantation were not in good psychological condition for the surgery, being referred to psychotherapy before the surgery.

Types of Penile Implant

There are two main types of penile prosthesis: inflatable penile implants (IPP) and semirigid or malleable implants (SR). The IPP mimics normal penile erection in terms of girth and axial rigidity and circumferential rigidity, as well as flaccidity. IPP consists of a pair of cylinders implanted in the corpora cavernosa, inflated by saline flow within a closed circuit. This operation is controlled by a scrotal pump. A reservoir holds the saline (three-piece inflatable implant). All components are connected by tubes. Two-piece implants do not have an external reservoir [11].

Repetitive squeezing and release of the pump inflates the cylinders with saline up to full rigidity. A one-way valve keeps saline from flowing back, unless manually released. The three-piece is the most popular among IPPs. All IPPs expand in girth when inflated. Some manufacturers offer girth- and length-expanding cylinders. Another variant is the downsized IPP for cases with corporal scarring, such as following refractory priapism or explantation of an infected prosthesis. The narrow rear ends of those implants allow insertion in the tight space that is developed with difficulty through fibrous tissue. A further important advancement is the low-profile reservoir, which is particularly relevant for submuscular placement within the anterior abdominal wall, rather than the retropubic space [11].

SR implants, on the other hand, are permanently rigid, though they can be bent (usually downwards) for concealment. They cannot mimic the flaccid state, and their axial rigidity differs from that of IPP, though circumferential rigidity is similar and their penetration ability is adequated. They consist of a pair of rods, usually in the form of a metal wire core wrapped in a fabric jacket, mostly silicone. SR implants come in different sizes as regards length as well as girth. Girth is determined by the maximum size of dilator that the corpora and crura can accommodate. Accordingly, girth may be somewhat less than with IPP. The length of the rods is trimmed to fit the collective length of the corpora and crura. The design of the core and jacket also varies from one manufacturer to the other, with some sporting a higher bending angle than others. Another variation is one type of SR implant featuring an external jacket in two layers of different densities, lending to a more natural tactile sensation. Some models of SR implant sport a narrower rear end, particularly useful in cases with fibrosis [11].

An important feature offered by some manufacturers is the antibacterial coating, whether preimpregnated with antibiotics, or as a hydrophilic coating that imbibes antibiotics on first contact. Since the introduction of this feature, there has been a dramatic decrease in infection rates [14]. IPP provides the higher satisfaction rate [11], being the closest possible to normal erection and flaccidity. On the other hand, malleable implants are the more cost-effective option and less prone to mechanical failure.

Patient Preparation for Surgery

In addition to the general pre-operative considerations for any surgery, special attention should be paid to eradication of septic foci. Patient history may point to an ongoing infection. Potential sources of infection include infected skin, urinary infections, prostatitis, pyospermia, dental infections, and an infected foot ulcer. Those should be cleared prior to surgery.

Cessation of smoking before surgery has also shown a positive impact on minimizing infection [11]. Diabetic control is mandatory since uncontrolled diabetes has been associated with higher prosthetic infection rates. In a retrospective analysis of 2363 cases that underwent virgin iPP implantation, it was demonstrated that the highest infection rates were among patients with high glycosylated hemoglobin (HbA1c). The overall IPP infection revision rate was 3.9% and the highest rate of 12.1% was seen in the highest HbA1c group (>10%) [15]. However, a systematic review failed to find conclusive evidence to support the role of HbA1c as a gauge [16]. Bleeding tendencies, such as the use of current anticoagulants, including aspirin, coumadin, or the direct oral anticoagulants, should be identified and corrected, particularly with the IPP and penoscrotal approach [11].

Perioperative Preparation

Every effort must be made towards minimizing infection rates. Preoperative antibiotic prophylaxis is recommended, commonly 24 h in advance, at least 1 h prior to incision [17]. Preoperative antibiotics, with gram-positive and gram-negative coverage, should be given, with therapeutic antibiotic levels attained before making the surgical incision. Furthermore, a fungal coverage should be considered in obese, diabetic patients and revision cases [11].

Operative site cleansing by alcohol-based antiseptic is recommended over practice. It may start several days before surgery [18]. Hair removal should be on the day of surgery, preferably with clippers. Sterilization is preferably with an alcohol-based antiseptic solution, which has been proven superior to iodine-based ones [11]. One study showed lower colonization upon urethral sterilization with chlorhexidine gel [19]. The use of the “no-touch technique” seems to be plausible. This technique minimizes contact between patient skin and the implant, personnel, or surgical instruments [20]. Further recommendations include waterproof gowns, double gloving, and frequent changes of gloves. Personnel traffic into the operating theater should be kept to a minimum during the surgery. A urethral catheter is generally required, particularly with IPP. Some experts operate without it in case of SR implant surgery.

Operative Techniques

Surgical Approaches for PPI

Penoscrotal Approach

This variant is the most used incision in the current era, with most surgeons getting their training in this approach. The penoscrotal incision has the advantage of exposure to the crural bodies, which helps dilatation/excavation in case of corporal scarring, allows low placement of the corporotomies and therefore burying the tubing, and avoids injury of the neurovascular bundle that courses dorsally. The incision can either be transverse in the scrotum or midline longitudinal along the median raphe. Advocates of a median raphe incision perceive an added benefit of preserving the end arteries of the penile skin, cutting along rather than across them [11].

Subcoronal Approach

This approach is popular with malleable penile prosthesis implantation. Recently it became recognized with inflatable implants as well, particularly if plaque management is to be performed in cases with Peyronie's disease. In such cases, the subcoronal incision with degloving of the skin allows extended exposure of the corporal bodies, while allowing access to the external inguinal ring for reservoir insertion, and scrotal placement of the pump through the same incision [21]. Special attention to skin vascularity is to be paid, particularly in diabetic cases.

Infrapubic Approach

Some surgeons implant penile prosthesis through infrapubic incisions. The proposed, but unproven, benefit is the lower infection rate, considering the damper and contamination-prone scrotal skin, a shorter operative time, and easier access to the external inguinal ring for reservoir placement. The pump can be inserted through the same incision. However, experience is required to avoid injury of the neurovascular bundle, which is the one reason it is not the mainstream approach; also, this approach is more difficult in obese patients with a large suprapubic fat [21].

Single Midline Corporotomy Infrapubic Approach

Recently, a modification of the infrapubic approach was proposed, with a single midline corporotomy being cut in the midline, in the bed of the deep dorsal vein. This allows avoiding any risk of injury to the dorsal nerves of the penis, which run laterally, and shortens operative time even further. The procedure was tested with malleable implants only [22].

Abdominal Crease Approach

With this approach, the incision is in the abdominal crease, the so-called bikini line. Redundant pubic skin and fat are excised to reveal the concealed penis. Scarpa's fascia is cut open at the base of the penis. Cylinder insertion and reservoir and pump placement are performed through the same incision [23, 24].

Surgical Steps for IPP

Access

Following a skin incision, the subsequent layers of dartos muscle and Buck's fascia are dissected down to the tunica albuginea of the corpora cavernosa. With the subcoronal and infrapubic approaches, every attempt should be made to avoid injury to the dorsal nerves of the penis and their tributaries, while injury of the corpus spongiosum is what to look out for with the penoscrotal approach. Stay sutures are placed into the tunica albuginea at the intended sites of corporotomy on either side. Corporotomies are incised longitudinally between the stay sutures. Corporotomy length depends on the type of implant, whether malleable (longer corporotomy), or inflatable (shorter). With an inflatable implant, the corporotomies should be as proximal as possible so that the implant tubes do not protrude, and that the least length of rear tip extenders is used.

Dilatation and Sizing

The corpora cavernosa and crura are dilated with blunt dilators (such as Hegar or Brook dilators), always staying laterally to avoid crossing over. Care should be taken not to perforate distally or proximally. With a malleable implant, serial dilation up to the maximum girth is needed. Cylinder girth is determined as per the maximum-girth dilator that can be inserted while making sure that the corporotomies can be closed without tension. This is not the case with IPP where serial dilation is unnecessary.

Total length is measured from the tips of the corpora cavernosa to the tips of the crura, thereby determining cylinder length. Rear-tip extenders can be fitted to the rear end of the implant, keeping the total length within the measured length. With an inflatable implant, it is preferable to use the minimum length of rear-tip extenders, which reflects positively on rigidity, and stability of erection.

Implantation

The dilated space is irrigated with antibiotics. Gloves are changed. Cylinders are then inserted. Insertion of IPP cylinders is guided by the Furlow inserter and Kieth needle. Corporotomies are closed by tying the stay sutures or oversewing. Tying the stay sutures is the common practice with IPP to avoid cylinder injury by the needle.

With a three-piece Inflatable penile implant, the reservoir is placed, whether retropubic in the space of Retzius, or in the anterior abdominal wall; ectopic or submuscular. Ectopic placement avoids the rare complications of retropubic placement [25]. In case of extensive prior abdominal surgery, reservoir placement can be under vision through a dedicated incision on the lower abdomen. IPP pump is inserted into scrotum. There are variable approaches to the site of pump placement, whether posterior for the sake of concealment, or an interior for easier maneuverability.

Many surgeons prefer to leave a closed-suction drain, particularly with the penoscrotal approach. Buck's fascia, dartos muscle, and skin are then closed. Snug—though not tight—compressive dressing can be used as an alternative to, or in conjunction with, the drain, called the *mummy wrap*. If this is to be used, caution should be taken against excessive skin compression against the rigid implant that may result in tissue devascularization.

Adjuvant Techniques

Additional procedures can be performed concomitantly with penile prosthesis implantation. They are either for correction of Peyronie's deformities, excavation of fibrosis from scarred corporal bodies, or for size enhancement.

Adjuvant Procedures for Peyronie's Disease

Peyronie's disease commonly results in curvature, narrowing (hourglass deformity), and/or shortening. Mild curvature can be corrected with manual modeling, designed by Wilson [26]. The implant cylinders are inserted, tubing to pump is clamped, and the penis is forcibly bent to the counter-direction of the curvature. Caution should be taken to avoid extrusion of the cylinder tips through fossa navicularis.

Plication (shortening techniques) can also be employed to correct mild to moderate curvature, or residual curvature following modeling [27]. This is at the expense of length, and may therefore not be suitable in a shorter penis. The plication sutures can be preplaced and tied after cylinder implantation.

In moderate to severe curvature, it may be necessary to perform plaque surgery, whereby the Peyronie's plaque is incised or excised, with grafting of the resultant defect. Collagen fleece serves to close the defect by adhering to the edges of the tunica albuginea without the need for suturing, thereby shortening operative time, and avoiding damage to the cylinders [28]. Slitting of the tunica albuginea has also been successful in correcting Peyronie's deformity [29]. Plaque surgery requires meticulous mobilization of the neurovascular bundle to avoid desensitization of the penis. Several techniques have emerged to release the plaque from within the corpora cavernosa, thereby obviating the need for mobilization of the neurovascular bundle. Those include the utility of a resectoscope (penoscopy) [30], the utility of punch forceps that are originally used to nibble vertebral protrusions [31], and a scalpel for reducing the plaque from within, between the blades of a speculum (the scratch technique) [32].

Adjuvant Procedures for Fibrosis

Following refractory ischemic priapism or explantation of an infected penile implant, penile prosthesis implantation in scarred corporal bodies is a challenge only worthy of experienced surgeons. Due to the resistance by the firm fibrous tissue, complications are not uncommon, such as urethral injury, anterior or posterior perforation, and a higher infection rate due to the lengthy procedure. The track created through scarred corporal bodies is in many cases too narrow to accommodate the rear end of an inflatable implant. Hence, the development of downsized inflatable cylinders that have a narrower rear end. It is, however, necessary to use enough rear-tip extenders such that the tubing will not have to course within the fibrosed crura. With a malleable implant, it is common to be limited to girth-9 malleable cylinders.

Several instruments are available to help excavate fibrous tissue. This group includes cavernotomes [33, 34] and Wilson's Backward-Cutting Scissors. Recently, creating a wide track in the fibrosed crura—up to girth 13.5 Hegar—became possible using Shaeer's cavernotome. This instrument is essentially a hollow corer. It grinds fibrous tissue by advancing in rotatory movements rather than forward thrusting, reportedly making the procedure safer. Thus, it creates a track through fibrous tissue that is wide enough to accommodate either full-size inflatable cylinders or malleable devices with a larger girth [35].

If dilatation fails, open excavation is possible through an extended skin incision and extended corporotomies. Corporeal reconstruction with mesh laid over the implant can also be performed.

Adjuvant Procedures for Size Enhancement

Among the reasons for dissatisfaction following penile prosthesis implantation is the size of the penis. This is particularly noticeable in patients with Peyronie's disease, obese patients, and those following radical prostatectomy. But it can also be met otherwise and may possibly be a result of a body dysmorphic disorder. Adjuvant procedures are available to enhance length and girth of the penis as well as the size of the glans in select patients. Those procedures can be performed before, during, or after implantation [36].

Release of the penile suspensory ligament can be performed in the same session [37]. Shaeer described tucking in the pubic fat to the pubis with nonabsorbable sutures to reveal the concealed penis in cases with a loose penopubic junction and moderate suprapubic fat pad (Dorsal Phalloplasty) [38]. In cases with a larger and overhanging pubic fat pad, dermolipectomy can be performed, and the penile prosthesis can be inserted through the same abdominal crease incision [23]. Carrion reported excision of the penoscrotal web to enhance cosmetic outcome (ventral phalloplasty) [39]. The sliding technique and its modification [40] distract the tunica albuginea with an interpositional graft. However, it carries some risk of glans necrosis. Autologous fat injection [41] or dermofat grafting [36] can be used for girth enhancement.

Postoperative Care

The AUA guidelines on antimicrobial prophylaxis for urologic procedures state that there is no evidence to support continued antibiotic prophylaxis beyond wound closure and that prophylaxis should be limited to the duration of the procedure itself with no subsequent dosing postoperatively, even in the presence of a drain [42]. However, this is disputed by other urologists, some who recommend the addition of anti-fungal agents [43] and others who favor post-operative antibiotic prophylaxis. "The North American Consensus Document on Infection of Penile Prostheses" recommends the use of intravenous antibiotics as long as the patient is hospitalized and for a minimum of 24 h, as well as oral antibiotic prophylaxis for 5–14 days postoperatively [18].

Pain, ecchymosis, and swelling of varying degrees are common following implantation. Supportive undergarments help decrease edema. Cycling the iPP should begin as soon as possible, provided there is no risk of disrupting the penoscrotal incision and the patient can tolerate the process. This typically occurs within an average of 4 weeks, but may happen earlier with subcoronal and infrapubic approaches. Coital relationship is postponed for several weeks following surgery.

Outcomes

Satisfaction Rate

Satisfaction rates following IPP are generally high in uncomplicated cases. This has been well-documented, though it utilizes different tools and questionnaires, ranging from 5-point satisfaction scales to specific questionnaires. Utilizing the "Satisfaction Survey for Inflatable Penile Implant" questionnaire, 89.8% of patients were satisfied with the surgery [44], positively correlating with postoperative penile size. In a study of 883 patients utilizing the "Erectile Dysfunction Inventory of Treatment Satisfaction" questionnaire, couples' satisfaction rates were significantly higher in the 3-piece IPP group than in the malleable group, yet with no significant difference between the 2-piece and 3-piece IPP groups. There was no difference in terms of couples' satisfaction according to the brand of the implants. Of the patients, 99.2% were satisfied or somewhat satisfied with the 3-piece IPP; however, 90.3% were satisfied or somewhat satisfied with the malleable. Partner's dissatisfaction rates were 3.3% with the 3-piece IPP, 3.8% with the 2-piece IPP, and 11.2% with the malleable implants [45].

Mechanical Failure

In a meta-analysis of studies evaluating long-term survival of IPP, median survival was approximately 20 years. In 12 studies covering 20,161 patients, device survival exceeded 90% in the first 3 years and was 87.2% at 5 years, 76.8% at 10 years, 63.7% at 15 years, and 52.9% at 20 years [46].

Patients with a failed IPP usually present with a failure to inflate, despite the ability to compress the pump. However, some will present with the "Sticky Pump Syndrome," where the pump cannot be compressed. Others may present with cylinder herniation. Auto-inflation of the implant is rather rare with the more recent IPP designs.

Revision for mechanical failure implies exchange of some or all components of IPP. It is preferable to perform a repetitive antiseptic wash of the device space before implanting the new components (salvage/mini-salvage), though its value has been disputed [47]. Extracapsular implantation was suggested to avoid activation of bacterial biofilm. Instead of inserting the new components in the same space, another space for implantation is created between the implant fibrous tissue capsule and tunica albuginea [48]. In the absence of infection, if reservoir removal is difficult or risky, it can be emptied and left behind, and a new reservoir can be implanted on the contralateral side.

On the other hand, fracture or breakage of malleable implant rods is rare, with only a few case reports in the literature [49]. This may manifest as instability or a loss of rigidity in the implant. Fractures in the metal core can be visualized by roentgenogram. One suggested reason for breaks was reported to be misplacement, with crossing over of the rods [50].

Complications

Intraoperative complications include anterior extrusion, posterior perforation, urethral injury, crossing-over, failure of dilatation, and needle puncture of IPP cylinders. The most grave intraoperative complication may be visceral injury upon retro-pubic placement of the reservoir. Post-operatively, device infection and tissue devascularization are the most horrid complications. Device herniation, or extrusion, whether distal or proximal, can manifest later following surgery.

Intraoperative extrusion is mostly due to aggressive dilatation, particularly in cases with corporal scarring. The surgeon can evaluate for anterior (distal) perforation by forceful irrigation of saline distally, where it will spurt out of the urethral meatus if perforation did occur. In rare cases, the dilator may emerge out of the meatus. Such an event is mostly a reason to terminate the procedure. Urinary diversion, through a Foley catheter, will provide a chance for healing, and implantation is performed later. Some surgeons advocate repair and proceed with implantation if the urethra is not compromised. Urethral injury can mostly be avoided by "staying lateral" upon dilatation. If injury does occur, the mainstream approach is to terminate, divert urine, and come back later for the implant. Some surgeons will perform primary repairs particularly if the injury is proximal [11]. Sterilization of the urethra with chlorhexidine gel perioperatively further enables the latter option [19]. Pending anterior perforation is a postoperative finding that is either due to oversizing or to aggressive coitus. It can be repaired by either re-routing the implant tip under the capsule [51] or primary repair of the defect with or without mesh [52].

Posterior (proximal) extrusion is diagnosed when the dilator sinks into the perineum rather than stopping at the pubic bone. It can be managed intraoperatively and is not a reason to abort. Several techniques were designed to repair proximal extrusion. Apart from a perineal incision and direct repair, the rear-tip extenders can be anchored by non-absorbable suture to the corporotomy, thereby holding the implant in place until fibrosis closes the defect. The same can be achieved with the "WindSock" technique, where the proximal end is wrapped in a mesh [53].

Crossing-over occurs when one dilator (and consequently cylinder) crosses the midline septum into the contralateral side. The "Goal Post" sign indicates a misshap when one dilator fully enters while the other does not, producing a characteristic metallic sound as it clicks against the first dilator. Crossing-over can be avoided by staying lateral during dilatation. If it does occur, redilation is necessary. Needle-puncture of the IPP can be avoided by tying the pre-placed stay sutures to close the corporotomy, rather than suturing it closed. This may come at the expense of possible bleeding through the corporotomy, hence draining and/or "mummy wrap." Finally, injury of the urinary bladder, bowl, or iliac vessels has promoted ectopic reservoir placement. Nevertheless, if retropubic placement is intended, the urinary bladder should be emptied, and entry to the space of Retzius should not be laterally directed to avoid the iliac vessels.

Glans or skin necrosis can be the result of compressive dressing, oversizing in length and girth, or neglected device infection, particularly if the neurovascular bundle and spongiosum are mobilized, and particularly in diabetic patients. Early removal of the device may control the damage.

Device infection rates have been dramatically reduced since the introduction of antibiotic/hydrophilic coating. It is currently less than 1% in expert hands. Patient-related factors that may predispose to infection include diabetes, degree of diabetic sugar control, presence of pathologic nasal flora, long-term steroid use, active smoking, HIV status, history of radiation therapy, virgin implantation versus redo, spinal cord injury, obesity, concomitant circumcision, and prior renal transplantation. Surgeon-related factors include experience, operative time, proper preoperative preparation as stated earlier, and minimizing contact between the patient's skin and the implant, the instruments, and the surgical gloves [11].

If infection does occur, it will almost always indicate explantation of all device components. The mainstream approach is to wait several weeks following explantation until resolution of infection and control of risk factors, then to re-implant (delayed replantation). In the meantime, fibrosis sets in, indicating the use of one of the previously described techniques for implantation in scarred corporal bodies. An alternative is immediate salvage, whereby all components are explanted, and the component spaces are irrigated with a series of antiseptic/antibacterial solutions. Rescrubbing and redraping are performed, and a replacement prosthesis is implanted [54]. The essence of salvage technique is to avoid fibrosis and the burden of a third surgery. Outcome reports are highly variable. Some experts advocate using a malleable implant as the replacement, either temporarily or permanently, because its surface area for colonization is smaller than that of IPP. A more recent trend is "Delayed Salvage," whereby the infected device is explanted, and reimplantation is performed within 3–4 weeks at most, giving a chance for resolution of the infection yet reimplanting before extensive fibrosis sets in. Another modification of salvage is to perform the wash-out and then implant the replacement prosthesis outside the original capsule [48]. A third modification is irrigation with 0.05% chlorhexidine gluconate (Irrisept®) following explantation, with corporal rechanneling where a new space is developed for implantation of a size 9 malleable prosthesis through a separate incision [55].

In the case of delayed replantation, two methods have been proposed to avoid or minimize fibrosis and maintain the cavity for the replacement cylinders. One is the use of a high-purity calcium sulfate (SHPCaSO$_4$) component that acts as a "spacer" [56], and the other is instilling mitomycin (an antifibrotic agent) [57].

Patient Dissatisfaction

Although penile prosthesis implants have a high rate of patient satisfaction [45], patient selection is very important in the process. Surgeons must spend time explaining the procedure and solving all patients and partners' doubts and bringing patients' expectations to reality. Most of malpractice claims against urologists who perform reconstructive procedures result from dissatisfaction and misunderstanding due to lack of communication between patient and doctor [11].

Vascular Surgery

Penile Arterial Revascularization

Penile arterial insufficiency and venous occlusive dysfunction are important causes of erectile dysfunction. The goal of restoring penile vascularization and/or improving venous occlusion alterations have led to the proposition of many surgical procedures. Despite these surgical procedures present the possibility of restoring the erectile they are still considered experimental in many cases, because of the lack of standardization in patient selection, diagnostic parameters surgical technique, and limited long-term outcome data using validated instruments [58].

The idea of increasing blood flow to the penis to treat erectile dysfunction began in 1973 with Michal's description of the anastomosis of the inferior epigastric artery to the corpus cavernosum [59]. Although the initial result was good, all anastomoses thrombosed. Michal then described the anastomosis of the inferior epigastric artery to the dorsal artery of the penis [60]. Virag then described the first anastomosis of the inferior epigastric artery to the dorsal vein, with the aim of increasing arterial blood supply retrogradely [61]. Fisher and Furlow [62] then perfected the arteriovenous anastomosis technique by tying the circumflex veins and avoiding the main complication, which was hyperemia of the glans.

Although penile vascular surgery ushered in a new era in the treatment of erectile dysfunction, attracting urologists and vascular surgeons, time showed that these operations had limited results, primarily due to the lack of standardized diagnosis of vasculogenic erectile dysfunction [63]. Furthermore, arterial anastomoses in the penis had a high rate of thrombosis due to the low-pressure gradient between the donor and recipient sites, given that in the flaccid penile state, the penile vessels have very low flow and high resistance.

According to the Guidelines of the European Association of Urology [64], penile revascularization is reserved for post-traumatic arteriogenic ED. In young patients with pelvic or perineal trauma. The stenosis must be confirmed by penile pharmaco-arteriography. Corporeal veno-occlusive dysfunction is a contraindication to revascularization and must be excluded.

Munarriz et al. [63] proposed that the ideal candidate for penile revascularization must be younger than 40 years old and should not have any of the following vascular risk factors (such as diabetes, hypertension, tobacco use, and hypercholesterolemia), neurologic causes of erectile dysfunction (including multiple sclerosis, pelvic surgery, lumbosacral, radiculopathies, peripheral neuropaties), hormonal abnormalities, psychogenic erectile dysfunction, the use of psychotropic drugs, Peyronie's disease or premature ejaculation.

Repair of Internal Iliac Artery Stenosis

The internal iliac artery is responsible for delivering blood to the pelvic region, encompassing the penis. Repairing internal iliac artery stenosis involves a precise method to rectify erectile dysfunction related to arterial insufficiency by mending or circumventing the narrowed portion of the internal iliac artery. The goal of this intervention is to reestablish adequate blood flow to the pelvic area and the penile arteries, which is intended to enhance erectile capability and overall sexual function. However, a personalized evaluation is essential to weigh the potential risks and decide if internal iliac artery stenosis repair is a suitable treatment for erectile dysfunction. There have been a limited number of studies that have identified erectile dysfunction as a consequence of external iliac steal syndrome. In such cases, treatments have included percutaneous transluminal angioplasty and stent placement targeting either the common iliac artery or the internal iliac artery [65–67]. Endovascular recanalization, which involves reopening blocked common iliac arteries or internal iliac arteries, has been shown to enhance sexual function. In fact, more than half of the patients with erectile dysfunction who underwent this endovascular procedure experienced improvements in their sexual performance [65, 67].

Venous Ligation Surgery

In 1981, Virag [68] described erectile dysfunction that occurred due to increased penile venous drainage, which became known as venous leak and later as veno-occlusive dysfunction of the corpora cavernosa. In this same article, Virag described dorsal vein ligation to treat this entity. In 1985, Wespes and Schulman [69] described cavernosometry as a method for diagnosing veno-occlusive dysfunction of the corpora cavernosa.

Since then, several techniques have been proposed to treat this entity: crural ligation of the penis, to treat the leakage through the crura [70]; a combination of both deep dorsal vein and penile crura ligation [71]; spongiosolysis, with the aim to ligate the shunts between distal corpora cavernosa and the corpus spongiosum [72]; penile venous stripping, a meticulous resection of the whole superficial venous drainage of the penis [73]; ligation of the internal pudendal vein [74]; and percutaneous veno-ablation [75].

However, venous surgery to treat venous occlusive of the corpora cavernosa is no longer recommended due to the poor results [64]. The poor results may be due to the lack of standardization of diagnostic methods for veno-occlusive dysfunction of the corpora cavernosa and the lack of characterization of this entity, since venous diseases are characterized by blood stasis and not by increased flow as would occur in penile venous leak [76, 77].

References

1. Tracy EE. Ligation of the dorsal vein of the penis for impotency. South Med Rec. 1897;27(12):616–8.
2. Lespinasse V. Impotency: its treatment by transplantation of the testicle. Surg Clin Chicago. 1918;2:281–8.
3. Stanley L. An analysis of one thousand testicular substance implantations. Endocrinology. 1922;6(6):787–94.
4. Lowsley O. Impotence in man. South Med J. 1935;28:1091–7.
5. Bogoras N. Über die volle plastische Wiederherstellung eines zum Koitus fähigen Penis (Peni plastica totalis). Zentralbl Chir. 1936;22:1271–6.
6. Goodwin WE, Scott WW. Phalloplasty. J Urol. 1952;68(6):903–8.
7. Beheri G. The problem of impotence solved by a new surgical operation. Kasr El Aini J Surg. 1960;1:50.
8. Beheri G. Surgical treatment of impotence. Plast Reconstr Surg. 1966;38(2):92–7.
9. Scott FB, Bradley WE, Timm GW. Management of erectile impotence. Use of implantable inflatable prosthesis. Urology. 1973;2(1):80–2.
10. Small MP, Carrion HM, Gordon JA. Small-Carrion penile prosthesis. New implant for management of impotence. Urology. 1975;5(4):479–86.
11. Köhler TS, Munarriz R, Parker J, et al. Penile prosthesis for erectile dysfunction: recommendations from the 5th International Consultation on Sexual Medicine. Sex Med Rev. 2025;13(2):144–71. https://doi.org/10.1093/sxmrev/qeaf001. PMID: 40072010.
12. Dos Reis MMF, Barros EAC, Pollone M, et al. Preoperative psychological evaluation for patients referred for penile prosthesis implantation. Sex Med. 2021;9(2):100311. https://doi.org/10.1016/j.esxm.2020.100311. Epub 2021 Mar 11. PMID: 33714883; PMCID: PMC8072176.
13. Barham DW, et al. Surgeon variations in the perioperative evaluation of penile prosthesis patients. Int J Impot Res. 2023;35(2):152–6.
14. Carson CC 3rd. Efficacy of antibiotic impregnation of inflatable penile prostheses in decreasing infection in original implants. J Urol. 2004;171(4):1611–4.
15. Chen T, Li S, Eisenberg ML. The association between hemoglobin A1c levels and inflatable penile prosthesis infection: analysis of US insurance claims data. J Sex Med. 2021;18(6):1104–9.
16. Dick BP, et al. Does lowering hemoglobin A1c reduce penile prosthesis infection: a systematic review. Sex Med Rev. 2021;9(4):628–35.
17. Wolf JS, et al. Best practice policy statement on urologic surgery antimicrobial prophylaxis. J Urol. 2008;179(4):1379–90.
18. Darouiche RO, et al. North American consensus document on infection of penile prostheses. Urology. 2013;82(4):937–42.
19. Shaeer O, et al. Urethral instillation of chlorhexidine gel is an effective method of sterilisation. Arab J Urol. 2021;19(3):419–22.
20. Eid JF. Penile implant: review of a "no-touch" technique. Sex Med Rev. 2016;4(3):294–300.
21. Otero JR, Manfredi C, Wilson SK. The good, the bad, and the ugly about surgical approaches for inflatable penile prosthesis implantation. Int J Impot Res. 2022;34(2):128–37.
22. Shaeer O, Shaeer K. Shaeer's infrapubic technique for penile prosthesis implantation through a single midline corporotomy: a single-center pilot study. J Sex Med. 2023;20(3):410–5.
23. Shaeer O, Shaeer K, AbdelRahman IF. Simultaneous suprapubic lipectomy and penile prosthesis implantation. J Sex Med. 2018;15(12):1818–23.
24. Baumgarten AS, et al. Suprapubic fat pad excision with simultaneous placement of inflatable penile prosthesis. J Sex Med. 2019;16(2):333–7.
25. Van Dyke M, et al. State of the reservoir: current concepts of penile implant reservoir placement and potential complications. Curr Urol Rep. 2021;22(4):20.

26. Wilson SK, Delk JR 2nd. A new treatment for Peyronie's disease: modeling the penis over an inflatable penile prosthesis. J Urol. 1994;152(4):1121–3.
27. Morey AF. Re: High patient satisfaction of inflatable penile prosthesis insertion with synchronous penile plication for erectile dysfunction and Peyronie's disease. J Urol. 2015;193(3):906.
28. Hatzichristodoulou G, et al. Multicenter experience using collagen fleece for plaque incision with grafting to correct residual curvature at the time of inflatable penile prosthesis placement in patients with Peyronie's disease. J Sex Med. 2020;17(6):1168–74.
29. Fernández-Pascual E, et al. Surgical technique for complex cases of Peyronie's disease with implantation of penile prosthesis, multiple corporeal incisions, and grafting with collagen fleece. J Sex Med. 2019;16(2):323–32.
30. Shaeer O, Shaeer A. Corporoscopic excavation of the fibrosed corpora cavernosa for penile prosethesis implantation: optical corporotomy and trans-corporeal resection, Shaeer's technique. J Sex Med. 2007;4(1):218–25.
31. Shaeer O, et al. Shaeer's punch technique: transcorporeal Peyronie's plaque surgery and penile prosthesis implantation. J Sex Med. 2020;17(7):1395–9.
32. Perito P, Wilson S. The Peyronie's plaque "scratch": an adjunct to modeling. J Sex Med. 2013;10(5):1194–7.
33. Rosselló Barbará M, Carrión H. Cavernotomy. Arch Esp Urol. 1991;44(2):185–6.
34. Mooreville M, et al. Implantation of inflatable penile prosthesis in patients with severe corporeal fibrosis: introduction of a new penile cavernotome. J Urol. 1999;162(6):2054–7.
35. Shaeer O, Shaeer K. Shaeer's cavernotome for penile prosthesis implantation in scarred corpora cavernosa. Urol Res Pract. 2023;49(2):116–9.
36. Shaeer O. Supersizing the penis following penile prosthesis implantation. J Sex Med. 2010;7(7):2608–16.
37. El Gharably MAF, et al. The efficacy of suspensory ligament release and pubic lipectomy via penopubic Z plasty during penile prosthesis implantation in improving sexual satisfaction: a prospective randomized controlled trial. J Sex Med. 2022;19(5):852–63.
38. Shaeer O, et al. Dorsal phalloplasty accompanying penile prosthesis implantation minimizes penile shortening and improves patient satisfaction. Int J Impot Res. 2019;31(4):276–81.
39. Miranda-Sousa A, et al. Concomitant ventral phalloplasty during penile implant surgery: a novel procedure that optimizes patient satisfaction and their perception of phallic length after penile implant surgery. J Sex Med. 2007;4(5):1494–9.
40. Egydio PH, Kuehhas FE, Valenzuela RJ. Modified sliding technique (MoST) for penile lengthening with insertion of inflatable penile prosthesis. J Sex Med. 2015;12(5):1100–4.
41. Salem AM, et al. Effect of girth supersizing on patient satisfaction after semi-rigid penile implant insertion: a prospective case-control study. Aesthet Surg J. 2019;39(7):np259–65.
42. Lightner DJ, et al. Best practice statement on urologic procedures and antimicrobial prophylaxis. J Urol. 2020;203(2):351–6.
43. Barham DW, et al. AUA-recommended antibiotic prophylaxis for primary penile implantation results in a higher, not lower, risk for postoperative infection: a multicenter analysis. J Urol. 2023;209(2):399–409.
44. Beirnaert J, et al. Evaluation of patient satisfaction using the validated French version of the SSIPI questionnaire after inflatable penile implantation. J Sex Med. 2023;21(1):67–71.
45. Çayan S, et al. Comparison of long-term results and couples' satisfaction with penile implant types and brands: lessons learned from 883 patients with erectile dysfunction who underwent penile prosthesis implantation. J Sex Med. 2019;16(7):1092–9.
46. Miller LE, et al. Long-term survival rates of inflatable penile prostheses: systematic review and meta-analysis. Urology. 2022;166:6–10.
47. Bartley J, Zimmerman WB, Dhabuwala CB. Inflatable penile prosthesis and salvage protocol for mechanical failure: is it really necessary? J Sex Med. 2012;9(8):2175–81.
48. Shaeer O, Shaeer K, Soliman AbdelRahman IF. Salvage and extracapsular implantation for penile prosthesis infection or extrusion. J Sex Med. 2019;16(5):755–9.

49. Pinheiro MA, et al. Multiple site fracture of both rods in a malleable penile implant. Case Rep Urol. 2016;2016:9564904.
50. Karakoyunlu N, et al. Malfunctioned and fractured penile prosthesis caused by cross placement: case report. Urol Case Rep. 2015;3(3):80–1.
51. Pe Leve PJP, et al. Cylinder rerouting for lateral extrusion after inflatable penile prosthesis implantation—surgical technique revision. Arch Ital Urol Androl. 2020;92(3):271–2. https://doi.org/10.4081/aiua.2020.3.271.
52. Shaeer O. Management of distal extrusion of penile prosthesis: partial disassembly and tip reinforcement by double breasting or grafting. J Sex Med. 2008;5(5):1257–62.
53. Pearlman AM, Terlecki RP. Proximal corporal perforation during penile prosthesis surgery: prevention, recognition, and review of historical and novel management strategies. J Sex Med. 2018;15(7):1055–60.
54. Swanton AR, et al. Penile prosthesis salvage: a historical look at the Mulcahy technique and a review of the latest literature. Int J Impot Res. 2023;35(2):90–4.
55. Razdan S, et al. Three piece penile prosthesis salvage with chlorhexidine gluconate and length preservation: our technique and outcomes. Am J Clin Exp Urol. 2023;11(2):155–9.
56. Swords K, et al. A preliminary report on the usage of an intracorporal antibiotic cast with synthetic high purity CaSO4 for the treatment of infected penile implant. J Sex Med. 2013;10(4):1162–9.
57. Shaeer O, Abdel Rahman IFS, Shaeer K. Shaeer's anti-scarring technique: a preventive measure against corporal fibrosis upon explantation of infected penile implants. Sex Med. 2019;7(3):357–60.
58. Argiolas A, Argiolas FM, Argiolas G, Melis MR. Erectile dysfunction: treatments, advances and new therapeutic strategies. Brain Sci. 2023;13(5):802.
59. Michal V, Kramar R, Pospichal J, et al. Direct arterial anastomosis to the cavernous body in the treatment of erectile impotence. Cesk Rozhl Chir. 1973;52:587–93.
60. Michal V, Kramer R, Hejhal L. Revascularization procedures of the cavernous bodies. In: Zorgniotti AW, Ross G, editors. Vasculogenic impotence: Proceedings of the first international conference on corpus cavernosum revascularization. Springfield: Charles C Thomas; 1980. p. 239–55.
61. Virag R, Zwang G, Dermange H, et al. Vasculogenic impotence: a review of 92 cases with 54 surgical operations. Vasc Surg. 1981;15:9–16.
62. Furlow WL, Fisher J. Deep dorsal vein arterialization: clinical experience with a new technique for penile revascularization. J Urol. 1988;139:298A. Abstr. 543
63. Munarriz R, Thirumavalavan N, Gross MS. Is there a role for vascular surgery in the contemporary management of erectile dysfunction? Urol Clin North Am. 2021;48(4):543–55.
64. Salonia A, Capogrosso P, Boeri L, et al. European Association of Urology guidelines on male sexual and reproductive health: 2025 update on male hypogonadism, erectile dysfunction, premature ejaculation, and Peyronie's disease. Eur Urol. 2025;88(1):76–102.
65. Gur S, et al. Impotence due to external iliac steal syndrome: treatment with percutaneous transluminal angioplasty and stent placement. Korean J Radiol. 2013;14(1):81–5.
66. Urigo F, et al. Role of arteriography and percutaneous transluminal angioplasty in the diagnosis and treatment of arterial vasculogenic impotence. Radiol Med. 1994;88(1–2):86–92.
67. Gur S, et al. The effect of endovascular revascularization of common iliac artery occlusions on erectile function. Cardiovasc Intervent Radiol. 2013;36(1):84–9.
68. Virag R. Syndrome d'érection instable par insuffisance veineuse. Diagnostic et correction chirurgicale. A propos de 10 cas avec un recul moyen de 12 mois [Unstable erection due to venous insufficiency. Diagnosis and surgical correction. 10 cases with a mean follow-up 12 months (author's transl)]. J Mal Vasc. 1981;6(2):121–4.
69. Wespes E, Schulman CC. Venous leakage: surgical treatment of a curable cause of impotence. J Urol. 1985;133(5):796–8.
70. Puech-Leão P, Reis JM, Glina S, Reichelt AC. Leakage through the crural edge of corpus cavernosum. Diagnosis and treatment. Eur Urol. 1987;13(3):163–5.

71. Hassan AA, Hassouna MM, Elhilali MM. Long-term results of penile venous ligation for corporeal venous occlusive dysfunction. Can J Surg. 1995;38(6):537–41.
72. Gilbert P, Stief C. Spongiosolysis: a new surgical treatment of impotence caused by distal venous leakage. J Urol. 1987;138(4):784–6.
73. Hsu GL, et al. Clinical experience of a refined penile venous stripping surgery procedure for patients with erectile dysfunction: is it a viable option? J Androl. 2010;31(3):271–80.
74. Shaeer O, et al. Sub-gluteal ligation of the internal pudendal vein for management of veno-occlusive erectile dysfunction (Shaeer's vein ligation-I): the cadaveric study. Int J Impot Res. 2024. https://doi.org/10.1038/s41443-024-00846-1.
75. Maiza D, et al. Preliminary results 6 months after embolization of the deep dorsal vein of the penis in erectile insufficiencies of venous origin. J Mal Vasc. 1984;9(4):327.
76. Glina S, Silva MF, Puech-Leão P, Reis JM, Lucon AM. Veno-occlusive dysfunction of corpora cavernosa: comparison of diagnostic methods. Int J Impot Res. 1995;7(1):1–10. discussion 11.
77. Glina S, Ghanem H. SOP: corpus cavernosum assessment (cavernosography/cavernosometry). J Sex Med. 2013;10(1):111–4.

Chapter 6
Regenerative Therapies for Erectile Dysfunction: How Far Are We with the Evidence?

Manaf Al Hashimi, Tuncay Toprak, and Rupin Shah

Introduction

ED is described as the incapability to obtain or maintain erections that are adequate for satisfactory sexual performance. Its prevalence increases with age, with 22.5% of men between 40 and 80 years old in the United States reporting ED [1].

ED can profoundly impact the psychosocial aspects of a man's life, causing a range of emotional and relational challenges. Men experiencing ED face frustration, loss of self-esteem, anxiety, depression, and even avoidance of intimate relationships. Additionally, ED may diminish overall quality of life, impacting social interactions, work productivity, and self-image [2].

Multiple ED treatment options are available. A common recommendation is to maintain a healthy lifestyle and manage any related comorbidities. Phosphodiesterase 5 Inhibitors (PDE5Is) continue to be preferred as an initial treatment choice due to their effectiveness and safety. However, it is clear that a portion of patients either do

M. Al Hashimi (✉)
Department of Urology, Burjeel Hospital, Abu Dhabi, UAE

Department of Clinical Urology, College of Medicine and Health Science, Khalifa University, Abu Dhabi, UAE

Global Andrology Forum, Moreland Hills, OH, USA

T. Toprak
University of Health Sciences, Hamidiye Faculty of Medicine, FSM Health Practice & Research Center, Deparment of Urology, Istanbul, Turkey

R. Shah
Department of Urology, Lilavati Hospital & Research Centre, Mumbai, India

R. Shah et al. (eds.), *Diagnosis and Treatment of Male Sexual Dysfunction*,
https://doi.org/10.1007/978-3-032-12423-4_6

not respond to or are non-compliant with PDE5 inhibitors. Data indicates that nearly half of these patients discontinue the use of PDE5 inhibitors within a year, with no single predominant factor contributing to the dropout rates [3, 4]. For these patients, intracavernosal injections or intraurethral alprostadil provide an alternative therapeutic option, although they are not without potential local adverse effects [3, 4].

When the aforementioned therapies prove ineffective, then penile prosthesis implants (PPI) emerge as the final recourse for addressing erectile dysfunction. Studies consistently report a patient satisfaction rate ranging between 80% and 90%, affirming the validity of penile implants as a viable option for motivated individuals grappling with ED. Nevertheless, before undergoing this irreversible surgical procedure, patients should be meticulously chosen and provided with counseling for possible surgical and technical complications [5].

Despite all available options for ED treatment, most men and their partners report that spontaneous erections are preferable to pharmacologic or surgical approaches to ED [6]. Therefore, experts have actively sought novel approaches like regenerative therapy (RT), which reverses organ dysfunction and restores the function of the penile vasculature.

RT for ED relies on the idea of repairing or substituting damaged tissue through the stimulation of the body's natural regenerative abilities. These approaches offer a hopeful alternative to existing treatment methods and signify a shift away from merely alleviating symptoms towards restoring the integrity and functionality of erectile tissue [7]. RT encompasses interventions like stem cell therapy (SCT) or platelet-rich plasma (PRP) treatments, as well as technologies grounded in regenerative principles, like low-intensity shock wave therapy (LISWT). These modalities aim to stimulate the natural erectile mechanisms in the penile tissues [8].

While numerous clinical trials have been conducted worldwide on the use of RT for ED, many of these studies involve small patient cohorts, lack randomization, and exhibit significant heterogeneity in both patient selection and application protocols. These factors create obstacles for societies in developing practical recommendations for ED specialists, leading to uncertainty about which practices to implement in their clinical approach [9]. Consequently, the aim of this review is to present an overview of studies on different RT modalities and existing guidelines from relevant societies, thereby offering guidance for optimal clinical practice in the treatment of ED.

Low-Intensity Shock Wave Therapy

LISWT is a non-invasive medical treatment aimed at improving ED by stimulating the growth of new blood vessels and enhancing blood flow to the penis. It involves the application of low-energy shockwaves, typically delivered to targeted areas of the penis using a specialized device. In the field of andrology and sexual medicine, Vardi et al. were the pioneers in introducing LISWT clinical research in treating

ED. They demonstrated, for the first time, the successful treatment of ED patients using LISWT [10].

Types of Shock Wave

Different types of shocks utilized in LISWT for addressing ED include electrohydraulic, electromagnetic, and piezoelectric methods.

In *electrohydraulic generators*, electrodes' tips are immersed in a fluid. Upon application of voltage, the fluid undergoes vaporization, leading to rapid expansion in the surrounding fluid and resulting in shockwave propagation.

Electromagnetic generators disturb a fluid by applying a voltage across metallic membranes, generating a magnetic field that induces sudden movement in a metallic membrane, consequently propagating shockwaves.

Piezoelectric generators incorporate piezoceramic elements within a spherical device submerged in a medium. Upon voltage application, the ceramic elements expand, causing a mechanical disturbance in the surrounding medium.

In electrohydraulic and most electromagnetic shockwave generators, a lens or reflector is utilized to focus the waves onto a specific target. However, certain electromagnetic generators and all piezoelectric generators are self-focusing due to the arrangement of the piezoelectric crystals [11].

Some other companies have introduced a range of devices known as linear shockwave generators, with the ability to direct shockwaves through an aperture to specifically align with the configuration of corpora and crura. Unlike traditional point-focused methods, these devices administer energy to a broader area of intended tissue simultaneously [11, 12].

The fourth type of waves is ballistic radial pressure waves, which represent a distinct category of acoustic waves. They arise from a controlled explosion, propelling a projectile into a probe, thus generating a wave upon impact. They objectively resemble "conventional" sound waves and exhibit lower peak pressure, a slower rise time, and propagation outward without a focal point. This type of wave and its producing machines are of questionable value in producing therapeutic effects for treating ED [11, 13].

Mechanisms of Action

It is postulated that LISWT causes repetitive shear stress (microtrauma) to target tissue, resulting in a cascade of biological reactions, including the release of various angiogenic factors, such as endothelial nitric oxide synthase [13]. LISWT provides low-intensity shock waves that are thought to induce beneficial effects in human tissues, possibly through the stimulation of mechanic sensors. The proposed therapeutic mechanisms of action for LISWT include neovascularization, tissue regeneration, and reduction of inflammation. These effects are thought to be mediated by enhanced expression of vascular endothelial growth factor, endothelial nitric oxide synthase, and proliferating cell nuclear antigen [14, 15]. Upregulation of chemoattractant factors and recruitment/activation of stem/progenitor cells may also play a role. Moreover, immunohistochemistry or immunefluorescence analyses indicated that LISWT led to an augmentation in the cavernosal smooth muscle/collagen ratio, enhanced elastin fiber presence, and a suppression of the transforming growth factor-ß1/Smad/connective tissue growth factor signaling pathway. Consequently, LIESWT exhibits anti-fibrotic tissue remodeling properties [14, 15]. Additionally, possible nerve regeneration by enhancing the recruitment and activation of progenitor Schwann cells has been suggested [15].

Clinical Studies of LISWT in ED Treatment

Due to the low risk associated with treatment and the increasing evidence for positive results, numerous specialists in ED are now presenting LISWT as an alternative treatment for ED in particular instances. However, a notable challenge exists in identifying the most efficient treatment regimen, primarily due to the significant heterogeneity present in the available studies. This heterogeneity pertains to various factors such as the type of shockwave, the frequency and duration of shockwave sessions, the intervals between sessions, and the criteria for selecting patients for this treatment approach [16–18].

Hayon S. et al. presented a review of literature focusing on randomized, sham-controlled trials of LISWT for ED published between 2012 and 2022. The review included only studies that specified device settings, number of shocks, treatment sessions, shock locations, etiology of ED, and concurrent medication usage. The review encompasses a total of 14 studies with 968 patients with different outcome measures, including both subjective and objective, like the International Index of Erectile Function (IIEF), erection hardness score (EHS), and peak systolic velocity (PSV). Across the reviewed studies, there was a consistent trend toward positive treatment outcomes. The most prevalent settings included an energy level of 0.09 mJ/mm^2 and a frequency of 5 Hz. Although shock numbers and locations varied, the typical protocol comprised 1500 shocks per session, with 900 directed to the penis (shaft, base, or hilum) and 600 to the proximal corpora/crura. The number of sessions ranged from 4 to 12, with variable intervals between treatments [17] (Table 6.1).

Lu Z et al. presented a meta-analysis of 14 studies published between 2005 and 2015 and involving 833 patients. Seven of these studies were randomized controlled trials (RCTs), and the others were cohort studies. The IIEF was the prevailing assessment tool for ED. The findings suggest that LISWT boosted the IIEF scores and enhanced erectile function in individuals with ED. The setup parameters for LISWT differed across various studies, and the quantity of shock wave pulses administered per treatment varied between 1500 and 5000. In the majority of

Table 6.1 The treatment protocols of LISWT for ED from variable studies [17]

Author (country year)	ED patient population	Patients (n)	Energy (mJ/mm^2)	Pulse frequency (Hz)	Total shocks (sessions)	Penile shocks (shaft/base/glans)	Proximal shocks (corpora/crura)	No. of sessions	Device	Outcome
Kaylaynaks (Turkey 2012)	ED: mixed	20	0.096	5	2000	2000	600	12	Aries 2 (OmniSpecMeditech)	IIEF: +, EHS: +
Vardi (Israel 2012)	ED: mixed	29	0.16	5	3000	3000	900	12	PiezoWave2 (Richard Wolf)	IIEF: +, EHS: +
Gruenwald (Israel 2013)	ED: mixed	29	0.15	5	4000	4000	1200	12	Duolith SD1 (Storz Medical)	IIEF: +, EHS: +
Kalyvianakis (Greece 2014)	ED: mixed	30	0.2	5	4000	4000	1800	12	CSW-400 (Chattanooga Intelect)	IIEF: +, EHS: +
Kitrey (Israel 2016)	ED: mixed	58	0.09	5	3000	3000	900	12	Renova (DirexGroup)	IIEF: +, EHS: +
Moayedifar (Iran 2018)	ED: mixed	28	0.2	5	5000	5000	1500	12	MT ONE (UrotechKorea)	IIEF: +, EHS: +
Fojecki (Denmark 2017)	ED: mixed	60	0.09	2.7	1500	1500	600	12	Aries 2 (OmniSpecMeditech)	IIEF: no change, EHS: no change
Vardi (Israel 2012)	ED: vasculogenic	20	0.096	5	2000	2000	600	12	Aries 2 (OmniSpecMeditech)	IIEF: +, EHS: +
Kalyvianakis (Greece 2017)	ED: vasculogenic	30	0.16	5	3000	3000	900	12	PiezoWave2 (Richard Wolf)	IIEF: +, EHS: +
Motil (Czech 2021)	ED: vasculogenic	60	0.15	5	4000	4000	1200	12	Duolith SD1 (Storz Medical)	IIEF: +, EHS: +

(continued)

Table 6.1 (continued)

Author (country year)	ED patient population	Patients (n)	Energy (mJ/mm^2)	Pulse frequency (Hz)	Total shocks (sessions)	Penile shocks (shaft/base/glans)	Proximal shocks (corpora/crura)	No. of sessions	Device	Outcome
Gupta (India 2017)	ED: vasculogenic	65	0.2	5	4000	4000	1800	12	CSW-400 (Chattanooga Intelect)	IIEF: +, EHS: +
Kitrey (Israel 2019)	ED: vasculogenic	50	0.09	5	3000	3000	900	12	Renova (DirexGroup)	IIEF: +, EHS: +
Kim (Korea 2020)	ED: vasculogenic	56	0.2	5	5000	5000	1500	12	MT ONE (UrotechKorea)	IIEF: +, EHS: +
Kitrey (Israel 2016)	ED: PDE5i non-responders	47	0.09	5	1500	1500	600	12	Aries 2 (OmniSpecMeditech)	IIEF: no change, EHS: no change
Kalyvianakis (Greece 2015)	ED: PDE5i non-responders	90	0.16	5	3000	3000	900	12	PiezoWave2 (Richard Wolf)	IIEF: +, EHS: +
Vardi (Israel 2015)	ED: PDE5i non-responders	55	0.15	5	4000	4000	1200	12	Duolith SD1 (Storz Medical)	IIEF: +, EHS: +
Vardi (Israel 2012)	ED: PDE5i non-responders	57	0.09	5	3000	3000	900	12	Renova (DirexGroup)	IIEF: +, EHS: +

Kalyvianakis (Greece 2016)	ED: PDE5i non-responders	46	0.2	5	4000	4000	1800	12	MT ONE (UrotechKorea)	IIEF: +, EHS: +
Lee (Korea 2013)	ED: PDE5i non-responders	50	0.09	5	3000	3000	900	12	Aries 2 (OmniSpecMeditech)	IIEF: +, EHS: +
Vardi (Israel 2010)	ED: mixed	20	0.096	5	2000	2000	600	12	Aries 2 (OmniSpecMeditech)	IIEF: +, EHS: +

studies, LISWT targeted multiple sites on the penis during each session. Most studies followed a treatment regimen lasting no more than 6 weeks, with only three studies extending the treatment duration to 9 weeks. The meta-analysis revealed a noteworthy enhancement in IIEF among patients classified under the mild ED category subsequent to LISWT. Conversely, individuals in the severe and moderate ED groups did not demonstrate a statistically significant elevation in their IIEF scores [18].

Another systematic review was done by Sokolakis et al. for pertinent clinical studies spanning from January 2010 to September 2018. The review included clinical studies that focused solely on investigating the effectiveness of LISWT for ED, with primary outcomes measured through IIEF-EF scores/questionnaires. Both randomized controlled trials (RCTs) and cohort studies were considered, though meta-analysis was specifically conducted for sham-controlled RCTs. Ten RCTs, comprising 873 patients, were chosen for the meta-analysis. The aggregated data from these studies demonstrated a significant enhancement in erectile function among men with ED, as indicated by both patient-reported outcomes (IIEF-EF: +3.97; 95% CI [2.09–5.84]; $p < 0.0001$, EHS $\geq$ 3: OR: 4.35; 95% CI [1.82–10.37]; $p = 0.0009$) and objective measures (peak systolic velocity: +4.12; 95% CI [2.30–5.94]; $p < 0.00001$). In summary, this meta-analysis underscores that LISWT yields a significant improvement in erectile function among patients afflicted with vasculogenic ED [19].

Yao et al. conducted a meta-nalysis to evaluate the efficacy of LISWT on studies published from July 2011 to June 2021 and selected 16 RCTs, including 1064 participants. Fifteen studies referenced the IIEF across three follow-up periods (1, 3 and 6 months), and the results favor LISWT. Eight out of the 16 trials provided data on the proportion of patients with a baseline EHS, and the LISWT group also demonstrated significantly better outcomes than the placebo group. Further, the results of this meta-analysis suggest that treatment plans with an energy density of 0.09 mJ/mm^2 and a pulse number of 1500–2000 are more beneficial to IIEF in ED patients. In addition, IIEF improvement was more pronounced in patients with moderate ED after LISWT [20].

Dong et al. conducted a significant meta-analysis covering seven RCTs released between January 2010 and June 2018, focusing on the effectiveness of LISWT in treating ED, with a total of 522 participants. The findings affirmed a notable increase in the IIEF-EF score across the treatment group in all seven studies and a significant improvement in the EHS within the treatment group in four studies. Moreover, individuals with moderate and/or severe ED exhibited notably improved mean IIEF scores [21].

The problem of heterogeneity in patient selection affects the quality of most studies, especially RCTs. Kalyvianakis et al. conducted a double-blind RTC that revealed a significant minimal clinically important difference in both the IIEF score and the Sexual Encounter Profile (SEP) score among men who underwent LISWT compared to those who received sham therapy. At both the 1- and 3-month follow-ups, there was an improvement of approximately 4 points in the IIEF score, while the SEP score showed enhancements of 18 and 22 points at the 1- and 3-month follow-ups, respectively. This study marked the first RCT examining the efficacy of LISWT in men with ED using a consistent sample in terms of baseline demographics and ED severity [22]. This type of study can provide better evidence if it has a larger number of patients.

The quality of these reviews and meta-analyses was explored by Yuan et al., as they conducted a compelling study examining eight meta-analyses and systematic reviews on the use of LISWT in ED. The objectives were to assess the quality of the studies, identify biases, evaluate recommendation grading, and others. The findings revealed that seven reviews were rated as having critically low overall confidence, while one review had low confidence according to the AMSTAR-2 (A Measurement Tool to Assess Systematic Reviews) appraisal tool. While the majority of the Preferred Reporting Items for Systematic Reviews and Meta-Analyses (PRISMA) criteria were satisfied, notable reporting deficiencies were observed, especially the lack of financial disclosures and protocol registrations. Three reviews were deemed to have low bias risk based on the ROBIS tool. According to the GRADE method, only one review provided high-quality evidence, with seven reviews offering evidence of moderate quality [23].

An intriguing umbrella review conducted by Medrano-Sánchez EM and colleagues examined a total of 25 clinical trials across five meta-analyses. These trials focused on assessing the effects of LISWT on vasculogenic ED, primarily using the IIEF-EF and EHS scale as key measures. The findings indicated a statistically significant increase in mean IIEF-EF scores in the experimental group. Furthermore, four out of five studies reported an elevation in EHS scores among those receiving LISWT compared to the placebo. Optimal treatment outcomes were associated with an energy density of 0.09 mJ/mm^2 and the application of 1500–2000 pulses. Additionally, a follow-up period of 6–12 months showed greater improvement in ED compared to a 3-month follow-up. Despite the challenges in obtaining conclusive results, the evidence suggests that LISWT presents a promising therapeutic option for vasculogenic ED due to its low risk and efficacy in improving erectile function [24].

Hartmut Porst extensively analyzed numerous published clinical studies on LISWT for ED treatment, highlighting numerous deficiencies in both the technical and clinical aspects of these studies. The trials exhibited a wide range of energy flux densities (EFDs), spanning from 0.09 to 0.25 mJ/mm^2, owing to considerable differences in device design, with a variance of almost 2000–3000 times. Notably, parameters such as the number of shockwaves per session and the total number of shockwaves varied significantly, with sessions ranging from 600 to 4000 shots and total shots administered over one treatment period ranging from 6000 to 36,000. Furthermore, the treated populations were heterogeneous, encompassing distinct target groups—PDE5Is responders and non-responders—yet were subjected to similar protocols. Despite these substantial variations in applied energies and patient demographics across study protocols, it is noteworthy that nearly all studies reported positive outcomes in the active arms following a short-term follow-up period of 1–3 months [25].

Choosing LISWT as per Etiology of ED

Most of the studies highlighted that the best responders to LISWT are those with vasculogenic etiology [19, 20, 26]. Furthermore, EAU guidelines affirm that patients with mild to moderate vasculogenic ED have better responses than those with severe ED. Another systematic review and meta-analysis were conducted to assess the efficacy of LIEWT in treating ED following radical prostatectomy (RP). The final analysis included five papers involving 460 patients. Results indicated that at 3–4 months post-LIESWT, the group receiving treatment demonstrated significantly better IIEF scores compared to the control group (WMD = −2.04; 95% CI, −3.72 to −0.35; $p = 0.02$). However, only two studies assessed outcomes at 9–12 months, revealing no significant difference between the groups (WMD = −5.37; 95% CI, −12.42 to 1.69; $p = 0.14$). These findings suggest that LISWT has a statistically significant impact on early recovery in penile rehabilitation following RP-induced ED. Nonetheless, the evidence level remains low, necessitating a cautious interpretation of the results [26].

The Indications of LISWT

Most of the studies have heterogeneous patient selection, and they were treated with LISWT either as first-line therapy or as a second-line therapy for non-responders to PDE5Is [18–20].

Non-responders to PDE5Is represent a significant patient population explored for alternative treatment with LISWT. A study conducted by Bechara et al. showed positive response rates in 60% of patients, with 91.7% of responders maintaining their positive responses throughout the 12-month study period [27]. In another study by Jose Vinay et al., a randomized, double-blind, sham-controlled trial was carried out involving 76 patients with vascular ED refractory to PDE5Is. Forty patients received LISWT treatment, while 36 received sham treatment. Baseline and post-treatment evaluations at 1, 3, and 6 months were conducted using validated erectile function questionnaires. The findings of this study suggested that LISWT could modestly improve erectile function in some PDE5I non-responders, providing an alternative for vascular ED patients who are averse to more invasive therapies [28].

Follow-Up After LISWT

The longest follow-up period to assess the maintenance of the efficacy of LISWT in treated ED patients was evaluated by research over a minimum follow-up period of 5 years. This extended analysis revealed a gradual decline in observed clinical enhancement in erectile function, which seemed to stabilize at approximately 40% efficacy between 48 and 60 months following the completion of LISWT. Furthermore, the absence of penile pain and deformity noted at the 5-year follow-up underscores the therapy's long-term safety [29].

In summary, LISWT is regarded as a promising alternative treatment for patients with ED. This modality of treatment has gained more popularity than other RT because of more extensive studies that showed significant responses. However, the evidence supporting LISWT is compromised by several factors, including a limited number of participants, short follow-up periods, reliance on subjective rather than objective outcome measures, variations in the application protocol, and heterogeneous patient selection criteria. Currently, LISWT is recommended as a possible option for men with mild to moderate vasculogenic ED.

Platelet-Rich Plasma Therapy

Platelet-rich plasma (PRP) is plasma obtained from whole blood that is rich in platelets (3–7 times higher than normal) [30]. It is a treatment approach that has been explored in the management of erectile dysfunction (ED) [30]. The basic idea behind PRP therapy is to use a patient's own blood components, specifically the platelets, to stimulate tissue repair and regeneration. The augmented levels of platelets have been demonstrated to introduce enlarged amounts of growth factors that provide stimulation for tissue repair, such as transforming growth factor β, insulin growth factor-1, platelet-derived growth factor, vascular endothelial growth factor, connective tissue growth factor, basic fibroblast growth factor, cytokines, and chemokines [31]. These factors carry out several roles, including collagen synthesis, myogenesis, angiogenesis, and proliferation and migration of endothelial and smooth muscle, as well as mesenchymal cells [32].

PRP injections have recently been marketed in regenerative medicine as a form of autologous cell therapy, although there is no clear scientific evidence for their use in treating ED [33]. There is a worldwide trend for many men to be advised to use PRP for the treatment of ED. However, despite the widespread use of this treatment, there is little evidence to support its use and guide the patient or clinician in the decision-making process [33]. Furthermore, the use of PRP is generally not supported by insurance. Therefore, men seeking regenerative medicine must bear the cost and uncertain risks of such treatments [30].

The Methods of Preparation

For preparation, a small amount of the patient's blood is drawn, similar to a routine blood test. The collected blood is then processed using a centrifuge for separating its components based on density. In this way, removal of RBCs is achieved and isolates the platelets and plasma from other blood component [34]. As a result, this process separates the blood into three components: RBCs, platelet-poor plasma, and PRP.

Commercial PRP separation systems vary widely. Today, there are many PRP preparation systems with FDA approval. Commercial PRP kits contain high concentrations of both PDGF and VEGF in the activated PRP.

The Mechanism of Actions

Platelets have an important role in clotting and accelerating wound healing after injury [32]. They contain various growth factors such as vascular endothelial growth factor (VEGF), platelet-derived growth factor (PDGF), insulin-like growth factor, and fibroblast growth factor (FGF), which are responsible for regenerative functions, including modulation of inflammatory responses, recruitment of stem cells, and stimulation of angiogenesis [30, 32]. Each factor has its impact. For example, FGF plays a role in increasing axonal myelination and nerve regeneration in the corpus cavernosum, VEGF stimulates angiogenesis and differentiation of mesenchymal stem cells, insulin-like growth factor plays a role in restoring smooth muscle integrity, and PDGF plays a role in the extracellular matrix and collagen synthesis. From this perspective, it is believed that such treatments may provide benefits that support the healing of damaged tissues and also play a role in restoring erectile function [30, 32]. PRP, an autologous product obtained from whole blood, contains high concentrations of platelet growth factor. It provides a fibrin framework on platelets that can support the regenerative matrix [35]. The advantage of PRP over recombinant human growth factors is that it releases multiple growth factors upon platelet activation [36].

The rationale behind using PRP in the management of erectile dysfunction is based on the belief that the growth factors and other bioactive substances present in platelets can stimulate tissue repair and regeneration. The idea is that by injecting PRP into the penis, it may promote the growth of new blood vessels, improve blood flow, and enhance overall tissue health.

Disadvantages of the PRP

Medical treatments are traditionally integrated into standard practice after extensive research and clinical practice. Although innovations offer the opportunity for medical progress, they can bring about unpredictability and harm. PRP can serve as an example in this respect. The biological properties of PRP and its effects in clinical applications are poorly understood [37]. Most current PRP systems are approved in orthopedic practice, so their use outside of orthopedics should be considered an "off-label" treatment [38]. Despite the lack of strong clinical evidence supporting the effectiveness of PRP, this practice continues to be widely used, and its unproven benefits in treating ED are frequently cited. In both the United States and Australia, clinicians may use such products off-label, provided certain conditions are met. Nonstandardized nomenclature, lack of adequate classification, and heterogeneous processing methods make comparison of available evidence difficult [39]. There are currently no multicenter, randomized, double-blind clinical studies published that provide generalizable clinical data with sufficient statistical power to demonstrate the effectiveness of PRP treatments in any of the medical disciplines. Clinical adoption of unproven medical treatments without scientific support creates an ethical concern that requires strong regulation of the practice. Additionally, practitioners of such treatments may not be held accountable for the validity of their therapeutic claims, leaving patients susceptible to emotional, physical, and financial burdens.

Another critical issue is the quality of the PRP used. There is no consensus on the criteria that the produced PRP should meet to be the most appropriate preparation for the treatment of ED (volume, number of platelets, growth factor concentrations). Closed systems clearly offer several benefits for the standardized preparation of PRP [40]. Moreover, the administration method is an issue of high clinical significance characterized by many points still to be resolved. The ideal number of sessions, the time interval between the treatment sessions, the ideal dosage per session, and if there is a minimum number of punctures per session—these are questions that currently lack a definitive answer. Finally, the profile of the patient (age, ED severity, comorbidities) that could get the most benefit from PRP treatment should be defined, and the potential synergistic effect of combinations with other treatment modalities for ED should be further explored. So, strict regulations should be implemented with appropriate testing protocols to address ethical and legal issues.

Evidence for PRP Therapy in ED

Emerging evidence suggests that growth factors and neurophilin ligands play important roles in nerve regeneration and upregulation of impaired nitric oxide synthesis, as well as in the recovery of erectile function after cavernous nerve (CN) injury [28, 41]. PRP has been shown to improve erectile function [28]. Experiments on rats have shown that PRP application provides an increase in intracavernous pressure and erectile function and a decrease in apoptotic markers and fibrosis [30, 42]. Wu et al. reported in their study that PRP treatments resulted in significant improvement of erectile function compared with the vehicle (normal saline) group alone, and that the PRP-treated group had significant protection of myelinated axons of CNs and a lower apoptotic index [28]. RNA expression of TGF-β1 in corpus cavernosum tissue was significantly lower in the PRP-treated group than in the other group. The same group also showed in another study that PRP provides a synergistic effect on the release of various growth factors to facilitate the recovery of erectile function in a rat model [43]. In another CN animal study, it was found that immediate PRP application resulted in significantly higher maximal intracavernosal pressure/mean arterial pressure (ICP/MAP) ratio and mean maximal ICP compared with those in the injured control group after 3 months of follow-up [41]. It was also demonstrated that direct PRP application on the suture site promotes the regeneration of injured CNs, as evidenced by a greater number of axons compared with sham operation and pure sutured groups [44]. Although animal studies indicate that PRP can improve erectile function, most of the studies have small sample sizes, and at the same time, studies have emphasized that clinical effects may vary depending on the preparation method, dosage, and application of PRP [43].

In humans, the use of PRP in orthopedic applications is a more established treatment. A meta-analysis including 16 randomized controlled trials concluded that PRP was more effective than a placebo injection for symptomatic tendinopathy [45]. There is currently no strong, convincing evidence to support the use of PRP in treating ED in humans. A randomized controlled human study reported increased concentrations of growth factors in ED and control, which was evaluated by the xMAP system (Luminex, Austin, TX) [46]. These findings confirm that the improvement of erectile function is due to the influence of these growth factors. Another human study highlighted platelet-rich fibrin matrix injection as a well-tolerated and safe treatment method for conditions such as Peyronie's disease (PD), stress urinary incontinence, and ED [47]. They reported an average improvement in the IIEF score of 4.14 points after the injections. Despite the current lack of data supporting its clinical effectiveness, PRP therapy is marketed as a "P-shot" therapy in many countries. The PRP procedure used to treat ED is registered as a "service mark" in the US Patent and Trademark Office [30]. Given the lack of control of medical advertising and the limited scientific evidence for PRP, PRP therapy is seen as a case of commercial interests despite its potential therapeutic benefit [30]. Reducing exploitative practices is essential for accurate scientific research. In this way, evidence-based and useful therapeutic innovations can be developed. Tables 6.2 and 6.3 provide a summary of animal and human studies that have applied PRP for ED.

It's important to note that while some studies and anecdotal reports suggest potential benefits, the use of PRP for ED is still an area of active research, and its efficacy is not universally accepted. Several preclinical and clinical trials were designated to use autologous PRP for treating ED, with a limitation of small groups and short follow-up periods [48]. The main outcome measures for those preclinical trials on ED were erectile function, evaluated with intracavernosal pressure and histopathology of the cavernous tissue [49, 50]. Besides, the main outcome measures for clinical trials included validated questionnaires as well as penile duplex Doppler ultrasound [30, 32, 42, 51]. Results can vary among individuals, and more high-quality clinical research is needed to establish its effectiveness, safety, and long-term outcomes. Before considering any form of treatment for erectile dysfunction, individuals should consult healthcare professionals who can provide personalized advice based on the individual's health status and medical history. It's also crucial to be aware that not all treatments, including PRP, may be appropriate or effective for everyone.

Table 6.2 Summary of animal studies that have applied PRP for ED

Study	Type of study	Animal	Sample size total (case/control)	Follow-up	Outcome
Ding et al. (2009) [41]	Prospective randomized controlled trial	Sprague-Dawley rats	(a) Sham group ($n = 8$) (b) CN dissection ($n = 8$) (c) CN dissection + PRP ($n = 8$)	*3 month*	The PRP-treated group had a higher maximal ICP and ICP/MAP ratio than the injured control group but a lower ICP/MAP ratio than the sham group
Wu et al. (2012) [28]	Prospective randomized controlled trial	Sprague-Dawley rats	(a) Sham group ($n = 8$) (b) BCNC injury + normal saline IC injection ($n = 8$) (c) BCNC injury + PRP ICI ($n = 8$)	*1 month*	PRP resulted in significant recovery of EF as compared with the normal saline group, successful nerve regeneration, significant preservation of CNs myelinated axons, and a lower apoptotic index
Wu et al. (2016) [43]	Prospective randomized controlled trial	Sprague-Dawley rats	(a) Sham group ($n = 6$) (b) BCNC injury + normal saline ICI ($n = 6$) (c) BCNC injury + general PRP ICI ($n = 6$) (d) BCNC injury + optimized PRP ICI ($n = 6$)	*1 month*	Optimized PRP had the largest amount of PDGF-AB and showed a synergistic effect on the release of growth factors. Functional improvement after bilateral CN injury when the optimized PRP was applied. Optimized PRP was more stable, and its injection in CC facilitated recovery of EF
Liao et al. (2018) [52]	Prospective comparative trial	Sprague-Dawley rats	(a) Control group ($n = 8$) (b) Normal saline ICI in diabetic rats with ED ($n = 7$) (c) PRP ICI in diabetic rats with ED ($n = 8$)	1 month	Group C showed an increase in all EF parameters at day 28. PRP showed tissue-protective effects in the corpus cavernosum

(continued)

Table 6.2 (continued)

Study	Type of study	Animal	Sample size total (case/control)	Follow-up	Outcome
Huang et al. (2014) [53]	RCT	Sprague-Dawley rats	(a) Control group ($n = 10$) (b) High-fat diet for 5 months and the 1 ICI of supernatant weekly for 4 week ($n = 10$) (c) Group H + PRP. Same as group H but received ICI of PRP ($n = 10$)	7 day	ICP/MAP was significantly higher in the control and PRP groups than in group H. IGF-1, BNF, and VEGF are significantly higher in the PRP group than in the control group and group H. CNNOS, ENOS, and ECs weakly expressed in group H compared with the other groups. Intracorporal oxidative stress and apoptotic index were significantly higher in group H than in the control and PRP groups
Wu et al. (2021) [50]	RCT	Sprague-Dawley rats	(a) BCNC injury + normal saline ICI ($n = 11$) (b) BCNC injury + PRP ICI ($n = 11$)	7, 14, 28 days	The EF parameters showed significant improvements at 14 and 28 days after the injury. cPRP injections simultaneously prevented the loss of neuronal NOS–positive neurons and nerve fibers in the MPG and CN, respectively, compared with saline injections

Stem Cell Therapy

Stem cells are undifferentiated cells that have the ability to develop into different types of specialized cells in the body [2]. They are characterized by their unique ability to self-renew and differentiate into various cell types, such as muscle cells, nerve cells, or blood cells [59]. Given their precursory nature, these cells harbor self-renewal potential and the ability to differentiate into other types of cells. Recently, studies have shown that these cells exhibit regenerative effects by releasing growth factors, cytokines, and chemokines; upregulating pathways to reduce inflammation, inhibiting apoptosis, improve wound healing; and driving angiogenesis and neuritogenesis [60]. They can also modulate other regenerative molecular pathways through paracrine effects such as neurogenesis, apoptosis, angiogenesis, and wound healing [61]. Stem cells play a crucial role in the development, growth, and repair of tissues and organs in the body. They can be found in various sources, including embryos, adult tissues, and certain organs [59]. Stem cell research holds great potential for medical advancements, as they can be used to study diseases, develop new therapies, and potentially regenerate damaged or diseased tissues. SCT

Table 6.3 Summary of human studies that have applied PRP for erectile dysfunction (ED)

Study	Type of study	Sample size total (case/control)	Number of PRP injection	PRP volume (ml)	ED duration, month (mean ± SD)	Age, year (Ave)	BMI, kg/m^2	Follow-up (month)	Increase in IIEF score	Adverse events
Poulios et al. et al. (2021) [49]	Double-blind RCT	60 (30/30)	2	5	78.7 ± 54.6	57.7	28.8	24	Yes	No
Zaghloul et al. (2021) [54]	Prospective study	34	8	1	26.5 ± 23.8	50.2	N/A	12	Yes	N/A
Taş et al. (2021) [55]	Prospective study	31	3	3	64.2 ± 46.6	54.4	30.8	24	Yes	No
Wong et al. (2021) [56]	Prospective study	30	3	1–2	25.7	54.9	25.7	12	Yes	No
Schirmann et al. (2022) [57]	Prospective study	15	3	6	N/A	56.1	N/A	24	Yes	No
Shaher et al. (2023) [58]	Double-blind RCT	100 (50/50)	3	6	43.5 ± 14.1	54.9	25	24	Yes	No

BMI body mass index, *ED* erectile dysfunction, *NA* not available, *PRP* platelet-rich plasma, *RCT* randomized clinical trial is an exciting application of restorative medicine with a theoretical promise of disease "cure" [62].

The Mechanism of Action

The precise mechanism by which stem cells exert their action is still unclear [63]. The mechanism of action of stem cells involves their unique properties and abilities to contribute to tissue repair and regeneration. Here are some key aspects of their mechanism of action:

1. Differentiation: Stem cells have the ability to differentiate into specialized cell types. They can transform into various cell lineages, such as muscle cells, nerve cells, or blood cells, depending on the signals they receive from their surrounding environment [63].
2. Self-renewal: Stem cells can divide and replicate themselves, maintaining a pool of undifferentiated cells. This self-renewal capacity allows them to continuously produce new cells and replenish the stem cell population [64].
3. Paracrine signaling: Stem cells secrete various bioactive molecules, such as growth factors, cytokines, and chemokines. These molecules act as signaling factors that can influence the behavior of nearby cells, promoting tissue repair, reducing inflammation, and stimulating the growth of new blood vessels [65].
4. Immunomodulation: Stem cells possess immunomodulatory properties, meaning they can regulate the immune response. They can modulate the activity of immune cells, such as T cells and macrophages, to promote tissue healing and reduce excessive inflammation.
5. Homing and migration: Stem cells have the ability to migrate to injured or damaged tissues. They can sense signals released by damaged tissues and navigate towards those areas, where they can exert their regenerative effects.

Overall, the mechanism of action of stem cells involves their ability to differentiate into specialized cells, self-renew, secrete bioactive molecules, modulate the immune response, and migrate to damaged tissues. These properties make them valuable in various fields, including regenerative medicine, tissue engineering, and therapeutic interventions.

Regulation of both nitric oxide and calcium intracellularly via the action of various transmembrane transport ionic channels is believed to be the therapeutic target of stem cell therapy in ED; however, the exact mechanism is still unknown [66].

Types of Stem Cells

Stem cells are classified as totipotent, pluripotent, multipotent, and unipotent stem cells. Totipotent stem cells are cells that have the ability to divide and develop into cells from all three germ layers and extraembryonic tissues (e.g., zygotes) [61]. Pluripotent stem cells can develop into all three germ layers; however, they cannot develop into extra-embryonic tissues (e.g., embryonic stem cells) [61]. Multipotent stem cells can only develop into a specific tissue or organ [e.g., mesenchymal stem cells (e.g., myocytes, osteoblasts, adipocytes)] [61].

Mesenchymal stem cells (MSCs) are a pluripotent adult stem cell population capable of both self-renewal and differentiation into multiple cell lines and represent the most widely studied and used cellular group for the treatment of ED [64]. MSC can be obtained from a variety of cellular populations present in the organism. Bone marrow-derived stem cells (BMSC), adipose-derived stem cells (ADSC), amniotic fluid stem cells (AFSC), placental stem cells (PSC), and urine-derived stem cells have all been used in animal or human research in the context of ED management [64].

Ethical Issues with the Use of Stem Cell Therapy

The use of stem cell therapy raises several ethical considerations that need to be carefully addressed. Here are some of the key ethical issues associated with the use of stem cells:

1. Source of stem cells: The source of stem cells can be a subject of ethical debate. Embryonic stem cells, derived from early-stage embryos, raise ethical concerns due to the destruction of the embryo during the extraction process. This raises questions about the moral status of the embryo and the potential for the commodification of human life. On the other hand, adult stem cells obtained from adult tissues or organs do not pose the same ethical concerns.
2. Informed consent: In any medical procedure, including stem cell therapy, obtaining informed consent from patients is crucial. Patients should be fully informed about the potential risks, benefits, and uncertainties associated with the treatment. Ensuring that patients have a clear understanding of the experimental nature of some stem cell therapies is essential to protect their autonomy and well-being.
3. Safety and efficacy: The safety and efficacy of stem cell therapies are still being extensively researched. Ethical concerns arise when unproven or inadequately tested stem cell treatments are offered to patients, potentially exposing them to unknown risks. It is important to conduct rigorous scientific studies and adhere to regulatory standards to ensure patient safety and avoid false or misleading claims.

4. Fair access and affordability: Stem cell therapies can be expensive, making them inaccessible to many individuals who could potentially benefit from them. Ensuring fair access to these therapies and addressing issues of affordability and equity are ethical considerations that need to be addressed.
5. Oversight and regulation: The field of stem cell research and therapy requires appropriate oversight and regulation to ensure ethical practices. This includes monitoring the quality and safety of stem cell products, enforcing ethical guidelines, and preventing the exploitation of vulnerable individuals.

Addressing these ethical issues requires a comprehensive and balanced approach that considers the potential benefits of stem cell therapy while also safeguarding the rights and well-being of patients and respecting ethical principles.

Evidence for Stem Cell Treatment in ED

The effect of stem cells on ED has been examined in animal models of diabetes, aging, and cavernous nerve injury [61]. First, in 2004, Bochinski et al. injected neural-derived embryonic stem cells into the corpus cavernosa of male rats with ED of neurogenic origin and found that it improved erectile function [67]. Since then, a large number of studies in a preclinical setting have aimed to prove the efficacy of stem cell therapy for the treatment of ED secondary to different etiologies: aging, diabetes mellitus, hypertriglyceridemia, cavernous nerve injury, and others.

In the bilateral cavernous compression injury rat model, injection of autologous ADSC into the cavernous cavernosal of rats could effectively prevent erectile dysfunction caused by cavernous nerve damage, promote neuronal nitric oxide synthase positive nerve regeneration, and increase the ratio of smooth muscle to collagen content [68, 69]. It has been shown that injection of ADSC can ameliorate intracavernous damage caused by hyperlipidemia or chronic tobacco exposure in rats [70]. It has also been shown that exosomes produced by stem cells can improve erectile dysfunction in rats [71]. Although many animal experiments show that stem cell therapy is effective in treating ED, clinical studies on this treatment are limited.

There are four published meta-analyses that cover the available evidence in a preclinical setting to this day [65, 72–74]. In the first work, the final analysis of the 12 included studies allowed Shan et al. to prove the efficacy of stem cell therapy in rat models with cavernous nerve injury (CNI) [73]. In 2017, Hou et al. further reviewed the available evidence on the use of ADSC in ED rat models other than CNI, including other etiologies such as diabetes mellitus, smoking, radiotherapy, and tunica albuginea injury. Meta-analysis results revealed that ADSC use can regenerate damaged erectile tissues and aid in the recovery of erectile function [65]. In line with previous research in the field, Park et al., in a meta-analysis published in 2019, analyzed 19 studies with the aim of evaluating the effects of ADSC in rat models with CNI-induced ED. The main findings revealed that ADSC therapy improved erectile function based on penile hemodynamic parameters, intracavernous pressure and mean arterial penile pressure proportion (ICP/MAP), and that ADSCs were able to regenerate damaged tissues following changes in measured levels of nitric oxide synthase (NOS), cyclic guanosine monophosphate (cGMP), and smooth muscle-to-collagen ratio [74]. Similar results are described in a recently published network meta-analysis by Wani et al. aimed at evaluating the role of stem cell therapy in erectile dysfunction secondary to cavernous nerve injury [72]. Results, including 29 animal studies and three human trials (post-RP patients), revealed a significant increase in histological and molecular parameters of response, including nNOS, smooth muscle content, and anti-apoptotic activity in rats, and an improvement in IEEF and EHS in human studies. Studies in a preclinical setting have not been able to elucidate the exact specific mechanism by which stem cell therapy exerts its therapeutical effect. However, a paracrine effect derived from their use with the secretion of growth factors with chemotactic, anti-inflammatory, regenerative, angiogenic, and antiapoptotic properties has been proposed, which favors the regeneration of damaged tissues [75]. Preclinical research studies have demonstrated an improvement in the vascular function of cavernous endothelium and the suppression of cavernous fibrosis with an increase in the proportion of smooth muscle derived from stem cell use [76]. Furthermore, the use of ADSC also leads to a neurological improvement at the level of cavernous bodies, which is crucial for the maintenance of erectile function [77] and a reduction in apoptotic and inflammatory response levels related to increasing ED risk factors such as diabetes mellitus or obesity [76].

The first human clinical trial published by Bahk et al. in 2010 used for the first time in an experimental setting allogenic umbilical cord stem cells in diabetes mellitus-derived ED. ICI with 1.5×10^7 cells was performed in seven men between the ages of 57 and 83. Most of the patients recovered matutine spontaneous erections in the period of a month, and these results were maintained over the period of 6 months of follow-up [78]. In a posterior phase I clinical trial published by Levy et al., eight patients suffering from complete PDEi non-responsive ED were followed up for 6 months. No serious adverse events were noted, and an improvement in mean penile arterial flow was maintained at 6 months after treatment initiation [79].

You et al. published a phase I/II clinical trial (INSTIN Study) in which they included a total number of 18 patients (12 in the first phase of the study) following radical prostatectomy. Dose-escalating ICI in BMSC was employed. Authors concluded that a single autologous BMSC ICI was safe and effective in patients with vasculogenic ED; further improvements in perceived erectile function and sexual satisfaction were observed at the 6-month follow-up and were maintained over a 1-year period. The complete mean follow-up period of 62.1 months confirmed a complete absence of treatment-derived adverse effects; however, a slight worsening in erectile function was observed with respect to results obtained in the first year following treatment. The authors additionally concluded that further ICI may be required over time for maintenance of the therapeutic effect [80, 81]. In the field of diabetes mellitus-derived ED, Al Demour et al. carried out two consecutive clinical trials in diabetic patients exploring the use of autologous BMSC and allogenic

Wharton's Jelly-derived stem cells (WJSC) to treat ED. In the first trial, ICI of BMSC was found to be safe and effective, with a significant improvement in International Index of Erectile Function (IIEF-15) and Erection Hardness Score (EHS) questionnaires [82]. In the second, the use of two consecutive ICI of WJSC was explored for the first time in a total sample of 22 diabetic patients with ED. Positive results regarding tolerability, safety, and efficacy measured via IIEF-15 and EHS questionnaires and duplex Doppler penile ultrasound imaging (DPE) were observed at the 12-month follow-up [83].

In a clinical study, 17 male patients with PDE5I and ICI-refractory ED after radical prostatectomy received autologous adipose-derived regenerative cell therapy. It was observed that 73% of the patients regained their erectile functions within 3 months after treatment [84]. Small phase 1 studies in humans have shown promising results in terms of tolerability, safety, and efficacy of use of intracavernosal stem cell transplant for the treatment of ED [82].

Table 6.4 details the type of human studies, number of patients included, the number of stem cells used, the regime, and outcomes.

Based on animal experiments and a small number of clinical studies, we can conclude that stem cell therapy is safe and reliable. However, despite the promising results, the lack of abundant and high-quality clinical evidence makes it difficult to determine the usefulness of stem cells in the clinical therapy of ED [61].

It is not yet clear which patients are the best candidates for stem cell therapy, where the stem cells should be taken from and how they will be administered, the number of stem cells to be injected, how many times the stem cells will be administered, and whether they should be given as a single treatment or as part of a multimodal treatment. Stem cell therapy should not be introduced into routine clinical practice until these data are completed.

Since stem cell treatments are not patentable, cost and patient recruitment become problems for future studies. This situation prevents sponsorship from pharmaceutical companies, as they have no economic interest. Therefore, such studies have to be economically supported by public or nonprofit organizations, and the high cost of stem cell therapy makes this situation difficult. Patient recruitment is another issue that limits the study on this subject.

Guidelines for RT in ED

Limitations of the Evidence

There are several limitations that need to be addressed prior to widespread acceptance of restorative therapies. A key element is standardizing measurable validated outcome instruments, which would quantify therapy efficacy as well as allow for comparison between studies. Important limitations to these future studies include costs and patient recruitment. With regard to funding, it is critical that patients are

Table 6.4 Summary of human studies that have applied stem cell therapy for ED

Study	Type of study	Sample size total (case/control)	Age, year, range (mean)	Stem cell origin	Stem cell volume (ml)	ED aetiology	Significant improvement	Follow-up (month)	Findings
Bahk et al. (2010) [78]	Non-randomised, single-blind	(7-3)	57–87 (69.5)	Umbilical cord	1.5×10^7	Diabetes	Yes	11	6/7 patients regained morning erections by 3 months; 2/7 regained enough rigidity for penetration with the aid of PDE5i
Levy et al. (2016) [79]	Non randomize, single arm-open label	(8-0)	40–70	Placental matrix	1.5	Organic	Yes	6	3/8 patients achieved erections at 3 months, and PSV increased from 50.7 to 73.9 cm/s at 6 months
Yiou et al. (2016) [80]	Non-randomised, single arm-open label	(12-0)	45–70 (63.6)	Bone marrow	Four doses used 2×10^7 2×10^8 1×10^9 2×10^9	Radical prostatectomy	Yes	6	Post-prostatectomy patients were in four groups, each group treated with a different dosage of cavernosal injected stem cells. There were no serious side effects reported. A significant improvement in IIEF-15 and EHS was observed at 6 months. A higher dosage of stem cells showed significant improvements in spontaneous erections

(continued)

Table 6.4 (continued)

Study	Type of study	Sample size total (case/control)	Age, year, range (mean)	Stem cell origin	Stem cell volume (ml)	ED aetiology	Significant improvement	Follow-up (month)	Findings
Haahr et al. (2016) [84]	Single arm-open label	(17-0)	49–69 (median: 63)	Autologous adipose-derived	2.2×10^7	Radical prostatectomy	Yes	6	Post-prostatectomy patients were treated with a single cavernosal injection. No major adverse events, only minor events related to liposuction and ecchymosis from injection. 8/17 patients recovered erectile functions to perform sexual intercourse. In the post-hoc stratification of continent men who underwent prostatectomy, 8 out of 11 recovered erectile function, while no incontinent men regained erectile function
Yiou et al. (2017) [81]	Single arm-open label	(6-0)	(59.9 ± 3.8)	Bone marrow	1×10^9	Radical prostatectomy	Yes	6	The study provided a more comprehensive update on the previous research, incorporating six additional post-prostatectomy patients who showed comparable improvements in IIEF-15 and EHS scores. There was no recurrence of prostate cancer in the first study after a follow-up period of 62.1 ± 11.7 months

Al Demour et al. (2018) [82]	Single arm-open label	(4-0)	49–60 (54.8)	Bone marrow	30×10^6	Diabetes	Yes	12	Diabetic ED patients are treated with two consecutive cavernosal injections. The study did not report any adverse effects. Significant improvement in IIEF-15 and EHS
You et al. (2020) [85]	Single arm-open label	(10-0)	(62 ± 13)	Bone marrow	3×10^7	Diabetes (*n* = 5) radical prostatectomy (*n* = 5)	Yes	N/A	
Al Demour et al. (2021) [83]	Single arm-open label	(22-0)	(59.2 ± 8.5)	Wharton's jelly-derived mesenchymal stem cell	20×10^6	Diabetes	Yes	12	
Mirzaei et al. (2021) [86]	Single-blind RCT	(10-10)	Case: (63.8 ± 7.4) Control (65.5 ± 5.1)	Autologous mesenchymal	50×10^6	Diabetes	Yes	6	

enrolled in studies at minimal additional cost to avoid financial incentives and reduce selection bias.

Additionally, most of the studies are limited by the small samples. Furthermore, the long-term efficacy of the therapies was not assessed because of the limited duration of the follow-up period. Double-blind RCTs with longer follow-up periods are needed to evaluate true therapeutic efficacy, duration of effect, and parameters such as optimal dose in various patient populations with erectile dysfunction. Additionally, the physiological mechanism of action and histopathological changes can be better elucidated with more animal and laboratory studies.

Available Guidelines

Despite the concerns mentioned above, regenerative therapies present a new avenue for treating patients with ED. These treatments hold the potential to restore lost erectile function while boasting improved safety and efficacy compared to current options. Currently, there appears to be stronger evidence supporting the use of LI-SWT over SCT and PRPT, as reflected in recommendations from the AUA, EAU, and SMSNA. However, many studies in this field lack consistent inclusion and exclusion criteria as well as defined endpoint goals [87]. Further research is imperative to comprehensively understand the effects of these therapies and to establish safe and universally effective protocols suitable for widespread adoption. Moreover, addressing challenges such as affordability and access to facilities offering these innovative modalities is essential. Additionally, the scarcity of clear protocols and broadly applicable evidence for these therapies fosters a concerning trend of commercializing sexual health without adequate standards [87] (Table 6.5).

Global Andrology Forum (GAF) Survey Study on RT in ED and Experts' Recommendation

This is the largest global survey study to explore the current practice of RT in ED until 2024. The survey garnered responses from a total of 479 participants hailing from 62 countries. One-third of them acknowledged using RT and shared their experiences and conclusions. Among the treatments, LISWT was predominant (54.6%), followed by PRP (24.5%) and a combination of both (14.7%). STC was the least utilized (3.7%). The primary reason for using RT was for cases refractory to or experiencing adverse effects from PDE5i. RT appeared most effective in middle-aged patients and those with mild-to-moderate ED, with respondents expressing confidence in its safety. Many non-users expressed interest in future RT adoption if supported by guidelines. Furthermore, in this study, GAF provides

Table 6.5 The societies guidelines about RT in ED

Society	Recommendation
American Urology Association (AUA) Guidelines—2018 [88]	Penile LISWT and intracavernosal SCT should be considered investigational conditional recommendation; (Grade C Evidence level). Intracavernosal PRP therapy is regarded as experimental (expert opinion)
Sexual Medicine Society of North America (SMSNA) Position Statement—2021 [9]	There is an absence of robust clinical data supporting the efficacy of RT for the treatment of ED. However, technologies such as LISWT have established relative safety
The Asia-Pacific Society for Sexual Medicine Guidelines—2021 [89]	The use of LISWT to improve penile erectile hemodynamics is supported by convincing basic science evidence (Level 2; Grade B). Correct patient selection is essential for treatment success; younger patients with mild-moderate ED, minimal cardiovascular comorbidities, and absence of diabetes or cavernous nerve injury are likely to have recovery and spontaneous erection (Level 2; Grade B). Adjunctive measures like combination with PDE5is may enhance LISWT effects and erectile function recovery (Level 2; Grade C). LISWT improves erectile function scores and penile hemodynamic parameters in men with vasculogenic ED (Level 1; Grade B). However, the long-term outcome is uncertain. Evidence suggests benefits up to 12 months after treatment (Level 2; Grade B). LISWT for treatment of ED should be restricted to men with mild-moderate vasculogenic ED, either responders or non-responders to PDE5is, and be performed in highly specialized centers (Level 2; Grade B). LISWT is a safe and well-tolerated procedure without clinically significant adverse events (Level 1; Grade A)
Canadian Urological Association (CUA) Guidelines—2021 [90]	Conditional recommendations against LISWT as a treatment for ED patients are also recommended. Additional studies are required
The Italian Society of Andrology and Sexual Medicine (SIAMS) Guidelines—2023 [91]	Suggest the use of LISWT in patients with mild vasculogenic ED not responding to PDE5is (Weak recommendation, very low-quality evidence). No clear recommendations on the use of SC and PRP therapies can be provided, given the limited data

(continued)

Table 6.5 (continued)

Society	Recommendation
European Association of Urology (EAU) Guidelines—2024 [92]	LISWT with/without PDE5Is can be used in patients with mild vasculogenic ED or as an alternative first-line therapy in well-informed patients who do not wish for or are not suitable for oral vasoactive therapy or desire a curable option (weak recommendations). LISWT with/without PDE5Is may be used in vasculogenic ED patients who are poor responders to PDE5Is (weak recommendations). Intracavernous injections of PRP have led to a mild improvement of EF among patients with organic ED, but the available evidence is still insufficient to provide a recommendation regarding its use. Its use should be limited to clinical trials (weak recommendations).
European Society for Sexual Medicine (ESSM) position statements—[93]	LISWT is a safe and well-tolerated procedure, but its efficacy for the treatment of ED is doubtful and deserves more investigation Cell therapy (CT) for ED should be considered a treatment under investigation and not offered outside of clinical trials. (Good Clinical Practice Statement) Patients should be informed regarding the limited evidence on the efficacy and safety of CT for ED. (Level 3, Grade C)
Urological Society of Australia and New Zealand—[94]	The use of LISWT regenerative technology and cellular-based therapy in ED should be cautioned due to unknown long-term outcomes and remains largely experimental (Level 3; Grade B) recommendation

statements of experts' recommendations about the use of RT in ED to guide the practitioners for the best clinical practice, as in Table 6.6 [95].

Table 6.6 GAF expert's recommendations about RT for the treatment of ED

RT should not be considered the standard of care for treating ED and should be offered to patients with informed consent according to its current limitations
RT appears to be more effective in patients with vasculogenic ED compared to other types of ED
RT appears to be most effective in men with mild to moderate ED
Young and middle-aged males appear to derive the most benefits from RT for the treatment of ED
RT can be used in combination with other ED treatment modalities or as a solo treatment for males for whom standard treatments have failed or who wish to try and regain natural erections
A limited proportion of patients treated with RT for ED report satisfaction with treatment
Current evidence is unclear as to the duration of significant improvement in erectile function after RT
Although RT is associated with high short-term safety and minimal adverse effects, its long-term safety is still unknown
Currently, there is more evidence to support the efficacy of low-intensity shock wave therapy compared to other modalities of RT

Table 6.7 GAF Expert's recommendations about the use of different modalities of RT for the treatment of ED

Currently, there is a lack of consensus regarding the effectiveness of RT in treating ED, and further large controlled studies are crucial to reach a definitive recommendation
There is no consensus on the available data for making direct comparisons of effectiveness between RT and PDE5is
Current data are uncertain about the expected duration of improvement of ED after treatment of each modality of RT
There is severe diversity in protocols and applications across different modalities of RT
There are limited data about the safety and better efficacy of combining different modalities of RT with each other or with PDE5is
There is overall good short-term safety data about using different modalities of RT, although the long-term safety data is still lacking
Due to lack of current evidence, intracavernosal PRP or SCT should only be considered within the context of clinical trials or experimental treatments
Despite limited studies demonstrating the effectiveness of LISWT in treating ED, further high-quality evidence is necessary to support its use as a routine therapeutic option

Another GAF international survey about the use of different modalities of RT in ED, involving 163 clinicians from 39 countries, reveals that RT is increasingly used for ED, with LISWT being the most commonly adopted modality (81%), followed by PRP (61%) and SCT (18%). While LISWT is generally perceived as safe and moderately effective, SCT was viewed by nearly half of its users as more effective than PDE5 inhibitors, despite limited usage. Protocols for PRP and SCT showed wide variability, and the supporting evidence for both was rated as poor to moderate. The study highlights significant heterogeneity in clinical practice, application protocols, and perceived efficacy, reinforcing the need for standardized guidelines and large-scale randomized controlled trials to optimize the use of RT in ED management [95]. Additionally, GAF provides statements of experts' recommendations about the use of different modalities of RT in ED to guide the practitioners for the best clinical practice, as in Table 6.7 [95].

Conclusion

It is a landmark progress to have the emergence of RT in ED with the aim of more sustainable and natural outcomes in treatment. However, these therapeutic methods are still in their early stages of development, with their pharmacological pathways and precise mechanisms yet to be fully elucidated. Current studies on regenerative therapy for erectile dysfunction face several shortcomings, including limited sample sizes, short follow-up periods, and a lack of standardized outcome measures. These limitations hinder the ability to draw definitive conclusions about the efficacy and long-term effects of regenerative therapies. To improve future research in this area, larger and more diverse study populations should be recruited, with longer follow-up periods to assess both short-term and long-term outcomes. Additionally, researchers should establish standardized protocols for treatment administration and outcome assessment to facilitate comparison between studies and ensure the reliability of results. Collaborative efforts among researchers and clinicians, as well as transparent reporting of study methodologies and results, are also essential for advancing our understanding of regenerative therapies for erectile dysfunction.

References

1. Laumann EO, Glasser DB, Neves RCS, Moreira E. A population-based survey of sexual activity, sexual problems and associated help-seeking behavior patterns in mature adults in the United States of America. Int J Impot Res. 2009;21:171–8.
2. McCabe MP, Althof SE. A systematic review of the psychosocial outcomes associated with erectile dysfunction: does the impact of erectile dysfunction extend beyond a man's inability to have sex? J Sex Med. 2014;11:347–63.
3. Hatzimouratidis K, Salonia A, Adaikan G, Buvat J, Carrier S, El-Meliegy A, et al. Pharmacotherapy for erectile dysfunction: recommendations from the Fourth International Consultation for Sexual Medicine (ICSM 2015). J Sex Med. 2016;13:465–88.
4. Corona G, Rastrelli G, Burri A, Serra E, Gianfrilli D, Mannucci E, et al. First-generation phosphodiesterase type 5 inhibitors dropout: a comprehensive review and meta-analysis. Andrology. 2016;4:1002–9.
5. Giraldi L, Felbo J, Sønksen J, Fode M. Penisimplantater er en god sidste behandlingsmulighed for erektil dysfunction. Ugeskr Læger. 2015;177:2–5.
6. Burri A, Porst H. Results from an online survey investigating ED patients' insights and treatment expectations. Int J Impot Res. 2015;27:191–6.
7. Campbell JD, Milenkovic U, Albersen M, Bivalacqua TJ. What is the future of erectile dysfunction therapy? Curr Sex Health Rep. 2018;10:169–76.
8. Campbell JD, Milenkovic U, Usta MF, Albersen M, Bivalacqua TJ. The good, bad, and the ugly of regenerative therapies for erectile dysfunction. Transl Androl Urol. 2020;9:S252.
9. Liu JL, Chu KY, Gabrielson AT, Wang R, Trost L, Broderick G, et al. Restorative therapies for erectile dysfunction: position statement from the Sexual Medicine Society of North America (SMSNA). Sex Med. 2021;9:100343.
10. Vardi Y, Appel B, Jacob G, Massarwi O, Gruenwald I. Can low-intensity extracorporeal shockwave therapy improve erectile function? A 6-month follow-up pilot study in patients with organic erectile dysfunction. Eur Urol. 2010;58:243–8.
11. McClure S, Dorfmüller C. Extracorporeal shock wave therapy: theory and equipment. Clin Tech Equine Pract. 2003;2:348–57.
12. Katz JE, Clavijo RI, Rizk P, Ramasamy R. The basic physics of waves, soundwaves, and shockwaves for erectile dysfunction. Sex Med Rev. 2020;8:100–5.
13. Ciampa AR, de Prati AC, Amelio E, Cavalieri E, Persichini T, Colasanti M, et al. Nitric oxide mediates anti-inflammatory action of extracorporeal shock waves. FEBS Lett. 2005;579:6839–45.
14. Sokolakis I, Dimitriadis F, Teo P, Hatzichristodoulou G, Hatzichristou D, Giuliano F. The basic science behind low-intensity extracorporeal shockwave therapy for erectile dysfunction: a systematic scoping review of pre-clinical studies. J Sex Med. 2019;16:168–94.
15. Liu T, Shindel AW, Lin G, Lue TF. Cellular signaling pathways modulated by low-intensity extracorporeal shock wave therapy. Int J Impot Res. 2019;31:170–6.

16. Young Academic Urologists Men's Health Group, Fode M, Hatzichristodoulou G, Serefoglu EC, Verze P, Albersen M. Low-intensity shockwave therapy for erectile dysfunction: is the evidence strong enough? Nat Rev Urol. 2017;14:593–606.
17. Hayon S, Panken EJ, Bennett NE. Variations in low intensity shockwave treatment protocols for erectile dysfunction: a review of the literature and guide to offering treatment. World J Mens Health. 2024;42:283.
18. Lu Z, Lin G, Reed-Maldonado A, Wang C, Lee Y-C, Lue TF. Low-intensity extracorporeal shock wave treatment improves erectile function: a systematic review and meta-analysis. Eur Urol. 2017;71:223–33.
19. Sokolakis I, Hatzichristodoulou G. Clinical studies on low intensity extracorporeal shockwave therapy for erectile dysfunction: a systematic review and meta-analysis of randomised controlled trials. Int J Impot Res. 2019;31:177–94.
20. Yao H, Wang X, Liu H, Sun F, Tang G, Bao X, et al. Systematic review and meta-analysis of 16 randomized controlled trials of clinical outcomes of low-intensity extracorporeal shock wave therapy in treating erectile dysfunction. Am J Mens Health. 2022;16:15579883221087532.
21. Dong L, Chang D, Zhang X, Li J, Yang F, Tan K, et al. Effect of low-intensity extracorporeal shock wave on the treatment of erectile dysfunction: a systematic review and meta-analysis. Am J Mens Health. 2019;13:1557988319846749.
22. Kalyvianakis D, Mykoniatis I, Pyrgidis N, Kapoteli P, Zilotis F, Fournaraki A, Hatzichristou D. The effect of low-intensity shock wave therapy on moderate erectile dysfunction: a double-blind, randomized, sham-controlled clinical trial. J Urol. 2022;208:388–95.
23. Yuan F, Wang Y, Ma Z, Jing M, You Y, Yu X, et al. Low-intensity extracorporeal shockwave therapy for erectile dysfunction: an overview of systematic reviews. Transl Androl Urol. 2021;10:3684.
24. Medrano-Sánchez EM, Peña-Cantonero B, Candón-Ballester P, Blanco-Díaz M, Díaz-Mohedo E. Effectiveness of low-intensity extracorporeal shock wave therapy in erectile dysfunction: an analysis of sexual function and penile hardness at erection: an umbrella review. J Pers Med. 2024;14:177.
25. Porst H. Review of the current status of low intensity extracorporeal shockwave therapy (Li-ESWT) in erectile dysfunction (ED), Peyronie's disease (PD), and sexual rehabilitation after radical prostatectomy with special focus on technical aspects of the different marketed ESWT devices including personal experiences in 350 patients. Sex Med Rev. 2021;9:93–122.
26. Rho BY, Kim SH, Ryu J-K, Kang DH, Kim JW, Chung DY. Efficacy of low-intensity extracorporeal shock wave treatment in erectile dysfunction following radical prostatectomy: a systematic review and meta-analysis. J Clin Med. 2022;11:2775.
27. Bechara A, Casabé A, De Bonis W, Ciciclia PG. Twelve-month efficacy and safety of low-intensity shockwave therapy for erectile dysfunction in patients who do not respond to phosphodiesterase type 5 inhibitors. Sex Med. 2016;4:e225–e32.
28. Vinay J, Moreno D, Rajmil O, Ruiz-Castañe E, Sanchez-Curbelo J. Penile low intensity shock wave treatment for PDE5I refractory erectile dysfunction: a randomized double-blind sham-controlled clinical trial. World J Urol. 2021;39:2217–22.
29. Chung E, Cartmill R. Evaluation of long-term clinical outcomes and patient satisfaction rate following low intensity shock wave therapy in men with erectile dysfunction: a minimum 5-year follow-up on a prospective open-label single-arm clinical study. Sex Med. 2021;9(4):100384.
30. Scott S, Roberts M, Chung E. Platelet-rich plasma and treatment of erectile dysfunction: critical review of literature and global trends in platelet-rich plasma clinics. Sex Med Rev. 2019;7:306–12.
31. Galliera E, Corsi M, Banfi G. Platelet rich plasma therapy: inflammatory molecules involved in tissue healing. J Biol Regul Homeost Agents. 2012;26:35S–42S.
32. Epifanova MV, Gvasalia BR, Durashov MA, Artemenko SA. Platelet-rich plasma therapy for male sexual dysfunction: myth or reality? Sex Med Rev. 2020;8:106–13.

33. Chung E. Stem-cell-based therapy in the field of urology: a review of stem cell basic science, clinical applications and future directions in the treatment of various sexual and urinary conditions. Expert Opin Biol Ther. 2015;15:1623–32.
34. Sumida E, Iwasaki Y, Akiyoshi K, Kasugai S. Platelet separation from whole blood in an aqueous two-phase system with water-soluble polymers. J Pharmacol Sci. 2006;101:91–7.
35. El-Sharkawy H, Kantarci A, Deady J, Hasturk H, Liu H, Alshahat M, Van Dyke TE. Platelet-rich plasma: growth factors and pro-and anti-inflammatory properties. J Periodontol. 2007;78:661–9.
36. Sánchez AR, Sheridan PJ, Kupp LI. Is platelet-rich plasma the perfect enhancement factor? A current review. Int J Oral Maxillofac Implants. 2003;18:93.
37. Murray I, LaPrade R. Platelet-rich plasma: renewed scientific understanding must guide appropriate use. Bone Joint Res. 2016;5:92–4.
38. Sastry A. Overview of the US FDA medical device approval process. Curr Cardiol Rep. 2014;16:1–5.
39. Chahla J, Cinque ME, Piuzzi NS, Mannava S, Geeslin AG, Murray IR, et al. A call for standardization in platelet-rich plasma preparation protocols and composition reporting: a systematic review of the clinical orthopaedic literature. J Bone Joint Surg. 2017;99:1769–79.
40. Kushida S, Kakudo N, Morimoto N, Hara T, Ogawa T, Mitsui T, Kusumoto K. Platelet and growth factor concentrations in activated platelet-rich plasma: a comparison of seven commercial separation systems. J Artif Organs. 2014;17:186–92.
41. Ding X-G, Li S-W, Zheng X-M, Hu L-Q, Hu W-L, Luo Y. The effect of platelet-rich plasma on cavernous nerve regeneration in a rat model. Asian J Androl. 2009;11:215.
42. Alkandari MH, Touma N, Carrier S. Platelet-rich plasma injections for erectile dysfunction and Peyronie's disease: a systematic review of evidence. Sex Med Rev. 2022;10:341–52.
43. Wu YN, Wu CC, Sheu MT, Chen KC, Ho HO, Chiang HS. Optimization of platelet-rich plasma and its effects on the recovery of erectile function after bilateral cavernous nerve injury in a rat model. J Tissue Eng Regen Med. 2016;10:E294–304.
44. Ding X, Li S, Zheng X, Hu L, Hu W, Luo Y. Effect of platelet-rich plasma on the regeneration of cavernous nerve: experiment with rats. Zhonghua Yi Xue Za Zhi. 2008;88:2578–80.
45. Miller LE, Parrish WR, Roides B, Bhattacharyya S. Efficacy of platelet-rich plasma injections for symptomatic tendinopathy: systematic review and meta-analysis of randomised injection-controlled trials. BMJ Open Sport Exerc Med. 2017;3:e000237.
46. Epifanova M, Chalyi M, Krasnov A. Investigation of mechanisms of action of growth factors of autologous platelet-rich plasma used to treat erectile dysfunction. Urologiia. 2017;4(4):46–9.
47. Matz EL, Pearlman AM, Terlecki RP. Safety and feasibility of platelet-rich fibrin matrix injections for treatment of common urologic conditions. Investig Clin Urol. 2018;59:61–5.
48. Chung E. Regenerative technology to restore and preserve erectile function in men following prostate cancer treatment: evidence for penile rehabilitation in the context of prostate cancer survivorship. Ther Adv Urol. 2021;13:17562872211026421.
49. Poulios E, Mykoniatis I, Pyrgidis N, Zilotis F, Kapoteli P, Kotsiris D, et al. Platelet-rich plasma (PRP) improves erectile function: a double-blind, randomized, placebo-controlled clinical trial. J Sex Med. 2021;18:926–35.
50. Wu Y-N, Liao C-H, Chen K-C, Chiang H-S. CXCL5 cytokine is a major factor in platelet-rich plasma's preservation of erectile function in rats after bilateral cavernous nerve injury. J Sex Med. 2021;18:698–710.
51. Raheem OA, Natale C, Dick B, Reddy AG, Yousif A, Khera M, Baum N. Novel treatments of erectile dysfunction: review of the current literature. Sex Med Rev. 2021;9:123–32.
52. Liao C, Wu Y, Chiang H. MP43-09 effects of platelet rich plasma on improving erectile dysfunction in streptozotocin-induced diabetic rats. J Urol. 2018;199:e582–e3.
53. Huang Y-C, Wu C-T, Chen M-F, Kuo Y-H, Li J-M, Shi C-S. Intracavernous injection of autologous platelet-rich plasma ameliorates hyperlipidemia-associated erectile dysfunction in a rat model. Sex Med. 2021;9:100317.

54. Zaghloul AS, Mahmoud ElNashar AER, GamalEl Din SF, Zaki Said S, Saad HM, Refaat Eldebs H, Abdel Latif Osman I. Smoking status and the baseline international index of erectile function score can predict satisfactory response to platelet-rich plasma in patients with erectile dysfunction: a prospective pilot study. Andrologia. 2021;53:e14162.
55. Taş T, Çakıroğlu B, Arda E, Onuk Ö, Nuhoğlu B. Early clinical results of the tolerability, safety, and efficacy of autologous platelet-rich plasma administration in erectile dysfunction. Sex Med. 2021;9:100313.
56. Wong S-M, Chiang B-J, Chen H-C, Wu Y-N, Lin Y-H, Liao C-H. A short term follow up for intracavernosal injection of platelet rich plasma for the treatment of erectile dysfunction. Urol Sci. 2021;32:171–6.
57. Schirmann A, Boutin E, Faix A, Yiou R. Pilot study of intra-cavernous injections of platelet-rich plasma (P-shot®) in the treatment of vascular erectile dysfunction. Prog Urol. 2022;32:1440–5.
58. Shaher H, Fathi A, Elbashir S, Abdelbaki SA, Soliman T. Is platelet rich plasma safe and effective in treatment of erectile dysfunction? Randomized controlled study. Urology. 2023;175:114–9.
59. Slack JM. What is a stem cell? Wiley Interdiscip Rev Dev Biol. 2018;7:e323.
60. Baraniak PR, McDevitt TC. Stem cell paracrine actions and tissue regeneration. Regen Med. 2010;5:121–43.
61. Milenkovic U, Albersen M, Castiglione F. The mechanisms and potential of stem cell therapy for penile fibrosis. Nat Rev Urol. 2019;16:79–97.
62. Hanson-Divers C, Jackson SE, Lue TF, Crawford SY, Rosen RC. Health outcomes variables important to patients in the treatment of erectile dysfunction. J Urol. 1998;159:1541–7.
63. Pérez-Aizpurua X, Garranzo-Ibarrola M, Simón-Rodríguez C, García-Cardoso JV, Chávez-Roa C, López-Martín L, et al. Stem cell therapy for erectile dysfunction: a step towards a future treatment. Life. 2023;13:502.
64. Zhang H, Albersen M, Jin X, Lin G. Stem cells: novel players in the treatment of erectile dysfunction. Asian J Androl. 2012;14:145.
65. Hou Q-L, Ge M-Y, Zhang C-D, Tian D-D, Wang L-K, Tian H-Z, et al. Adipose tissue-derived stem cell therapy for erectile dysfunction in rats: a systematic review and meta-analysis. Int Urol Nephrol. 2017;49:1127–37.
66. Song J, Sun T, Tang Z, Ruan Y, Liu K, Rao K, et al. Exosomes derived from smooth muscle cells ameliorate diabetes-induced erectile dysfunction by inhibiting fibrosis and modulating the NO/cGMP pathway. J Cell Mol Med. 2020;24:13289–302.
67. Bochinski D, Lin GT, Nunes L, Carrion R, Rahman N, Lin CS, Lue TF. The effect of neural embryonic stem cell therapy in a rat model of cavernosal nerve injury. BJU Int. 2004;94:904–9.
68. Xu Y, Guan R, Lei H, Li H, Wang L, Gao Z, et al. Therapeutic potential of adipose-derived stem cells-based micro-tissues in a rat model of postprostatectomy erectile dysfunction. J Sex Med. 2014;11:2439–48.
69. Chen Z, Han X, Ouyang X, Fang J, Huang X, Wei H. Transplantation of induced pluripotent stem cell-derived mesenchymal stem cells improved erectile dysfunction induced by cavernous nerve injury. Theranostics. 2019;9:6354.
70. Huang Y-C, Ning H, Shindel AW, Fandel TM, Lin G, Harraz AM, et al. The effect of intracavernous injection of adipose tissue-derived stem cells on hyperlipidemia-associated erectile dysfunction in a rat model. J Sex Med. 2010;7:1391–400.
71. Chen F, Zhang H, Wang Z, Ding W, Zeng Q, Liu W, et al. Adipose-derived stem cell-derived exosomes ameliorate erectile dysfunction in a rat model of type 2 diabetes. J Sex Med. 2017;14:1084–94.
72. Wani MM, Rai BP, Webb WR, Madaan S. Is there a role for stem cell therapy in erectile dysfunction secondary to cavernous nerve injury? Network meta-analysis from animal studies and human trials. Ther Adv Urol. 2022;14:17562872221086999.
73. Shan H, Chen F, Zhang T, He S, Xu L, Wei A. Stem cell therapy for erectile dysfunction of cavernous nerve injury rats: a systematic review and meta-analysis. PLoS One. 2015;10:e0121428.

74. Park HJ, Jeong H, Park YH, Yim HW, Ha U-s, Hong S-H, et al. Adipose tissue-derived stem cell therapy for cavernous nerve injury-induced erectile dysfunction in the rat model: a systematic review and meta-analysis using methodological quality assessment. Int J Stem Cells. 2019;12:206–17.
75. Zhang H-Y, Jin X-B, Lue TF. Three important components in the regeneration of the cavernous nerve: brain-derived neurotrophic factor, vascular endothelial growth factor and the JAK/STAT signaling pathway. Asian J Androl. 2011;13:231.
76. Zhou F, Hui Y, Xu Y, Lei H, Yang B, Guan R, et al. Effects of adipose-derived stem cells plus insulin on erectile function in streptozotocin-induced diabetic rats. Int Urol Nephrol. 2016;48:657–69.
77. Lu J, Xin Z, Zhang Q, Cui D, Xiao Y, Zhuo J, et al. Beneficial effect of PEDF-transfected ADSCs on erectile dysfunction in a streptozotocin-diabetic rat model. Cell Tissue Res. 2016;366:623–37.
78. Bahk JY, Jung JH, Han H, Min SK, Lee YS. Treatment of diabetic impotence with umbilical cord blood stem cell intracavernosal transplant: preliminary report of 7 cases. Exp Clin Transplant. 2010;8:150–60.
79. Levy JA, Marchand M, Iorio L, Cassini W, Zahalsky MP. Determining the feasibility of managing erectile dysfunction in humans with placental-derived stem cells. J Osteopath Med. 2016;116:e1–5.
80. Yiou R, Hamidou L, Birebent B, Bitari D, Lecorvoisier P, Contremoulins I, et al. Safety of intracavernous bone marrow-mononuclear cells for postradical prostatectomy erectile dysfunction: an open dose-escalation pilot study. Eur Urol. 2016;69:988–91.
81. Yiou R, Hamidou L, Birebent B, Bitari D, Le Corvoisier P, Contremoulins I, et al. Intracavernous injections of bone marrow mononucleated cells for postradical prostatectomy erectile dysfunction: final results of the INSTIN clinical trial. Eur Urol Focus. 2017;3:643–5.
82. Al Demour S, Jafar H, Adwan S, AlSharif A, Alhawari H, Alrabadi A, et al. Safety and potential therapeutic effect of two intracavernous autologous bone marrow derived mesenchymal stem cells injections in diabetic patients with erectile dysfunction: an open label phase I clinical trial. Urol Int. 2018;101:358–65.
83. Al Demour S, Adwan S, Jafar H, Rahmeh R, Alhawari H, Awidi A. Safety and efficacy of 2 intracavernous injections of allogeneic Wharton's jelly-derived mesenchymal stem cells in diabetic patients with erectile dysfunction: phase 1/2 clinical trial. Urol Int. 2021;105:935–43.
84. Haahr MK, Jensen CH, Toyserkani NM, Andersen DC, Damkier P, Sørensen JA, et al. Safety and potential effect of a single intracavernous injection of autologous adipose-derived regenerative cells in patients with erectile dysfunction following radical prostatectomy: an open-label phase I clinical trial. EBioMedicine. 2016;5:204–10.
85. You D, Jang MJ, Song G, Shin HC, Suh N, Kim YM, et al. Safety of autologous bone marrow-derived mesenchymal stem cells in erectile dysfunction: an open-label phase 1 clinical trial. Cytotherapy. 2021;23:931–8.
86. Mirzaei M, Bagherinasabsarab M, Pakmanesh H, Mohammadi R, Teimourian M, Jahani Y, Farsinejad A. The effect of intracavernosal injection of stem cell in the treatment of erectile dysfunction in diabetic patients: a randomized single-blinded clinical trial. Urol J. 2021;18:675.
87. Gryzinski GM, Hammad MAM, Barham DW, Yafi FA. Regenerative therapy in sexual medicine: the hard facts. J Urol. 2023;209:1048–50.
88. Burnett AL, Nehra A, Breau RH, Culkin DJ, Faraday MM, Hakim LS, et al. Erectile dysfunction: AUA guideline. J Urol. 2018;200:633–41.
89. Chung E, Lee J, Liu C, Taniguchi H, Zhou H, Park HJ. Clinical practice guideline recommendation on the use of low intensity extracorporeal shock wave therapy and low intensity pulsed ultrasound shock wave therapy to treat erectile dysfunction: the Asia-Pacific Society for Sexual Medicine Position Statement. World J Mens Health. 2020;39(1):1–8.
90. Domes T, Najafabadi BT, Roberts M, Campbell J, Flannigan R, Bach P, et al. Canadian Urological Association guideline: erectile dysfunction. Can Urol Assoc J. 2021;15:310.

91. Corona G, Cucinotta D, Di Lorenzo G, Ferlin A, Giagulli V, Gnessi L, et al. The Italian Society of Andrology and Sexual Medicine (SIAMS), along with ten other Italian Scientific Societies, guidelines on the diagnosis and management of erectile dysfunction. J Endocrinol Investig. 2023;46:1241–74.
92. Salonia A, Bettocchi C, Carvalho J, Corona G, Jones T, Kadioglu A, et al. EAU guidelines on sexual and reproductive health. European Association of Urology; 2022. https://d56bochluxqnz.cloudfront.net/documents/full-guideline/EAU-Guidelines-on-Sexual-and2020.
93. Capogrosso P, Frey A, Jensen CFS, Rastrelli G, Russo GI, Torremade J, et al. Low-intensity shock wave therapy in sexual medicine—clinical recommendations from the European Society of Sexual Medicine (ESSM). J Sex Med. 2019;16:1490–505.
94. Chung E, Lowy M, Gillman M, Love C, Katz D, Neilsen G. Urological Society of Australia and New Zealand (USANZ) and Australasian Chapter of Sexual Health Medicine (AChSHM) for the Royal Australasian College of Physicians (RACP) clinical guidelines on the management of erectile dysfunction. Med J Aust. 2022;217:318–24.
95. Al Hashimi M, Pinggera GM, Mostafa T, Shah R, Sahin B, Chung E, Rambhatla A, Cayan S, Alipour H, Ragab M, Raheem O, Arafa M, Alnajjar H, Kadioglu A, Hegde AV, Harraz A, Agarwa A. The role of different modalities of regenerative therapies in the treatment of erectile dysfunction: a global survey and global andrology forum expert recommendations. World J Mens Health. 2025;43:875–91. https://doi.org/10.5534/wjmh.240214. Epub ahead of print. PMID: 39743219.

Chapter 7
Advances in the Management of Peyronie's Disease

Hyun Jun Park, Hussain Alnajjar, and Eric Chung

Introduction

Peyronie's disease (PD) is characterized by the development of fibrous plaque within the tunica albuginea, which prevents the tunica albuginea from expanding during an erection, resulting in a characteristic penile curvature. Clinically, this penile curvature is most problematic, as it often leads to sexual difficulties. In severe cases, it can also result in a penis deformity such as a collar or hourglass penis during erection, which can add to the patient's psychological distress.

The disease primarily affects middle-aged men and is increasing in prevalence, with a prevalence of 0.4%–20% of adult men [1–3]. The prevalence is estimated to be much higher if asymptomatic patients are included. Recently published studies often report higher prevalence rates than in the past, likely due to the underestimation of previous prevalence rates and increased awareness and interest in Peyronie's disease in recent years.

H. J. Park (✉)
Department of Urology, Pusan National University Hospital, Pusan National University School of Medicine, Busan, Korea (Republic of)

H. Alnajjar
Department of Urology, University College London Hospital NHS Foundation Trust, London, UK

Division of Surgery and Interventional Science, University College London (UCL), London, UK
e-mail: Hussain.alnajjar@nhs.net

E. Chung
Department of Urology, Princess Alexandra Hospital, University of Queensland, Brisbane, QLD, Australia

AndroUrology Centre, Brisbane, QLD, Australia

R. Shah et al. (eds.), *Diagnosis and Treatment of Male Sexual Dysfunction*,
https://doi.org/10.1007/978-3-032-12423-4_7

Table 7.1 Definitions of Peyronie's disease

EAU [4]	A connective tissue disorder, characterized by the formation of a fibrotic lesion or plaque in the tunica albuginea, which leads to penile deformity
AUA [5]	An acquired penile abnormality characterized by fibrosis of the tunica albuginea, which may be accompanied by pain, deformity, erectile dysfunction (ED), and distress
ICSM [6]	Psychosexual condition characterized by the presence of penile pain, curvature, and deformity, with a potential palpable plaque and concomitant sexual dysfunction

Currently, the most widely accepted and used guidelines for PD are the guidelines published by the European Association of Urology (EAU), the American Urological Association (AUA), and the International Consultation on Sexual Medicine (ICSM), respectively [4–6]. The definition of PD in each guideline is listed in Table 7.1.

Pathophysiology and Etiology

The exact pathogenesis of PD is unclear, but it can be described as the result of chronic microtrauma to the penis, which results in improper wound healing. When microscopic damage is caused by ongoing behaviors such as sexual activity, blood leaks from the microvessels of the corpora cavernosa tissue and pools in the subtunical layer of the tunica albuginea. Here, fibrin deposits, macrophages, neutrophils, etc. gather, causing an inflammatory response. These cells secrete cytokines and vasoactive factors that accelerate the fibrosis process, most notably transforming growth factor-β1 (TGF-β1), which increases the synthesis of collagen. Over time, defects in tissue recombination, i.e., dysregulation of collagen synthesis and inadequate dissolution of nodules, develop [7, 8]. In addition to trauma, genetic predispositions such as HLA-B27 and autoimmune abnormalities are also involved in the pathogenesis of Peyronie's disease [9].

Commonly reported risk factors or comorbidities include hypertension, diabetes, dyslipidemia, ischemic heart disease, autoimmune disease, erectile dysfunction, smoking, alcohol consumption, low testosterone levels, and a history of pelvic surgery [10–12].

Symptoms and Clinical Manifestations

The clinical course can be divided into active and stable phases, and treatment is differentiated accordingly [13].

Active Disease

This phase is characterized by rapidly changing symptoms, and pain in the penis or glans during erection or in a flaccid state is common. The onset of these symptoms may coincide with an injury to the penis during sexual activity, although in the vast majority of cases there is no etiological history of penile injury. At this stage, a tender fibrous plaque may be palpable with a concomitant de novo penile curvature. During this period, the symptoms are dynamic and largely progressive. This results in increased anxiety and mental distress. Erectile function may be normal or decrease as the disease progresses.

Stable Disease

This is when clinical symptoms no longer change and are stable, usually 12–18 months after the first symptoms. Characteristically, the penile pain tends to subside. Penile curvature is common, which is independent of the size or extent of the fibrous plaque. Penile deformity is common in the ventral, dorso-lateral, and dorsal regions (e.g., wasting, S shape, hourglass).

Penis curvature resolves spontaneously in 3%–13% of cases, becomes fixed in 36%–67% of cases, and continues to progress in 21%–48% of cases. Erectile pain is present in 20%–70% of patients and gradually decreases; it disappears in 90% of patients after 12 months [1–3].

Erectile dysfunction is present in as many as half of cases (8%–52%), and Dupuytren's contracture is reported in 4%–26% [14, 15].

Diagnostics

A diagnosis of PD can often be made based on medical history and physical examination alone. It is important to determine whether the disease is progressive or stable, which is essential in determining when and how to treat it. In addition, a history of penile surgery, mechanical manipulation of the urethra, penile injury, medications, Dupuytren's contracture/plantar fascial contracture, family history of fibrotic disease, smoking, dyslipidemia, hypertension, diabetes, and cardiovascular disease are all risk factors for erectile dysfunction. Abnormalities of the penis during erection, such as pain, fibrous plaque, hourglass deformity, penis shortening, distal flaccidity, hinge effect, direction and degree of penile curvature, and the degree of erectile dysfunction, should be evaluated. When assessing the penis, the size, location, intensity, and number of the fibrous plaques should be noted. The patient may take a picture of their erect penis from two angles at home to document their distorted erection. Additionally, an erection may be induced in the clinic, using intracavernosal injection, to assess the curvature in the erect state and to judge whether there is significant ED. In some cases, an artificially induced erection and a penile duplex ultrasonography [16] are necessary; these tests can help delineate calcified plaques and their nature. Doppler ultrasound is helpful in assessing erectile function and hemodynamics in the penis. An MRI of the penis can occasionally be requested to assess a detailed anatomy of the erect penis.

Treatment

In the early stages of PD, or the active phase, penile pain is common, especially during erections, and treatment with nonsteroidal anti-inflammatory drugs is recommended. Psychological distress is common during this active phase due to the pain, development of penile plaque, and rapid progression of penile deformity, so psychological counseling or therapy is also recommended to alleviate this distress.

Once the pain has subsided and the penile plaque or deformity is no longer problematic, various treatment options are available, depending on the severity of the symptoms and the patient's wishes. Over time, multiple penile deformities or side effects commonly develop. The distinction between active and stable phases can be a continuum, and at times, they can revert from one to the other. Pain can be an issue in the stable phase due to the torque of the penis during sexual intercourse. In general, treatment is usually started when penile pain appears or penile curvature becomes problematic. Specific treatments include oral medications that act systemically or locally, injectable drugs that are injected directly into the lesion, and surgical treatments. The current recommendations from the European Association of Urology (EAU) [4], American Urological Association (AUA) [6], and International Consultation on Sexual Medicine (ICSM) [5] guidelines are summarized in Table 7.2.

Nonsurgical Treatment

Conservative, or nonsurgical, treatment of Peyronie's disease is an adjunctive, supportive treatment that is usually performed to relieve symptoms and control disease progression in patients in the early stages of the disease [17, 18].

Intralesional Therapy

This method is an attractive treatment alternative as it increases the drug concentration locally in the area of constriction of the lesion and avoids systemic side effects [19]. The main indications for this treatment are when the penile curvature is not severe ($\leq$30), the size of the penile fibrous plaque is small and it is not calcified, the

Table 7.2 Treatment recommendations for Peyronie's disease

Treatment methods	EAU	AUA	ICSM
Oral nonsteroidal anti-inflammatory medications	N.A.	O	N.A.
Oral phosphodiesterase type 5 inhibitors	X	N.A.	O
Oral potassium para-aminobenzoate	O	X	O
Oral vitamin E, tamoxifen	X	X	X
Oral acetyl esters of carnitine, pentoxifylline, colchicine	X	X	X
Intralesional treatment with steroids	O	O	O
Intralesional interferon	O	O	O
Intralesional verapamil	O	O	O
Topical verapamil	O	O	X
Electromotive therapy with verapamil	O	X	X
Penile traction devices, vacuum devices	O	O	O
Extracorporeal shockwave for curvature and plaque	X	X	X
Extracorporeal shockwave for pain	O	O	O
Intralesional collagenase clostridium histolyticum	O	O	O
Tunical shortening procedures	O	O	O
Grafting techniques	O	O	O
Penile prosthesis implantation	O	O	O
Radiotherapy	N.A.	X	N.A.

N.A. no comments in the guidelines, *O* recommended or possible, *X* not recommended, *EAU* European Association of Urology, *AUA* American Urological Association, *ICSM* International Consultation on Sexual Medicine

deformity of the penis is minimal, and especially when the patient wants to avoid surgical treatment.

In the past, several nonspecific therapeutic drugs had been used, but their efficacy has been unclear. Recently, collagenase clostridium histolyticum (Xiaflex®, Auxilium Pharmaceuticals, Inc.) has been developed as an injectable therapy to reduce curvature without the need for surgery.

Collagenase Clostridium Histolyticum

Collagenase clostridium histolyticum (CCH) (Xiaflex®) is an injectable drug that contains a mixture of two enzymes, class I and class II collagenase, which cleave collagen at different sites, making it easier to break down fibrous plaques [20].

With the recent demonstration of the drug's intralesional efficacy in Dupuytren's contracture, its efficacy in Peyronie's disease has also been demonstrated, making it the only FDA-approved treatment for Peyronie's disease. Its primary effect is to reduce penile curvature in Peyronie's disease at rest.

The use of CCH is contraindicated in hourglass deformity, ventral curvature, calcified fibrous plaques, and fibrous plaques at the base of the penis.

The treatment regimen consists of two Xiaflex® injections administered into the Peyronie's plaque, 3 days apart, with gentle penile stretching and modeling to help break the collagen. The process is repeated at 6 weeks, up to a maximum of four treatment cycles. The price for a treatment cycle can range between $8000 and $12,000 in the United States. Each vial of Xiaflex® costs around $4000–$5000. Xiaflex® was fully withdrawn from the European market in March 2020 due to commercial reasons.

Ecchymosis of the penis, penile swelling, and penile pain occurred in almost all patients, but most resolved spontaneously. Rupture of the body of the penis is rare, but intercourse should be avoided for 4 weeks after injection to prevent this. Based on the results of previous studies [21–23], improvement in penis curvature is consistent, with 31.4%–42.9% of patients showing improvement, with an average improvement of 17°, and 50%–60% of cases reported improved ability to have intercourse. However, there was no improvement in pain, nodule size, or ED [24].

Interferon

Theoretically, it may improve penis curvature by decreasing fibroblast production of collagen and increasing collagenase production [25]. In clinical studies, it has been shown to help relieve penile pain and improve penile blood flow [26, 27]. Side effects such as sinusitis, penis swelling, and flu-like symptoms occurred in 40%–100% of patients but were usually mild and rarely required further treatment. Currently, this treatment modality is not widely utilized due to its poor efficacy, practical drawbacks, and side effects.

Verapamil

It is a typical calcium channel blocker that controls fibroblast function and fibrous tissue production and inhibits inflammatory responses and has been used as a typical intralesional treatment for Peyronie's disease in the past. However, in recent years, it has been reported that the improvement in penile curvature is not as pronounced as in the early clinical results. Therefore, verapamil 10 mg injected into the plaques every 2–4 weeks may be used to reduce the size and intensity of penile fibrous plaque. It has no significant side effects and is inexpensive to utilize, so it may still play a role in the treatment of this condition [28].

Oral Medications

The effectiveness of oral therapy in treating Peyronie's disease remains largely uncertain, with existing studies showing only minimal impact on reducing penile deformity. This is likely due to variations in the studies, such as small sample sizes, different stages of the disease, and limited measurable outcomes [5, 6]. Although vitamin E, tamoxifen, carnitine, colchicine, L-arginine, and pentoxifylline have been tried in the past for their antioxidant, anti-inflammatory, and antifibrotic properties, none have successfully corrected penile curvature. While randomized trials have found that oral treatments like vitamin E, colchicine, carnitine, potassium aminobenzoate, and tamoxifen are mostly ineffective, more recent research suggests that pentoxifylline and low-dose tadalafil may offer some benefits in managing Peyronie's disease [29–31]. Oral therapy might be especially useful in the early stages of the disease, particularly for men experiencing unstable or worsening penile curvature and painful erections, or for those who are not ready or willing to pursue surgical options.

Other Therapies

Penile Traction Therapy and Vacuum Erection Device (VED)

It involves wearing a device that physically elongates the penis for a certain number of hours per day to stretch it, provide additional length, reduce curvature, or shorten it. It can be applied during both the active and stable phases of the disease and is particularly effective when combined with intralesional drug injection therapy or as an adjunctive procedure before or after radical penile surgery. However, traction of the penis for a prolonged period of time can be uncomfortable for the patient and should be performed selectively [32]. Martinez-Salamanca et al. demonstrated that in a study of 55 men with acute-phase Peyronie's disease, those who used PTT for 6 months experienced an improvement in curvature from 33° to 15° at 6 months and to 13° at 9 months, compared to 41 untreated controls [33]. Macdonald et al. reviewed 20 men with Peyronie's using VED 10 min twice daily with a mean curvature improvement of 23° with a mean follow-up period of 14 months [34].

Extracorporeal Shock Wave Therapy

In theory, it is thought to disrupt fibrous plaque and induce its dissolution and resorption [33, 34]. Taken together, clinical studies have shown that it is helpful in relieving pain during erection, but not in reducing the size or curvature of penile fibrous plaque [35, 36]. It may be considered as a treatment for pain in Peyronie's disease, but the benefit-cost ratio should be considered [37].

Surgical Treatments

In patients with Peyronie's disease, the goal of surgery is to correct the penile curvature to the point where sexual activity is not impaired and erectile function is maintained at preoperative levels. In general, the younger the patient, the more likely it is that the penile curvature will cause mental distress in addition to physical disability. In addition, if there is a ventral curvature, vaginal penetration is more difficult. Therefore, the following cases of Peyronie's disease, i.e., (1) severe penile curvature, (2) deformity such as hourglass or wasting, which causes difficulty in sexual penetration, (3) severe penis shortening, (4) erectile dysfunction, and (5) a combination of the above factors, are indications for surgery. On the other hand, patients who have unrealistically high expectations or those with early-stage Peyronie's disease are not suitable candidates for surgical treatment. It is also important to determine the timing of surgery, which should only be performed when the disease is stable, usually around 12 months after the first symptoms. A detailed examination for penile vascular disorders or sexual dysfunction should be performed prior to surgery, and the appropriate surgical procedure should be selected after evaluation of all factors. Peyronie's disease corrective surgery can be categorized into three types: penile tunical shortening procedure, penile tunical lengthening procedure, and insertion of penile prosthesis. Penile tunical shortening and penile tunical lengthening procedures are recommended for patients who have normal erections or for whom oral pharmacotherapy is effective. Penile implants are a viable option for patients with severe erectile dysfunction who have failed medications [38, 39]. The treatment algorithm is summarized in Fig. 7.1.

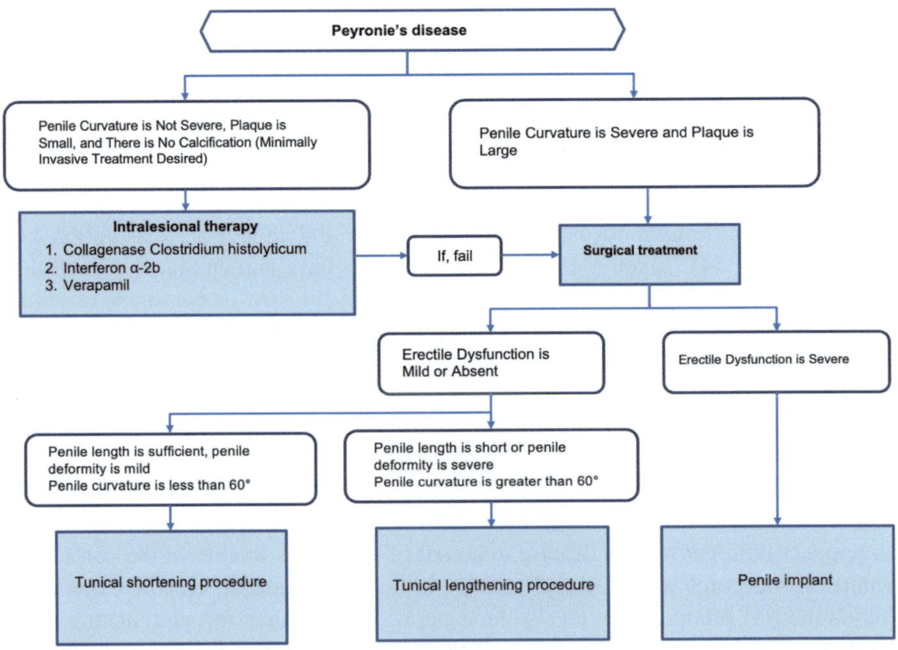

Fig. 7.1 Algorithm for surgical treatment of Peyronie's disease

Preoperative Preparation

The basic principle when considering surgery is that it should be performed when Peyronie's disease is in a stable phase. Surgery is usually considered at least 6–12 months after onset, when there is no change in fibrous plaque or curvature for 3–6 months, or when there is severe deformity that interferes with or makes intercourse difficult [40]. Surgery may also be considered when conservative treatment fails, when penile fibrous plaque is extensive to begin with, or when the patient wants quick results. It is also possible to skip nonsurgical treatment and proceed directly to surgery, but patients should be fully informed of the potential side effects of surgery and give informed consent [29, 41].

It is of utmost importance that patients considering surgery are fully counseled and informed of realistic expectations for the outcome of surgery. Patients often have unrealistic expectations, which can lead to postoperative difficulties for both patients and healthcare providers.

Components of informed consent should include a discussion of possible treatment options and their advantages and disadvantages and an explanation of how they apply to the patient's current state of Peyronie's disease. Realistic expectations and potential complications of the proposed surgery should be fully explained and agreed upon [40, 42].

Tunical Shortening Procedure

The tunica albuginea shortening procedure is a surgical technique to straighten the penis by shortening the long and convex part of the penis to equalize with the opposite side. In patients with good erectile function, moderate penile length, and without complicated deformities such as hourglass deformity or hinge effect and/or severe curvature (e.g., >60°), the tunica albuginea shortening procedure may be an appropriate surgical option. Although various methods and variations have been described, no one method is superior to the others, and each should be tailored to the individual patient.

The *Nesbit procedure* involves removing a portion of the tunica albuginea opposite the point of curvature and suturing it [43, 44]. The traditional Nesbit procedure with excision of an ellipse of tunica may sometimes increase the risk of ED secondary to postoperative veno-occlusive dysfunction [45]. However, several modifications of the Nesbit procedure have been published recently, which is considered the safer option and preferred method nowadays since it does not cause veno-occlusive ED. The *Yachia technique*, instead of removing a portion of the tunica albuginea, involves making a longitudinal incision and suturing it in a transverse direction. The *penile plication technique* involves shortening the tunica albuginea by passing sutures through an appropriate range of the tunica albuginea and tying them in a knot, rather than resection or incision of the tunica albuginea [46–48].

In general, tunical shortening procedures are successful in correcting the curvature in more than 85% of patients. Recurrence of curvature and penis hypoesthesia are uncommon (~10%), and the risk of postoperative ED is low. Disadvantages include penis shortening, and it does not resolve hinge or hourglass deformity and may even worsen it. Other complications may include persistent penile pain, persistence or recurrence of penile curvature (>30°, 8%–11%), penile hematoma (0%–9%), requirement for circumcision, palpable suture knots, and decreased penile sensation. These are rarely the cause of postoperative sexual dysfunction, but patients may perceive penis shortening to be greater than it actually is. Therefore, measuring and recording stretched penile length intraoperatively before and after surgery, regardless of the technique used, is paramount for both patient information and medico-legal cases [49–53].

Tunical Lengthening Procedure

The tunica albuginea lengthening procedure is a surgical method that involves incision or partial excision of the fibrous plaque or concavity of the penis, followed by the use of a graft to cover the defect. In patients with satisfactory erectile function, the tunica albuginea lengthening procedure may be an appropriate option if there is severe penis shortening, complex curvature, and simple curvature greater than 60°, a large fibrous plaque, or a complex deformity such as an hourglass or hinge effect.

The ideal graft should be traction-resistant, easy to suture and manipulate, flexible, readily available, cost-effective, and minimize infection, especially when using autografts (Table 7.3). However, no graft meets all of these requirements. In the case of the tunica albuginea lengthening procedure, structures within the deep penile

Table 7.3 Summary of grafts used in plaque incision and grafting, and their advantages versus disadvantages

Graft	Type	Advantages	Disadvantages
Saphenous vein	Autologous	Easily available, good handling characteristics	Additional operative time, donor site morbidity
Buccal mucosa	Autologous	Easily available, excellent take	Donor site morbidity, limited size for larger defects
Tunica vaginalis	Autologous	Thin and pliable, single operative field	Limited structural strength, limited surface area
Dermal grafts	Autologous	Pliable and readily available	Donor site scar, variable thickness, quality, lack of anchorage
Cadaveric human pericardium	Allograft	Readily available off the shelf, good handling	High cost, risk of contracture, risk of disease transmission
Fascia lata	Allograft	Strong, durable	Limited availability, cost
Small intestinal submucosa (SIS)	Xenograft	Excellent remodeling properties	Potential for calcification, cost
Bovine/porcine pericardium	Xenograft	Good strength and tensile properties	Contraction and possible immune reaction
Synthetic	PTFE/ Dacron	Unlimited supply, consistent	Higher infection risk, poor long-term outcomes

fascia, such as the neurovascular bundle, are mobilized and temporarily retracted; hence, there is a risk of temporary neuropraxia or even permanent numbness. Although damage to the cavernous artery is rare, the likelihood of postoperative erectile dysfunction is reported to be higher (10%–50%) than in the tunica albuginea shortening procedure for a variety of reasons. The presence of preoperative erectile dysfunction, the use of larger grafts, age over 60 years, and dorsal curvature are considered poor prognostic factors for surgical outcome [54].

There are four main types of grafts: autograft, allograft, xenograft, and synthetic graft, each with its own advantages and disadvantages, and there is no consistent evidence that any one graft is superior to the others [55].

For autografts, venous grafts, mainly saphenous vein, are commonly used, and recently buccal mucosal grafts have also been used. Dermal grafts are rarely used due to their lack of anchorage and potential for venogenic erectile dysfunction [56, 57]. Tunica albuginea grafts are the most histologically suitable, but caution should be exercised due to the limited size that can be obtained and the possibility of weakening penile support [58, 59].

For allografts, cadaveric pericardium is commonly used. Cadaveric dura mater is no longer used due to concerns about possible infection [60].

For xenografts, type I collagen-based xenografts such as small intestinal submucosa, or bovine pericardium, are commonly used. Recently, grafting with collagen fleece (TachoSil©) has been increasingly used due to several key advantages, such as shorter surgical time, ease of application, and hemostatic effect [61].

For synthetic grafts, polyester (Dacron®) and polytetrafluoroethylene (Gore-Tex®) have been introduced but are not recommended due to the potential for infection, inflammation, and allergic reactions and significant fibrosis [62–64].

The tunica albuginea lengthening procedure does not actually lengthen the penis but rather extends the fibrous plaque to the length of the original tunica albuginea. Nevertheless, postoperative penile shortening has been reported, with rates ranging from around 30% for saphenous vein grafts, 23%–30% for allografts, and 13%–20% for xenografts, depending on the type of graft used to cover the fibrous plaque [4]. The exact cause of penile shortening after tunica albuginea lengthening procedures has not been reported.

In tunica albuginea lengthening procedures, the risk of erectile dysfunction is greater than in tunica albuginea shortening procedures, with rates of up to 50% reported.

Recurrence of curvature occurs due to failure to wait for the disease to stabilize, reactivation of the condition after stable disease has occurred, or use of absorbable sutures, which lose their hold before healing, is complete. Therefore, it is recommended that non-absorbable sutures or slowly resorbing absorbable sutures (e.g., polydioxanone) be used. If nonabsorbable sutures are used, the knots should be buried to avoid irritation of the penile skin, but the use of slow resorbable sutures (e.g., polydioxanone) may reduce the likelihood of this occurring [65]. Changes in penile sensation are associated with damage to the neurovascular bundle, the degree of dissection required to remove fibrous plaque, and postoperative inflammation and fibrosis at the graft site. Reduction in penile sensation has been reported in rates up to 25%, but most studies report 5% or less [55].

Penile Prosthesis Implantation with Penile Reconstruction

For men with ED who want to preserve penile size, penile prosthesis implantation is advised [54]. The inflatable penile prosthesis generally provides higher functional outcomes and greater patient satisfaction compared to malleable implants [5, 6]. Although penile prosthesis implantation alone is usually adequate to correct minor penile curvature, patients with a residual curvature greater than 30° may require additional procedures such as repeated manual modeling, penile plication, or plaque incision with grafting during surgery [4–6]. However, using graft material is linked to an increased risk of prosthetic infection [5]. New surgical methods aimed at enhancing penile length and girth during prosthesis implantation, utilizing various modified sliding techniques, [38] have shown high rates of patient satisfaction but carry serious risks, including glans necrosis and penile gangrene [66].

Novel Pharmacological Treatments

Recent advancements in the treatment of Peyronie's disease have introduced novel therapeutic options that show promise in improving patient outcomes. Among these, stem cell therapy and platelet-rich plasma (PRP) injections are gaining attention for their potential to promote tissue repair and reduce fibrosis [67]. Stem cells, particularly mesenchymal stem cells, have demonstrated antifibrotic and regenerative properties in early studies, suggesting their potential to reverse the effects of Peyronie's disease [68]. PRP therapy, which utilizes a concentration of the patient's own platelets, is believed to release growth factors that can facilitate tissue healing and decrease plaque formation. In addition to these injectable therapies, H100 topical gel has emerged as a non-invasive treatment option [69]. This gel contains a combination of verapamil, a calcium channel blocker with antifibrotic effects, along with other active ingredients that aim to soften the plaques and improve penile curvature. Preliminary studies on H100 gel have shown promising results in reducing penile curvature and improving patient-reported outcomes. These novel therapies, though still under investigation, offer exciting new avenues for the management of Peyronie's disease, potentially improving efficacy while minimizing invasiveness compared to traditional surgical approaches.

Conclusion

Peyronie's disease is one of the most difficult conditions to treat in the field of andrology. Patients vary in the nature and severity of their symptoms, their level of psychological distress, and their desires and expectations for treatment. Treatment for this condition must take these variables into account. In general, in the acute phase of the disease, oral pharmacotherapy, such as anti-inflammatory medications, is indicated, along with psychological counseling. In the stable phase of the disease, a variety of treatment options are available to relieve the patient's sexual dysfunction. Various surgical treatments have been developed to correct penile curvature and they have become the mainstay of treatment. However, each of these surgical procedures has its disadvantages and should be used judiciously in properly selected patients. The recent development of collagenase clostridium histolyticum as an intralesional injection has opened up a new therapeutic option for nonsurgical treatment to reduce penile curvature, but cost is a concern. Advances in intralesional injections and newer drugs may alter the treatment in the future and lead to optimal management of the disease.

References

1. Mulhall JP, Schiff J, Guhring P. An analysis of the natural history of Peyronie's disease. J Urol. 2006;175(6):2115–8; discussion 2118.
2. Grasso M, Lania C, Blanco S, Limonta G. The natural history of Peyronie's disease. Arch Esp Urol. 2007;60(3):326–31.
3. Berookhim BM, Choi J, Alex B, Mulhall JP. Deformity stabilization and improvement in men with untreated Peyronie's disease. BJU Int. 2014;113(1):133–6.
4. Hatzimouratidis K, Eardley I, Giuliano F, Hatzichristou D, Moncada I, Salonia A, et al. EAU guidelines on penile curvature. Eur Urol. 2012;62(3):543–52.
5. Chung E, Ralph D, Kagioglu A, Garaffa G, Shamsodini A, Bivalacqua T, et al. Evidence-based management guidelines on Peyronie's disease. J Sex Med. 2016;13(6):905–23.
6. Nehra A, Alterowitz R, Culkin DJ, Faraday MM, Hakim LS, Heidelbaugh JJ, et al. Peyronie's disease: AUA guideline. J Urol. 2015;194(3):745–53.
7. Somers KD, Dawson DM. Fibrin deposition in Peyronie's disease plaque. J Urol. 1997;157(1):311–5.
8. Mulhall JP. Expanding the paradigm for plaque development in Peyronie's disease. Int J Impot Res. 2003;15(Suppl 5):S93–102.
9. Mitsui Y, Yamabe F, Hori S, Uetani M, Kobayashi H, Nagao K, et al. Molecular mechanisms and risk factors related to the pathogenesis of Peyronie's disease. Int J Mol Sci. 2023;24(12):9583.
10. Sommer F, Schwarzer U, Wassmer G, Bloch W, Braun M, Klotz T, et al. Epidemiology of Peyronie's disease. Int J Impot Res. 2002;14(5):379–83.
11. Rhoden EL, Riedner CE, Fuchs SC, Ribeiro EP, Halmenschlager G. A cross-sectional study for the analysis of clinical, sexual and laboratory conditions associated with Peyronie's disease. J Sex Med. 2010;7(4 Pt 1):1529–37.
12. Mitsui Y, Kobayashi H, Yamabe F, Nakajima K, Nagao K. ABO blood type and risk of Peyronie's disease in Japanese males. World J Mens Health. 2022;40(3):509–16.

13. Di Maida F, Cito G, Lambertini L, Valastro F, Morelli G, Mari A, et al. The natural history of Peyronie's disease. World J Mens Health. 2021;39(3):399–405.
14. Arafa M, Eid H, El-Badry A, Ezz-Eldine K, Shamloul R. The prevalence of Peyronie's disease in diabetic patients with erectile dysfunction. Int J Impot Res. 2007;19(2):213–7.
15. Shindel AW, Sweet G, Thieu W, Durbin-Johnson B, Rothschild J, Szabo R. Prevalence of Peyronie's disease-like symptoms in men presenting with Dupuytren contractures. Sex Med. 2017;5(3):e135–41.
16. McCauley JF, Dean RC. Diagnostic utility of penile ultrasound in Peyronie's disease. World J Urol. 2020;38(2):263–8.
17. Lee HY, Pyun JH, Shim SR, Kim JH. Medical treatment for Peyronie's disease: systematic review and network Bayesian meta-analysis. World J Mens Health. 2024;42(1):133–47.
18. Joice GA, Burnett AL. Nonsurgical interventions for Peyronie's disease: update as of 2016. World J Mens Health. 2016;34(2):65–72.
19. Cai T, Tiscione D, Favilla V, Puglisi M, Palumbo F, Zucchi A, et al. Oral administration and intralesional injection of hyaluronic acid versus intralesional injection alone in Peyronie's disease: results from a phase III study. World J Mens Health. 2021;39(3):526–32.
20. Cocci A, Di Maida F, Russo GI, Di Mauro M, Cito G, Falcone M, et al. How atypical penile curvature influences clinical outcomes in patients with Peyronie's disease receiving collagenase Clostridium histolyticum therapy. World J Mens Health. 2020;38(1):78–84.
21. Gelbard M, Lipshultz LI, Tursi J, Smith T, Kaufman G, Levine LA. Phase 2b study of the clinical efficacy and safety of collagenase Clostridium histolyticum in patients with Peyronie's disease. J Urol. 2012;187(6):2268–74.
22. Gelbard M, Hellstrom WJ, McMahon CG, Levine LA, Smith T, Tursi J, et al. Baseline characteristics from an ongoing phase 3 study of collagenase Clostridium histolyticum in patients with Peyronie's disease. J Sex Med. 2013;10(11):2822–31.
23. Zhang F, Xiong Y, Wang W, Wu C, Qin F, Yuan J. The efficacy and safety of intralesional injection of collagenase Clostridium histolyticum for Peyronie's disease: a meta-analysis of published prospective studies. Front Pharmacol. 2022;13:973394.
24. Sun AJ, Li S, Eisenberg ML. The impact of Clostridium histolyticum collagenase on the prevalence and management of Peyronie's disease in the United States. World J Mens Health. 2019;37(2):234–9.
25. Duncan MR, Berman B, Nseyo UO. Regulation of the proliferation and biosynthetic activities of cultured human Peyronie's disease fibroblasts by interferons-alpha, -beta and -gamma. Scand J Urol Nephrol. 1991;25(2):89–94.
26. Kendirci M, Usta MF, Matern RV, Nowfar S, Sikka SC, Hellstrom WJ. The impact of intralesional interferon alpha-2b injection therapy on penile hemodynamics in men with Peyronie's disease. J Sex Med. 2005;2(5):709–15.
27. Hellstrom WJ, Kendirci M, Matern R, Cockerham Y, Myers L, Sikka SC, et al. Single-blind, multicenter, placebo controlled, parallel study to assess the safety and efficacy of intralesional interferon alpha-2B for minimally invasive treatment for Peyronie's disease. J Urol. 2006;176(1):394–8.
28. Cocci A, Di Maida F, Cito G, Verrienti P, Laruccia N, Campi R, et al. Comparison of intralesional hyaluronic acid vs. verapamil for the treatment of acute phase Peyronie's disease: a prospective, open-label non-randomized clinical study. World J Mens Health. 2021;39(2):352–7.
29. Smith JF, Walsh TJ, Lue TF. Peyronie's disease: a critical appraisal of current diagnosis and treatment. Int J Impot Res. 2008;20(5):445–59.
30. Brant WO, Dean RC, Lue TF. Treatment of Peyronie's disease with oral pentoxifylline. Nat Clin Pract Urol. 2006;3(2):111–5; quiz 6.
31. Chung E, Deyoung L, Brock GB. The role of PDE5 inhibitors in penile septal scar remodeling: assessment of clinical and radiological outcomes. J Sex Med. 2011;8(5):1472–7.
32. Chung E, Gillman M, Tuckey J, La Bianca S, Love C. A clinical pathway for the management of Peyronie's disease: integrating clinical guidelines from the International Society of Sexual

Medicine, American Urological Association and European Urological Association. BJU Int. 2020;126(Suppl 1):12–7.

33. Martínez-Salamanca JI, Egui A, Moncada I, Minaya J, Ballesteros CM, Del Portillo L, et al. Acute phase Peyronie's disease management with traction device: a nonrandomized prospective controlled trial with ultrasound correlation. J Sex Med. 2014;11(2):506–15.
34. MacDonald LP, Armstrong ML, Lehmann KJ, Acker MR, Langille GM. Outcome analysis of patients with Peyronie's disease who elect for vacuum erection device therapy. Can Urol Assoc J. 2020;14(9):E428–31.
35. Husain J, Lynn NN, Jones DK, Collins GN, O'Reilly PH. Extracorporeal shock wave therapy in the management of Peyronie's disease: initial experience. BJU Int. 2000;86(4):466–8.
36. Kim KS, Choi YS, Bae WJ, Cho HJ, Ha US, Hong SH, et al. Efficacy of low-intensity extracorporeal shock wave therapy for the treatment of chronic pelvic pain syndrome IIIb: a prospective-randomized, double-blind, placebo-controlled study. World J Mens Health. 2022;40(3):473–80.
37. Chitale S, Morsey M, Swift L, Sethia K. Limited shock wave therapy vs sham treatment in men with Peyronie's disease: results of a prospective randomized controlled double-blind trial. BJU Int. 2010;106(9):1352–6.
38. Hatzichristodoulou G, Meisner C, Gschwend JE, Stenzl A, Lahme S. Extracorporeal shock wave therapy in Peyronie's disease: results of a placebo-controlled, prospective, randomized, single-blind study. J Sex Med. 2013;10(11):2815–21.
39. Di Mauro M, Russo GI, Della Camera PA, Di Maida F, Cito G, Mondaini N, et al. Extracorporeal shock wave therapy in Peyronie's disease: clinical efficacy and safety from a single-arm observational study. World J Mens Health. 2019;37(3):339–46.
40. Chung E. Penile reconstructive surgery in Peyronie disease: challenges in restoring normal penis size, shape, and function. World J Mens Health. 2020;38(1):1–8.
41. Segal RL, Burnett AL. Surgical management for Peyronie's disease. World J Mens Health. 2013;31(1):1–11.
42. Matsushita K, Stember DS, Nelson CJ, Mulhall JP. Concordance between patient and physician assessment of the magnitude of Peyronie's disease curvature. J Sex Med. 2014;11(1):205–10.
43. Kadioglu A, Kucukdurmaz F, Sanli O. Current status of the surgical management of Peyronie's disease. Nat Rev Urol. 2011;8(2):95–106.
44. Taylor FL, Levine LA. Surgical correction of Peyronie's disease via tunica albuginea plication or partial plaque excision with pericardial graft: long-term follow up. J Sex Med. 2008;5(9):2221–8; discussion 9–30.
45. Nesbit RM. Congenital curvature of the phallus: report of three cases with description of corrective operation. J Urol. 1965;93:230–2.
46. Sokolakis I, Schonbauer P, Mykoniatis I, Kubler H, Gschwend J, Lahme S, et al. Long-term results after surgical treatment of congenital penile curvature using a modified Nesbit technique. World J Mens Health. 2020;38(4):564–72.
47. Carson CC, Levine LA. Outcomes of surgical treatment of Peyronie's disease. BJU Int. 2014;113(5):704–13.
48. Sassine AM, Wespes E, Schulman CC. Modified corporoplasty for penile curvature: 10 years' experience. Urology. 1994;44(3):419–21.
49. Licht MR, Lewis RW. Modified Nesbit procedure for the treatment of Peyronie's disease: a comparative outcome analysis. J Urol. 1997;158(2):460–3.
50. Yachia D. Modified corporoplasty for the treatment of penile curvature. J Urol. 1990;143(1):80–2.
51. Nooter RI, Bosch JL, Schroder FH. Peyronie's disease and congenital penile curvature: long-term results of operative treatment with the plication procedure. Br J Urol. 1994;74(4):497–500.
52. Klevmark B, Andersen M, Schultz A, Talseth T. Congenital and acquired curvature of the penis treated surgically by plication of the tunica albuginea. Br J Urol. 1994;74(4):501–6.
53. Thiounn N, Missirliu A, Zerbib M, Larrouy M, Dje K, Flam T, et al. Corporeal plication for surgical correction of penile curvature. Experience with 60 patients. Eur Urol. 1998;33(4):401–4.

54. Chahal R, Gogoi NK, Sundaram SK, Weston PM. Corporal plication for penile curvature caused by Peyronie's disease: the patients' perspective. BJU Int. 2001;87(4):352–6.
55. Geertsen UA, Brok KE, Andersen B, Nielsen HV. Peyronie curvature treated by plication of the penile fasciae. Br J Urol. 1996;77(5):733–5.
56. Mulhall J, Anderson M, Parker M. A surgical algorithm for men with combined Peyronie's disease and erectile dysfunction: functional and satisfaction outcomes. J Sex Med. 2005;2(1):132–8.
57. Langston JP, Carson CC 3rd. Peyronie disease: plication or grafting. Urol Clin North Am. 2011;38(2):207–16.
58. Devine CJ Jr, Horton CE. Surgical treatment of Peyronie's disease with a dermal graft. J Urol. 1974;111(1):44–9.
59. Garcia-Gomez B, Ralph D, Levine L, Moncada-Iribarren I, Djinovic R, Albersen M, et al. Grafts for Peyronie's disease: a comprehensive review. Andrology. 2018;6(1):117–26.
60. Teloken C, Grazziotin T, Rhoden E, Da Ros C, Fornari A, Soares FC, et al. Penile straightening with crural graft of the corpus cavernosum. J Urol. 2000;164(1):107–8.
61. Da Ros CT, Graziottin TM, Ribeiro E, Averbeck MA. Long-term follow-up of penile curvature correction utilizing autologous albugineal crural graft. Int Braz J Urol. 2012;38(2):242–7; discussion 8–9.
62. Collins JP. Experience with lyophilized human dura for treatment of Peyronie disease. Urology. 1988;31(5):379–81.
63. Lahme S, Gotz T, Bichler KH. Collagen fleece for defect coverage following plaque excision in patients with Peyronie's disease. Eur Urol. 2002;41(4):401–5.
64. Schiffman ZJ, Gursel EO, Laor E. Use of Dacron patch graft in Peyronie disease. Urology. 1985;25(1):38–40.
65. Faerber GJ, Konnak JW. Results of combined Nesbit penile plication with plaque incision and placement of Dacron patch in patients with severe Peyronie's disease. J Urol. 1993;149(5 Pt 2):1319–20.
66. Ganabathi K, Dmochowski R, Zimmern PE, Leach GE. Peyronie's disease: surgical treatment based on penile rigidity. J Urol. 1995;153(3 Pt 1):662–6.
67. Ralph DJ, al-Akraa M, Pryor JP. The Nesbit operation for Peyronie's disease: 16-year experience. J Urol. 1995;154(4):1362–3.
68. Warner JN. A contemporary evaluation of Peyronie's disease during penile prosthesis placement: MOST, MUST, and more. Curr Urol Rep. 2019;20(2):9.
69. Asmundo MG, Durukan E, von Rohden E, Thy SA, Jensen CFS, Fode M. Platelet-rich plasma therapy in erectile dysfunction and Peyronie's disease: a systematic review of the literature. World J Urol. 2024;42(1):359.

Chapter 8
Comprehensive Management of Premature Ejaculation

Eric Chung, Vineet Malhotra, and Du Geon Moon

Introduction

Premature ejaculation (PE) is a common male sexual problem and has been called early ejaculation or rapid ejaculation. It is estimated to affect around 20–30% of men in the sexually active age group [1–4]. Published literature shows that PE adversely impacts not only psychological stress and loss of self-esteem per se, but also significantly affects various quality-of-life domains, such as relationship dynamics, work productivity, and social intimacy [5, 6].

Despite the high prevalence of PE, this sexual disorder remains undertreated and represents an area of unmet therapeutic need, since it is often neglected by clinicians due to a combination of many factors, including poor rates of seeking treatment because of embarrassment or shame, confusion with other male sexual complaints, lack of effective clinical treatment, and misperception on what constitutes normal time to ejaculation [7–9]. Psychological issues like depression, stress, or anxiety about sexual performance, can also trigger and/or worsen PE, resulting in a vicious cycle of sexual dysfunction [10].

The following chapter provides a narrative review of the different PE definitions, neurobiology, clinical assessment, and treatment options, including psychosexual, pharmacological, surgical, and combined treatments. The emphasis is placed on

E. Chung (✉)
Department of Urology, Princess Alexandra Hospital, University of Queensland, Brisbane, QLD, Australia

AndroUrology Centre, Brisbane, QLD, Australia

V. Malhotra
VNA Hospital, New Delhi, India

D. G. Moon
Department of Urology, Korea University College of Medicine, Seoul, South Korea

R. Shah et al. (eds.), *Diagnosis and Treatment of Male Sexual Dysfunction*,
https://doi.org/10.1007/978-3-032-12423-4_8

providing a holistic and multidisciplinary approach with the incorporation of various treatment strategies, including a better understanding of the neurophysiology and psychosocial impacts of PE on the man and his partner.

Definitions of PE

While PE was initially defined in the 1970s by Masters and Johnson as "the inability of a man to delay ejaculation long enough for his partner to reach organism in 50% of intercourse attempts" [11], its scientific definitions have changed over the years, and its exact terminology can vary depending on the scientific organizations.

The *American Urology Association* defined PE as "ejaculation occurring sooner than desired, causing distress to one or both partners" [4]. The *International Society for Sexual Medicine (ISSM)* and, subsequently, the International Consultation on Sexual Medicine (ICSM) classified PE more specifically into two main categories as "a male sexual dysfunction characterized by ejaculation which always or nearly always occurs prior to or within about one minute of vaginal penetration (lifelong PE), or a clinically significant and bothersome reduction in latency time, often to about 3 minutes or less (acquired PE); inability to delay ejaculation on all or nearly all vaginal penetrations; and negative personal consequences, such as distress, bother, frustration, and/or the avoidance of sexual intimacy" [1, 12]. The separation between lifelong and acquired PE is based largely on the initial presentation of PE and time to ejaculation, in which a patient with lifelong PE ejaculated within about 1 minute of vaginal penetration from his first sexual experience, while patients with acquired PE reported a clinically significant reduction compared to previous ejaculation latency (often to about 3 minutes or less). This distinction is made to reflect that PE is not a homogenous sexual disorder across populations, and perhaps there is a need to further define PE as variable and subjective too [3].

On the other hand, the *Diagnostic and Statistical Manual of Mental Disorders (DSM)* outlines the criteria for PE based on latency time, perceived control over ejaculation, and personal distress and interpersonal difficulty related to this condition [13]. The *American Psychiatric Association's* Diagnostic and Statistical Manual of Mental Disorders 5th edition (DSM-V), defines PE as "a persistent or recurrent pattern of ejaculation occurring during partnered sexual activity within approximately 1 minute following vaginal penetration and before the individual wishes it" [14]. The disorder must be present in 75% or more of sexual encounters and persistent over at least the last 6 months. To qualify as a dysfunction, the man must experience personal distress related to the dysfunction, and the condition cannot be better explained by a comorbid or concomitant diagnosis. The DSM-V definition permits the categorization of PE into lifelong versus acquired and generalized versus situational subtypes. The *World Health Organization's* International Classification of Diseases 11th edition (ICD-11) defines male early ejaculation as "ejaculation that occurs prior to or within a very short duration of the initiation of vaginal penetration or other relevant sexual stimulation, with no or little perceived control over ejaculation [15]. The pattern of early ejaculation has occurred episodically or persistently over a period of at least several months and is associated with clinically significant distress." This definition has the advantage of being flexible and inclusive but lacks quantitative criteria and is nebulous in terms of the chronicity and frequency of disturbance required for the diagnosis. It mirrors the definition of the DSM-V.

Patients with lifelong PE may suffer from other forms of male sexual dysfunction, such as the timing of erection (early erections), detumescence (inability to maintain erections), and arousal (hypererotic state) cycles [16]. Some studies suggest a possible familial tendency and genetic polymorphisms in those with lifelong PE [17]. In contrast, patients with acquired PE often suffer from other medical (such as urinary, endocrine, and neurological conditions), psychological, and interpersonal causes, resulting in reduced ejaculatory latency [18], and often exhibit other forms of sexual disorders such as erectile dysfunction.

Despite these (minor but) distinct variations in definitions, there is common ground in key criteria in PE, namely the short time to ejaculation [namely the intravaginal ejaculation latency time (IELT)], lack of ejaculatory control, and negative personal consequences, such as distress, bother, frustration, and the avoidance of sexual intimacy. However, this current definition has limitations because the data used to develop it were based on studies of vaginal intercourse, making it specifically applicable to coitus and possibly irrelevant in today's sociocultural climate of gender fluidity.

Pathophysiology of PE

It is important to understand the various neurobiological mechanisms involved in male ejaculation to better characterize the pathophysiology of PE.

The normal male sexual response is often categorized into four main sequential stages [18]. This process begins with sexual excitement, in which penile tumescence and subsequent erection occur after sexual interest and stimulation. This stage is followed by a plateau period, in which ejaculation is delayed and during which sexual intercourse may occur. Ejaculation and orgasm usually occur after this plateau stage, followed by sexual resolution and associated postejaculatory penile detumescence. It is postulated that these four stages are significantly condensed in patients with PE, causing a steep excitement period, followed by reduced latency during the plateau phase and rapid ejaculation [1, 3, 18].

Ejaculation is a highly coordinated spinal reflex involving emission and expulsion. The ejaculatory reflex comprises sensory receptors and areas, afferent pathways, cerebral sensory areas, cerebral motor centers, spinal motor centers, and efferent pathways. Cerebral control of ejaculation is achieved by a complex ejaculatory network—comprising several groups of interconnected neurons found at various levels of the brain, such as the posteromedial part of the bed nucleus of the stria terminalis, the posterodorsal area of the medial amygdala, the parvicellular part of the subparafascicular thalamus, the posterodorsal preoptic nucleus, and the nuclei of the ventral medulla [19]. The ejaculatory process involves these supraspinal centers in various roles, such as sensory/integrative, excitatory, and inhibitory actions. Recent research has identified a group of lumbar spinothalamic neurons in rats that may lead to synchronization in these spinal centers [20]. This group of neurons is known as the spinal generator of ejaculation (SGE).

A normal antegrade ejaculation consists of emission and expulsion with an ensuing orgasm, a process that involves key neurohumoral components and relevant pelvic structures [21, 22]. The pelvic organs that are involved in the emission phase are the ejaculatory apparatus (epididymis, vas deferens, seminal vesicles, and prostate gland), the prostatic urethra, and the bladder neck. These structures are supplied by both sympathetic and parasympathetic nerves derived from the pelvic plexus. The closure of the bladder neck during the emission phase prevents retrograde ejaculation. Emission and closure of the bladder neck are mediated by thoracolumbar sympathetic events, which are mainly alpha-adrenergic in innervation. The rhythmic contraction of the smooth muscle of the bladder neck, pelvic floor, bulbospongiosus, and ischiocavernosus are responsible for the expulsion phase and receive both sympathetic and parasympathetic supply (from the pelvic plexus) as well as somatic nerve supply (by the pudendal nerve and the motor neurons located in the nucleus of Onuf).

Diagnostic Evaluation

The diagnosis of PE can be made on the basis of the patient's sexual and medical history only. The use of a validated questionnaire and a focused physical exam can contribute to the final confirmation [1–4, 12, 18, 23].

ISSM recommends the following questions for elucidating a meaningful clinical diagnosis of PE [1, 9, 12].

Recommended questions for a diagnosis of PE:

1. What is the time between penetration and ejaculation?
2. Can you delay ejaculation?
3. Do you feel bothered, annoyed, and/or frustrated by your premature ejaculation?

Optional questions:

4. Differentiate lifelong and acquired PE: When did you first experience premature ejaculation?
5. Have you experienced premature ejaculation during almost every sexual attempt and with every partner since your first sexual experience?
6. Assess erectile function: Is your erection hard enough to penetrate?
7. Do you have difficulty in maintaining your erection until you ejaculate during intercourse?
8. Do you ever rush intercourse to prevent loss of your erection?

9. Assess relationship impact: How upset is your partner with your premature ejaculation?
10. Does your partner avoid sexual intercourse?
11. Is your premature ejaculation affecting your overall relationship?
12. Previous treatment: Have you received any treatment for your premature ejaculation previously?
13. Impact on quality of life: Do you avoid sexual intercourse because of embarrassment?
14. Do you feel anxious, depressed, or embarrassed because of your premature ejaculation?

With the above set of questions, one can diagnose PE, differentiate between lifelong and acquired PE, rule out ED as a cause of PE, and also assess the impact of PE on interpersonal relationships and QOL.

Intravaginal Ejaculatory Latency Time (IELT)

The IELT serves as a guide for assessing premature ejaculation (PE). The calibrated stopwatch IELT is an objective diagnostic criterion that is easier to use in a trial or study setting. Its use in clinical settings is impractical and not recommended, as it is disruptive and impacts spontaneity [24].

The pitfalls of IELT in practical settings include the overlap in IELT measurements between men with and without premature ejaculation (PE). It is not applicable to non-vaginal intercourse, masturbation, and male-to-male sex [24–26]. MELT, OELT, and AELT have been proposed to assess ejaculatory latency in the case of masturbation, oral sex, and anal sex, respectively, to overcome these shortcomings [27]. Standard population-based values of these parameters are yet to be elucidated and are not in clinical use.

It has been found that self-reported latency times are useful and practical, as they correlate well with the more objective stopwatch IELT [28, 29], although it is possible to self-estimate ejaculatory latency in determining IELT in clinical practice [1, 4].

The role of physical examination is relatively less in lifelong PE, which is more likely to be essentially normal. Despite this, hands-on physical examination can be reassuring for patients with lifelong PE. On the other hand, in acquired PE, a systematic physical examination is important for identifying underlying penile deformities and/or plaques, prostatitis, and picking up clues on risk factors and etiology [9, 10, 12].

Validated Questionnaires (Table 8.1)

Most of the available questionnaires are designed to assess patient-related treatment outcome measures and a few are designed to aid in diagnosing PE. Most guidelines suggest their use for research purposes. Validated questionnaires can be considered an adjunct in the diagnosis of PE [1–4, 12–15].

Specific Investigations and Tests

For the "Diagnosis" of PE and for "evaluation" of lifelong PE, standard guidelines do not recommend any investigations [1, 10, 12]. In the case of acquired PE, investigations can be performed based on clinical suspicion or clinical findings

Table 8.1 Questionaries in the diagnosis and evaluation of PE

Questionnaire	Utility	Validity	Comment/advantages
The Premature Ejaculation Profile (PEP) [30]	Characterizes PE and determines treatment effects	Extensive databases and meet most of the criteria for test development and validation	Assesses outcome Brief, easy to administer Evaluates the subjective and clinically relevant component domains
Index of Premature Ejaculation (IPE) [31]	Characterizes PE and determines treatment effects	Extensive databases and meets most of the criteria for test development and validation	Assesses outcome Brief, easy to administer Evaluates the subjective and clinically relevant component domains
Premature Ejaculation Diagnostic Tool (PEDT) [32]	Screening questionnaire for the diagnosing PE	Validated externally	Cut off scores Brief, easy to administer
Arabic Index of Premature Ejaculation (AIPE) [33]	Diagnose PE	Small sample size	PE severity is classified into five categories based on scores
Chinese Index of Premature Ejaculation questionnaire (CIPE-5) [34]	Diagnose PE	Small sample size	
Male Sexual Health Questionnaire Ejaculatory Dysfunction (MSHQ-EjD) [35]	Characterize ejaculatory dysfunction	Large database	Not specific for PE. Validated on a database composed mostly of "men with LUTS"
Masturbatory Premature Ejaculation Diagnostic Tool (MPEDT) [36]	Diagnose PE based on self-masturbatory ejaculation times	Small sample size, needs further validation	Help evaluate the presence of PE symptoms during self-masturbation/ non-vaginal coitus, or MSM

(concomitant ED, male hypogonadism, diabetes mellitus, prostatitis, urinary tract infection, hypothyroidism etc.).

Societal guidelines state that laboratory tests for assessing hypothalamic-pituitary-testicular axis, glycemic control, thyroid, and local infections and inflammatory conditions, such as prostatitis and pelvic pain syndromes, should be performed as deemed necessary [1, 4, 12].

Penile biothesiometry and penile electrophysiological tests have been used in the past [9, 10, 21, 23]. These tests were researched to objectively assess and quantify thresholds for penile stimulation and neurological conductivity in PE. Due to the complex nature of the tests and the absence of standard protocols, these tests are not in clinical use. Standardization of these tests may lead to the development of an objective test for making a diagnosis of PE [21, 23, 37].

Clinical Management for PE

Non-Surgical Management: Psychosexual Counselling, Behavioral Modifications and Pharmacological Agents

Psychosexual and behavioral modifications have a significant role in achieving good and consistent patient outcomes in men or couples suffering from PE.

They serve to achieve two goals [4, 7, 12]:

1. Help the man learn and develop sexual skills to delay ejaculation.
2. Correcting or reversing the "snowball effects" of PE. This includes loss of self-confidence; performance anxiety; modification of rigid sexual repertoires, and psychological and interpersonal problems that may have caused, maintained or worsened PE for the man and partner.

PE treatment entails utilizing the short-term psychotherapy model with the integration of multiple approaches—namely, behavioral, cognitive, systems, and psychodynamic approaches (Table 8.2).

To achieve effective psychotherapy, the following factors need to be kept in mind [38].

Table 8.2 Different theoretical schools of thought among clinicians treating PE [7]

Behavioral clinicians	Consider that PE arises due to a lack of sensory awareness, inability to understand levels of sexual excitement, and/or previous experiences conditioning their responses
Cognitive therapists	Look for and corrects distortions in thoughts that may contribute to worsening or maintaining PE
Psychodynamic clinicians	Highlight unconscious hostile emotional states towards women
Family/relationship therapists	Looks at the relationship dynamics, including managing emotional and sexual intimacy issues, as well as power and control dynamics

1. To provide the patient with the impression that they are capable of influencing external circumstances and bringing about change.
2. To offer a secure and compassionate space in which the patient can investigate the reasons behind his behavioral and psychological problems; and.
3. To project optimism and reasonable expectations for the future.

Behavioral Techniques

Men with PE are afraid to concentrate on their sexual arousal because they think it will make them ejaculate faster. Behavioral techniques try to correct this. The male partner needs to identify the point when one feels that ejaculation is imminent during intercourse, or in other terms, identify a mid-level range of excitement. They learn to stay in a moderate state of arousal, which delays ejaculation, starting with masturbation and progressing during foreplay and intercourse [4, 12, 39].

Some of the commonly used behavioral techniques are described below

1. *Squeeze technique*

According to the method proposed by Masters and Johnson, the man's partner stimulates the penis until he feels the need to ejaculate. At this point, the glans is squeezed until the sensation passes. This is repeated multiple times before ejaculation is allowed.

Internal squeeze: Reduced ejaculatory urgency may also be achieved without applying external manual pressure by stopping sexual thrusting movements and contracting the pelvic floor muscles for a prolonged period. This technique is often known as "internal squeeze" [40].

2. *Start and stop technique*

Using Semans' "stop-start" approach, a man or his partner stimulates the penis until he feels the urge to ejaculate, then stops until the sensation subsides. This process is repeated several times before permitting ejaculation to take place [41].

3. *Sensate focus technique*

The male and his partner engage in sensate focus, which involves focusing on touch instead of breasts, genitalia, or intercourse. This helps to reduce performance anxiety and promote body awareness. Genital touching is then gradually reintroduced, and finally, full intercourse [42].

4. *Pelvic floor exercises*

Exercises for the rehabilitation of the pelvic floor muscles, such as Kegel exercises, can help with ejaculatory control [43].

5. *Penile root masturbation training*

This technique is based on the hypothesis that regular penis-root masturbation may delay ejaculation, and this might have a therapeutic effect in patients with primary PE [44].

Cognitive Techniques

Cognitive distortions in thinking can ensure that PE persists or even worsens over time. Rosen et al. identified and described some common forms of distortions that require correction [45].

Cognitive distortions
All-or-nothing thinking
Overgeneralization
Disqualifying the positive
Mind reading
Fortune telling
Emotional reasoning
Categorical imperatives
Catastrophizing

Interpersonal Techniques

Therapists work to lessen animosity and withdrawal from one another while assisting couples in regaining their emotional and sexual closeness. The main objectives of relationship therapy for PE are to assist couples in overcoming these challenges, resolving their disputes rationally, and collaborating to discover solutions [9, 12].

Mindfulness Techniques

By practising mindfulness, one develops the capacity to observe emotions, feel their body, and live in the present moment without passing judgment. By reducing some of the established obstacles to sexual functioning (self-judgement; depression, and anxiety), mindfulness has been shown to promote interoceptive awareness, which can improve attention to sexual cues. Unlike sensate focus training, which necessitates a partner, mindfulness training allows patients to train in a group or alone. The intervention has not been tried in an individual setting yet [46].

Pharmacotherapy

A wide range of pharmacotherapeutic agents have been used in various forms for the treatment of PE [40]. Established treatment agents are selective serotonin reuptake inhibitors, tricyclic antidepressants, and topical anaesthetic agents. Alpha-blockers and PDE5i are utilized in concomitant cases of LUTS, prostate enlargement, and ED.

(a) *SSRIs*

The treatment of PE has changed dramatically with the advent of the SSRIs—paroxetine, sertraline, fluoxetine, citalopram—and the tricyclic antidepressant (TCA), clomipramine. SSRIs increase 5-HT neurotransmission and stimulate post-synaptic membrane 5-HT receptors by preventing axonal reuptake of serotonin from the synaptic cleft of central serotonergic neurons by blocking 5-HT transporters [47].

Dapoxetine is an SSRI with a brief half-life of 19 hours. Dapoxetine is licensed for the on-demand treatment of PE in numerous nations. Thirty to sixty milligrams of dapoxetine should be taken 1–3 hours before engaging in sexual activity [48]. Comparably efficacious in both men with LPE and APE, dapoxetine led to 2.5 and 3.0-fold increases in IELT, increased ejaculatory control, decreased distress, and enhanced pleasure [49, 50]. Side effects were rare and dose-dependent, and included headache, dizziness, nausea, and diarrhoea [50, 51]. There was minimal evidence of withdrawal symptoms following an abrupt stop of dapoxetine, and there was no indication of an elevated risk of suicidal ideation or suicide attempts [52]. Dapoxetine is safer as compared to off-label antidepressants used in the management of PE [53]. PDE5Is and dapoxetine together are well tolerated, and the safety profile of the combination is similar to that of earlier phase 3 trials using dapoxetine alone [54]. When compared to dapoxetine or sildenafil alone, an RCT with PE patients without ED showed that a combination of the two could dramatically improve IELT values with tolerable adverse effects [55]. A high discontinuation rate has been noted due to unsatisfactory patient-perceived outcomes and adverse events, which was also the case with other off-label SSRIs being used [56, 57].

(b) *Off label SSRIs*

SSRIs have been used as an off-label treatment of PE since the 1990s [47]. SSRIs that are frequently used include sertraline (50–200 mg), citalopram (20–40 mg), fluoxetine (20–40 mg), fluvoxamine, and paroxetine (10–40 mg). While all of these medications are effective, paroxetine is known to cause the greatest amount of ejaculation delay [58, 59]. According to many meta-analyses, SSRIs may cause a 2.6–13.2-fold rise in the geometric mean IELT [60]. After initiating treatment, ejaculation delay normally happens 5–10 days later. However, it may take 2–3 weeks for the whole therapeutic benefit to take effect, and long-term use is usually required to maintain it [61].

Typically mild adverse effects develop within the first week of treatment and may go away eventually in 2–3 weeks. They consist of drowsiness, sweating, light nausea, diarrhoea, and yawning. There is some evidence to suggest that ED and decreased libido are less common in nondepressed PE men receiving SSRI treatment than in depressed men receiving the same medication [8, 9]. Men with a history of bipolar depression should not receive SSRI medication, as it is known to cause neurocognitive adverse effects [62]. When administering SSRIs to men with PE who also have a concomitant depressive illness, or to adolescents with PE who are 18 years of age or younger, one should be cautious especially if there is a history of suicidal thoughts [63].

Men desiring to conceive should be told that SSRIs may alter the motility of spermatozoa and, therefore, should not begin treatment with an SSRI. If already on an SSRI, it should be discontinued [64]. It has been demonstrated that clomipramine, a mixed serotonin-norepinephrine reuptake inhibitor, is safe and effective when taken off-label either daily or for on-demand use. It increases IELT by four to six times [65].

Clomipramine has been used in doses ranging from 12.5 to 50 mg and the most common side effects include nausea and dizziness [60, 61, 66]. Individual patient needs should be evaluated to decide whether to treat PE with a daily off-label SSRI dose or on-demand dapoxetine treatment. Men in established relationships may prefer the convenience of daily medicine; on the other hand, men with PE who have irregular intercourse might prefer on-demand treatment [60, 61].

(c) *Topical local anaesthetics*

One of the oldest forms of pharmacotherapy, local topical anaesthetics desensitize the glans penis, thereby delaying ejaculation [4, 8, 67]. Three local anesthetics—benzocaine, prilocaine, and lidocaine—have been shown to be effective in treating PE. They come in gel, cream, or spray form. These drugs are applied on the glans penis 5–10 minutes before sexual activity [67]. In comparison to the placebo, the lidocaine-prilocaine mixed anesthetic spray was associated with significant improvements in ejaculation control and satisfaction [68]. A metered-dose aerosol spray containing lidocaine (150 mg/mL) and prilocaine (50 mg/mL) deposits a fixed dose of medication and produces minimal numbing and maximal neural blockage with no absorption through shaft skin [69, 70].

Topical anesthetics can lead to numbness and increased genital irritation in partners and penile hypoesthesia in men. To prevent these side effects, it is important to wipe off the anesthetic agent before intercourse, alternatively, condoms can be considered [68, 69]. In a meta-analysis by Shah et al., four topical agents were reviewed—namely, SS-cream (a mixture of Bufonis veneum extract, Asiasari radix extract, Caryophylli flos extract, Cinnamomi cortex extract, and Ginseng Radix Alba fructose), TEMPE or PSD502 (a combination of 7.5 mg prilocaine eutectic mixture and 22.5 mg lidocaine), EMLA (a cream consisting of 2.5 g prilocaine eutectic and 2.5 g lidocaine), and lidocaine spray 5%. They concluded that topical anesthetics produce a greater improvement in IELT compared to sildenafil, tadalafil, paroxetine, and dapoxetine [71].

(d) *Tramadol*

Due to its dual activation of opioid receptors and inhibition of serotonergic and noradrenergic reuptake, the opiate analgesic tramadol has been thoroughly researched for the treatment of PE. Oral formulations of tramadol—oral disintegrating tablets (62 and 89 mg) and tramadol hydrochloride (25, 50, and 100 mg)—have shown a median improvement of IELT of 2.5 times and >4.5 times, respectively [72, 73]. Tramadol is known to cause constipation, dry mouth, and sedation at doses used for analgesia. It is recommended as a second-line drug in the management of PE owing to its potential to cause addiction and a lack of data on its long-term safety [4, 7, 9]. Furthermore, tramadol should not be combined with SSRIs as it increases the risk of serotonin syndrome, which can be fatal [74].

(e) *Phosphodiesterase type 5 inhibitor (PDE5i)*

PDE5i is indicated in cases of acquired PE due to ED. These medications may help men with PE focus on controlling arousal and lessen their fear of losing an erection by lowering performance anxiety [54, 55, 75]. Several open-label studies have demonstrated the superiority of PDE5I/SSRI combination therapy over SSRI monotherapy [76, 77]. In males with normal erectile function, treating LPE with PDE5is is not advised.

(f) *Other and novel drugs*

- Oxytocin receptor antagonists: Epelsiban and cligosiban were found to be mildly effective in increasing IELT and relatively safe. Further trials will be needed before they can be included in the PE treatment regimen [78, 79]
- Modafinil: Given that d-modafinil tends to increase serotoninergic and decrease dopaminergic activity, it has been investigated for usage as an on-demand medication in the context of LPE. Large-scale trials are necessary to determine its utility in the management of PE [80]
- Caffeine: On-demand caffeine consumption has been shown to improve IELT by an unknown mechanism [81]
- Resiniferatoxin: A capsaicin analogue is known to reduce the sensitivity and excitability of peripheral sensory nerves via secretion of substance P. It is under evaluation for possible use in PE [82]
- Alfa-adrenergic blockers [83, 84]
- Botulinum toxin injections into the bulbospongiosus muscle [85, 86]

Surgical Treatment of PE

Current management strategies for PE include behavioral exercises and psychotherapy, use of topical anesthetic agents, and medication, with surgical interventions not currently widely adopted or endorsed—especially by major international guidelines—due to the lack of convincing evidence, high risk of complications, and unknown long-term clinical efficacy and safety outcomes [3, 4, 87, 88]. Nonetheless, surgical treatments may provide a "definitive" treatment that does not rely on treatment adherence and allows for more sexual spontaneity [88–90].

Biomaterial

A uniquely designed surgery called Inner Condom Technique involves implanting a "condom" made of acellular dermal matrix (ADM), which is used extensively in cosmetic augmentation surgery, under the skin of the penis [91]. The ADM condom works by reducing penile skin sensitivity. A published study showed a statistically significant increase in IELT, from 0.67 to 2.37 min ($p = 0.009$), with patients able to resume sexual activity 6 weeks postoperatively, and there were no reported serious perioperative complication, or adverse psychosexual effects.

Circumcision

Circumcision is perhaps a "safe" surgical option for uncircumcised men who may suffer from glans hypersensitivity that results in PE. The prepuce (foreskin) is highly innervated and serves as erogenous tissue. Systematic reviews and meta-analyses investigating the effects of circumcision on male sexual function found no difference between ejaculation latency time in circumcised and uncircumcised men during intercourse [92, 93], highlighting that male circumcision is not an effective modality in patients with PE.

Focal Therapy

Various focal therapies, such as cryoablation and radiofrequency, have been utilized to target the dorsal penile nerve to reduce hypersensitivity in the penis and responses to sexual input signals. The limited data on these focal therapies have found an improvement in ejaculation latency time although longer-term data showed a gradual decline in clinical efficacy and potentially less rigidity in penile erections [94, 95].

Bulking Agents

The use of bulking agents such as hyaluronic acid (HA) gel in penile glans augmentation has also been reported with some successes, and it is thought that HA under the skin creates a "physical" barrier and blocks signals to the dorsal nerve to prolong ejaculation. Studies on HA injections have reported longer-lasting ejaculation with higher sexual satisfaction [96–99].

Neurotomy and Neuromodulation

The roles of selective dorsal neurotomy and neuromodulation have been described over the years, albeit with reasonable success, by blocking hypersensitive peripheral sexual stimulation signals, inhibiting penile hypersensitivity and central excitability, and increasing ejaculation time and threshold [100–103]. The use of intraoperative neurophysiological monitoring (IONM) for penile sensory-evoked potentials could potentially improve clinical efficacy and lower postoperative complications [104]. However, there is a lack of clear standardization of techniques, potential recurrence of PE, and importantly, the ensuing risk of erectile dysfunction and glans complications—such as numbness or pain—which adversely impact overall sexual satisfaction and orgasm.

Future Directions

PE is a highly prevalent male sexual disorder that is largely an unmet therapeutic need. The current definition(s) of PE should be validated outside of the current heterosexist context and revised to take into consideration the current sociopolitical gender fluidity movement.

While patients with PE are characterized as having short ejaculation latency time, lacking control over ejaculation, and suffering from negative personal consequences, PE is more than just a psychosexual condition given our understanding of the underlying neurobiology and the fact that a single treatment modality is often not effective. As the causes and/or effects of PE are multifactorial, a holistic patient management plan composed of pharmacological management, psychological support, and psychosexual behavioral therapy is likely to produce the best outcomes for patients, and perhaps surgical intervention(s) may have a role in carefully selected patients.

At present, the ideal PE therapy remains elusive, since contemporary nonsurgical treatments do not guarantee complete clinical efficacy and only provide a temporary delay in ejaculation latency time, with PE recurring when the treatment is stopped. Newer generation and novel neurotransmitter blockers and more super-selective SSRIs may provide better pharmacological targets to address PE. Safer surgical interventions and neuromodulation technology may hold promise as a definitive treatment option for PE.

References

1. Serefoglu EC, McMahon CG, Waldinger MD, Althof SE, Shindel A, Adaikan G, et al. An evidence-based unified definition of lifelong and acquired premature ejaculation: report of the second International Society for Sexual Medicine Ad Hoc Committee for the Definition of Premature Ejaculation. J Sex Med. 2014;11:1423–41.
2. Porst H, Montorsi F, Rosen RC, Gaynor, Grupe S, Alexander J. The premature ejaculation prevalence and attitudes (PEPA) survey: prevalence, comorbidities, and professional help-seeking. Eur Urol. 2007;51:816–24.
3. Salonia A, Bettochi C, Boeri L, et al. European Association of Urology guidelines on sexual and reproductive health-2021 update: male sexual dysfunction. Eur Urol. 2021;80(3):333–57.
4. Shindel AW, Althof SE, Carrier S, Chou R, McMahon CG, Mulhall JP, et al. Disorders of ejaculation: an AUA/SMSNA guideline. J Urol. 2022;207(3):504–12.
5. Rosen RC, Althof S. Impact of premature ejaculation: the psychological, quality of life, and sexual relationship consequences. J Sex Med. 2008;5(6):1296–307.
6. Graziottin A, Althof S. What does premature ejaculation mean to the man, the woman, and the couple? J Sex Med. 2011;8(Suppl 4):304–9.
7. Althof S. The psychology of premature ejaculation: therapies and consequences. J Sex Med. 2006;3(Suppl 4):324–31.
8. Rowland DL. Psychological impact of premature ejaculation and barriers to its recognition and treatment. Curr Med Res Opin. 2011;27(8):1509–18.
9. Althof SE, McMahon CG, Rowland DL. Advances and missteps in diagnosing premature ejaculation: analysis and future directions. J Sex Med. 2022;19(1):64–73.
10. Gillman N, Gillman M. Premature ejaculation; aetiology and treatment strategies. Med Sci (Basel). 2019;7(11):E102.
11. Masters WH, Johnson VE. Human sexual inadequacy. London; Boston: Churchill; Little Brown; 1970.
12. Sadovsky R, Waldinger E, Becher E, et al. International Society for Sexual Medicine's guidelines for the diagnosis and treatment of premature ejaculation. J Sex Med. 2010;7:2947–69.
13. Waldinger MD, Schweitzer DH. The use of old and recent DSM definitions of premature ejaculation in observational studies: a contribution to the present debate for a new classification of PE in the DSM-V. J Sex Med. 2005;5:1079–89.
14. American Psychiatric Association, DSM-5 Task Force. Diagnostic and statistical manual of mental disorders: DSM-5. 5th ed. Arlington: American Psychiatric Publishing, Inc.; 2013. https://doi.org/10.1176/appi.books.9780890425596. Last accessed 1 Jan 2025.
15. International Classification of Diseases, Eleventh Revision (ICD-11), World Health Organization (WHO) 2019/2021. https://icd.who.int/browse11. Last accessed 1 Jan 2025.
16. McMahon CG, Jannini EA, Serefoglu EC, Hellstrom WJG. The pathophysiology of acquired premature ejaculation. Transl Androl Urol. 2016;5:434–49.
17. Janssen PK, Schaik RV, Olivier B, Waldinger MD. The 5-HT2C receptor gene Cys23Ser polymorphism influences the intravaginal ejaculation latency time in Dutch Caucasian men with lifelong premature ejaculation. Asian J Androl. 2014;16:607–10.
18. Buvat J. Pathophysiology of premature ejaculation. J Sex Med. 2011;8:316–27.
19. Holstege G, Georgiadis JR, Paans AMJ, et al. Brain activation during human male ejaculation. J Neurosci. 2003;23(27):9185–93.
20. Borgdorff AJ, Bernabé J, Denys P, Alexandre L, Giuliano F. Ejaculation elicited by microstimulation of lumbar spinothalamic neurons. Eur Urol. 2008;54:449–56.
21. Clement P, Giuliano F. Physiology and pharmacology of ejaculation. Basic Clin Pharmacol Toxicol. 2016;119:18–25.
22. Alwaal A, Breyer BN, Lue TF. Normal male sexual function: emphasis on orgasm and ejaculation. Fertil Steril. 2015;104:1051–60.
23. Jannini E, Maggi M, Lenzi A. Evaluation of premature ejaculation. J Sex Med. 2011;8:328–34.

24. Giuliano F, Patrick DL, Porst H, et al. Premature ejaculation: results from a five-country European observational study. Eur Urol. 2008;53(5):1048–57.
25. Shindel AW, Vittinghoff E, Breyer BN. Erectile dysfunction and premature ejaculation in men who have sex with men. J Sex Med. 2012;9(2):576–84.
26. Barbonetti A, D'Andrea S, Cavallo F, Martorella A, Francavilla S, Francavilla F. Erectile dysfunction and premature ejaculation in homosexual and heterosexual men: a systematic review and meta-analysis of comparative studies. J Sex Med. 2019;16(5):624–32.
27. Waldinger MD. Four measures of investigating ejaculatory performance. J Sex Med. 2007;4:520.
28. Pryor JL, Broderick GA, Ho KF, Jamieson C, Gagnon D. Comparison of estimated versus measured intravaginal ejaculatory latency time in men with and without premature ejaculation. J Sex Med. 2005;3:54.
29. Rosen R, McMahon C, Niederberger C, Broderick G, Jamieson C, Gagnon DD. Correlates to the clinical diagnosis of premature ejaculation: results from a large observational study of men and their partners. J Urol. 2007;177:1059–64.
30. Patrick DL, Giuliano F, Ho KF, Gagnon DD, McNulty P, Rothman M. The premature ejaculation profile: validation of self-reported outcome measures for research and practice. BJU Int. 2008;103:358–67.
31. Althof S, Rosen R, Symonds T, Mundayat R, May K, Abraham L. Development and validation of a new questionnaire to assess sexual satisfaction, control and distress associated with premature ejaculation. J Sex Med. 2006;3:465–75.
32. Symonds T, Perelman M, Althof S, Giuliano F, Martin M, May K, Abraham L, Crossland A, Morris M. Development and validation of a premature ejaculation diagnostic tool. Eur Urol. 2007;52:565–73.
33. Arafa M, Shamloul R. Development and validation of the Arabic Index of Premature Ejaculation (AIPE). J Sex Med. 2007;4:1750–6.
34. Yuan Y, Xin ZC, Jiang J, Guo YJ, Liu WJ, Tian L, Zhu JC. Sexual function of premature ejaculation patients assayed with the Chinese Index of Premature Ejaculation. Asian J Androl. 2004;6:121–6.
35. Rosen RC, Catania JA, Althof SE, Pollack LM, O'Leary M, Seftel AD, Coon DW. Development and validation of four-item version of Male Sexual Health Questionnaire to assess ejaculatory dysfunction. Urology. 2007;69(5):805–9.
36. Xi Y, Colonnello E, LimonCin E, Jannini EA, Zhang Y. The masturbatory premature ejaculation diagnostic tool (MPEDT): a novel psychometric tool to evaluate premature ejaculation during masturbation. Andrology. 2022;10(2):333–9.
37. Wei S, Wu C, Yu B, Ma M, Qin F, Yuan J. Advantages and limitations of current premature ejaculation assessment and diagnostic methods: a review. Transl Androl Urol. 2020;9(2):743–57.
38. Donahey KM, Miller SD. What works in sex therapy: a common factors perspective. In: Kleinplatz PJ, editor. New directions in sex therapy: innovations and alternatives. Philadelphia: Bruner Routledge; 2001. p. 210–33.
39. Veettil Raveendran A, Agarwal A. Premature ejaculation – current concepts in the management: a narrative review. Int J Reprod BioMed. 2021;19(1):5–22.
40. Siegel AL. Pelvic floor muscle training in males: practical applications. Urology. 2014;84:1–7.
41. Melnik T, Althof S, Atallah AN, Puga MEDS, Glina S, Riera R. Psychosocial interventions for premature ejaculation. Cochrane Database Syst Rev. 2011;(8):CD008195.
42. Richardson D, Goldmeier D, Green J, Lamba H, Harris JRW. Recommendations for the management of premature ejaculation: BASHH Special Interest Group for Sexual Dysfunction. Int J STD AIDS. 2006;17:1–6.
43. Pastore AL, Palleschi G, Leto A, Pacini L, Iori F, Leonardo C, et al. A prospective randomized study to compare pelvic floor rehabilitation and dapoxetine for treatment of lifelong premature ejaculation. Int J Androl. 2012;35:528–33.

44. Ma GC, Zou ZJ, Lai YF, Zhang X, Zhang Y. Regular penis-root masturbation, a novel behavioral therapy in the treatment of primary premature ejaculation. Asian J Androl. 2019;21(6):631–4.
45. Rosen RC, Leiblum SR, Spector IP. Psychologically based treatment for male erectile disorder: a cognitive interpersonal model. J Sex Marital Ther. 1994;20:67–85.
46. Krieger JF, Kristensen E, Marquardsen M, Ofer S, Mortensen EL, Giraldi A. Mindfulness in sex therapy and intimate relationships: a feasibility and randomized controlled pilot study in a cross-diagnostic group. Sex Med. 2023;11(3):qfad033.
47. Giuliano F, Clement P. Pharmacology for the treatment of premature ejaculation. Pharmacol Rev. 2012;64:621–44.
48. McMahon CG, Jannini E, Waldinger M, et al. Standard operating procedures in the disorders of orgasm and ejaculation. J Sex Med. 2013;10:204–29.
49. Porst H, McMahon C, Althof S, Sharlip I, Bull S, Rivas DA. Baseline characteristics and treatment outcomes for men with acquired or lifelong premature ejaculation with mild or no erectile dysfunction: integrated analysis of two phase III dapoxetine trials. J Sex Med. 2010;7:2231–42.
50. McMahon CG, Althof SE, Kaufman JM, Buvat J, Levine SB, Aquilina JW, Tesfaye F, Rothman M, Rivas DA, Porst H. Efficacy and safety of dapoxetine for the treatment of premature ejaculation: integrated analysis of results from five phase 3 trials. J Sex Med. 2011;8:524–39.
51. Pryor JL, Althof SE, Steidle C, Rosen RC, Hellstrom WJ, Shabsigh R, Miloslavsky M, Kell S. Efficacy and tolerability of dapoxetine in treatment of premature ejaculation: an integrated analysis of two double-blind, randomised controlled trials. Lancet. 2006;368:929–37.
52. Li J, Liu D, Wu J, Fan X, Dong Q. Dapoxetine for the treatment of premature ejaculation: a meta-analysis of randomized controlled trials with trial sequential analysis. Ann Saudi Med. 2018;38(5):366–75.
53. Verze P, Cai T, Magno C, et al. Comparison of treatment emergent adverse events in men with premature ejaculation treated with dapoxetine and alternate oral treatments: results from a large multinational observational trial. J Sex Med. 2016;13(2):194–9.
54. McMahon CG, Giuliano F, Dean J, et al. Efficacy and safety of dapoxetine in men with premature ejaculation and concomitant erectile dysfunction treated with a phosphodiesterase type 5 inhibitor: randomized, placebo-controlled, phase III study. J Sex Med. 2013;10(9):2312–25.
55. Abu El-Hamd M, Abdelhamed A. Comparison of the clinical efficacy and safety of the on-demand use of paroxetine, dapoxetine, sildenafil and combined dapoxetine with sildenafil in treatment of patients with premature ejaculation: a randomised placebo-controlled clinical trial. Andrologia. 2018;50(1):e12829.
56. Park HJ, park NC, Kim TN, Baek SR, Lee KM, Choe S. Discontinuation of dapoxetine treatment in patients with premature ejaculation: a 2-year prospective observational study. Sex Med. 2017;5(2):e99–e105.
57. Jern P, Johansson A, Piha J, Westberg L, Santtila P. Antidepressant treatment of premature ejaculation: discontinuation rates and prevalence of side effects for dapoxetine and paroxetine in a naturalistic setting. Int J Impot Res. 2015;27(2):75–80.
58. Zhang D, Cheng Y, Wu K, Ma Q, Jiang JH, Yan Z. Paroxetine in the treatment of premature ejaculation: a systematic review and meta-analysis. BMC Urol. 2019;19(1):2.
59. Waldinger MD. Emerging drugs for premature ejaculation. Expert Opin Emerg Drugs. 2006;11:99.
60. Sathianathen NJ, Hwang EC, Mian R, et al. Selective serotonin re-uptake inhibitors for premature ejaculation in adult men: a cochrane systematic review. World J Mens Health. 2022;40(2):257–63.
61. McMahon CG. Long term results of treatment of premature ejaculation with selective serotonin re-uptake inhibitors. Int J Impot Res. 2002;14:S19.
62. Marangell L, Dennehy E, Wisniewski S, Bauer MS, Miyahara S, Allen MH, Martinez M, Al Jurdi RK, Thase ME. Case control analyses of the impact of pharmacotherapy on

prospectively observed suicide attempts and completed suicides in bipolar disorder: findings from STEP-BD. J Clin Psychiatry. 2008;69:916–22.
63. Khan A, Khan S, Kolts R, Brown WA. Suicide rates in clinical trials of SSRIs, other antidepressants, and placebo: analysis of FDA reports. Am J Psychiatry. 2003;160:790–2.
64. Tanrikut C, Feldman AS, Altemus M, Paduch DA, Schlegel PN. Adverse effect of paroxetine on sperm. Fertil Steril. 2010;94:1021–6.
65. Waldinger MD, Zwinderman AH, Schweitzer DH, et al. Relevance of methodological design for the interpretation of efficacy of drug treatment of premature ejaculation: a systematic review and meta-analysis. Int J Impot Res. 2004;16:369–81.
66. Choi JB, Kang SH, Lee DH, et al. Efficacy and safety of on demand clomipramine for the treatment of premature ejaculation: a multicenter, randomized, double-blind, phase III clinical trial. J Urol. 2019;201:147–53.
67. Martin-Tuite P, Shindel AW. Management options for premature ejaculation and delayed ejaculation in men. Sex Med Rev. 2020;8(3):473–85.
68. Dinsmore WW, Wyllie MG. PSD502 improves ejaculatory latency, control and sexual satisfaction when applied topically 5 min before intercourse in men with premature ejaculation: results of a phase III, multicentre, double-blind, placebocontrolled study. BJU Int. 2009;103:940–9.
69. Porst H, Burri A. Fortacin spray for the treatment of premature ejaculation. Urologia. 2017;82(2 Suppl):1–10.
70. Henry R, Morales A, Wyllie MG. TEMPE: topical eutectic-like mixture for premature ejaculation. Expert Opin Drug Deliv. 2008;5(2):251–61.
71. Shah MDA, Shah S, Nusrat NB, Zafar N, Rehman AU. Topical anesthetics and premature ejaculation: a systematic review and meta-analysis. Cureus. 2023;15(8):e42913.
72. Lu Y, Zhou Z, Zhang X, Cui Y, Zhang Y, Wang Y. The influence of tramadol on intravaginal ejaculatory latency time and sexual satisfaction score in treating patients with premature ejaculation: a network meta-analysis. Am J Mens Health. 2021;15(5):15579883211057713.
73. Tan H, Zhou Z, Cui Y, Feng F, Zhang Y. A systematic review and meta-analysis of randomized controlled trials of "on-demand" use of tramadol vs "on-demand" use of paroxetine in the management of patients with premature ejaculation. Int J Clin Pract. 2021;75(11):e14825.
74. Takeshita J, Litzinger M. Serotonin syndrome associated with tramadol. Prim Care Companion J Clin Psychiatry. 2009;11:273.
75. Asimakopoulos AD, Miano R, Agrò EF, et al. Does current scientific and clinical evidence support the use of phosphodiesterase type 5 inhibitors for the treatment of premature ejaculation? A systematic review and meta-analysis. J Sex Med. 2012;9:2404–16.
76. Liu H, Zhang M, Huang M, Cai H, Zhang Y, Liu G, et al. Comparative efficacy and safety of drug treatment for premature ejaculation: a systemic review and Bayesian network meta-analysis. Andrologia. 2020;52(11):e13806.
77. Zhang X, Chi N, Sun M, Shan Z, Zhang Y, Cui Y. Phosphodiesterase-5 inhibitors for premature ejaculation: systematic review and meta-analysis of placebo-controlled trials. Am J Mens Health. 2020;14(3):1557988320916406.
78. McMahon C, Althof S, Rosen R, et al. The oxytocin antagonist cligosiban prolongs intravaginal ejaculatory latency and improves patient-reported outcomes in men with lifelong premature ejaculation: results of a randomized, double-blind, placebo-controlled proof-of-concept trial (PEPIX). J Sex Med. 2019;16(8):1178–87.
79. Althof S, Osterloh IH, Muirhead GJ, et al. The oxytocin antagonist cligosiban fails to prolong intravaginal ejaculatory latency in men with lifelong premature ejaculation: results of a randomized, double-blind, placebo controlled phase IIb trial (PEDRIX). J Sex Med. 2019;16(8):1188–98.
80. Tuken M, Kiremit MC, Serefoglu EC. On-demand modafinil improves ejaculation time and patient-reported outcomes in men with lifelong premature ejaculation. Urology. 2016;94:139–42.

81. Saadat S, Ahmadi K, Panahi Y. The effect of on-demand caffeine consumption on treating patients with premature ejaculation: a double-blind randomized clinical trial. Curr Pharm Biotechnol. 2015;16:281–7.
82. Shi B, Li X, Chen J, et al. Resiniferatoxin for treatment of lifelong premature ejaculation: a preliminary study: resiniferatoxin is efficient for PE treatment. Int J Urol. 2014;21:923–6.
83. Bhat GS, Shastry A. Effectiveness of 'on demand' silodosin in the treatment of premature ejaculation in patients dissatisfied with dapoxetine: a randomized control study. Cent Eur J Urol. 2016;69(3):280–4.
84. Fauzan MI, Daryanto B, Budaya TN, Makkaraka MAG, Fakhri M, Rahman IA. Promising selective alpha-1 blocker silodosin as a new therapeutic strategy for premature ejaculation and analysis of its drug adverse effect: a systematic review and meta-analysis of randomized controlled trials. Arch Ital Urol Androl. 2024;96(4):12984.
85. Elshahid AR, Taher AOA, Nouh AH. Evaluation of efficacy and safety of botulinum toxin-A injection at three deferent sites in treatment of premature ejaculation. Urologia. 2024;91(4):824–9.
86. Almekaty K, Ghaith A, Ragab M, Rashed A, Hagras A, Ghoneem A, et al. Effect of bulbospongiosus muscle injection with botulinum-A toxin for treatment of lifelong premature ejaculation: a randomized controlled trial. Int J Impot Res. 2024;36(8):864–8.
87. Gul M, Bocu K, Serefoglu EC. Current and emerging treatment options for premature ejaculation. Nat Rev Urol. 2022;19(11):659–80.
88. Chung E, Gilbert B, Perera M, Roberts MJ. Premature ejaculation: a clinical review for the general physician. Aust Fam Physician. 2015;44(10):737–43.
89. Hu QB, Zhang D, Ma L, Ng DM, Haleem M, Ma Q. Progresses in pharmaceutical and surgical management of premature ejaculation. Chin Med J (Engl). 2019;132(19):2362–72.
90. Deger MD, Gul M, Serefoglu EC. Surgical treatment of premature ejaculation: a narrative review. Int J Impot Res. 2023. https://doi.org/10.1038/s41443-023-00771-9.
91. Wang H, Bai M, Zhang HL, Zeng A. Surgical treatment for primary premature ejaculation with an inner condom technique. Medicine (Baltimore). 2019;98(3):E14109.
92. Tian Y, Liu W, Wang JZ, et al. Effects of circumcision on male sexual functions: a systematic review and meta-analysis. Asian J Androl. 2013;15:662–6.
93. Yang Y, Wang X, Bai Y, et al. Circumcision does not have effect on premature ejaculation: a systematic review and meta-analysis. Andrologia. 2018;50(2):e12851.
94. David PJ, Snyder LL, Cherullo E, Passalacqua M, Pirasteh A, Corn D. Percutaneous CT-guided cryoablation of the dorsal penile nerve for treatment of symptomatic premature ejaculation. J Vasc Interv Radiol. 2013;24:214–9.
95. Basal S, Goktas S, Ergin A, Yildirim I, Atim A, Tahmaz L, et al. A novel treatment modality in patients with premature ejaculation resistant to conventional methods: the neuromodulation of dorsal penile nerves by pulsed radiofrequency. J Androl. 2010;31:126–30.
96. Kwak TI, Jin MH, Kim JJ, Moon DG. Long-term effects of glans penis augmentation using injectable hyaluronic acid gel for premature ejaculation. Int J Impot Res. 2008;20:425–8.
97. Abdallah H, Abdelnasser T, Hosny H, Selim O, Al-Ahwany A, Shamloul R. Treatment of premature ejaculation by glans penis augmentation using hyaluronic acid gel: a pilot study. Andrologia. 2012;44:650–3.
98. Littara A, Palmieri B, Rottigni V, Iannitti T. A clinical study to assess the effectiveness of a hyaluronic acid-based procedure for the treatment of premature ejaculation. Int J Impot Res. 2013;25:117–20.
99. Du GM, Kwak TI, Kim JJ. Glans penis augmentation using hyaluronic acid gel as an injectable filler. World J Mens Health. 2015;33:50–61.
100. Shi WG, Wang XJ, Liang XQ, Liu ZQ, Huang MJ, Li SQ, et al. Selective resection of the branches of the two dorsal penile nerves for primary premature ejaculation. Natl J Androl. 2008;14:436–8.

101. Zhou XJ, Zhang ZG, Hao L, Zhang WD, Dong BZ, Han CH. Elective microscopic resection of dorsal penile nerves for primary premature ejaculation: a clinical observation. Natl J Androl. 2013;19:1003–6.
102. You HS. The partial neurectomy of the dorsal nerve of the penis for patients with premature ejaculation. Korean J Androl. 2000;18:143–8.
103. Liu Q, Li S, Zhang Y, Cheng Y, Fan J, Jiang L, et al. Anatomic basis and clinical effect of selective dorsal neurectomy for patients with lifelong premature ejaculation: a randomized controlled trial. J Sex Med. 2019;16:522–30.
104. Tang QL, Song T, Han YF, et al. The application of intraoperative neurophysiological monitoring in selective dorsal neurotomy for primary premature ejaculation: a prospective single-center study. Asian J Androl. 2023;25:137–42.

Chapter 9
Post-Orgasmic Illness Syndrome: Systematic Review of the Literature

Omer A. Raheem, Marwan Alkassis, and Ayman Rashed

Definition

Post-orgasmic Illness Syndrome (POIS) is a rare, poorly understood condition that is characterized by a cluster of flu-like and allergic symptoms after ejaculation.

Historical Background

Waldinger and Schweitzer first described a post-ejaculatory state of flu-like symptoms and myalgias in 2002. This constellation of symptoms had never been associated with an ejaculatory stimulus. They coined the condition Post orgasmic Illness Syndrome (POIS). Since then, scholars and clinicians have been trying to elucidate the pathophysiology, symptoms, diagnostic criteria, and management. This chapter will summarize the leading consensus on etiology, clinical diagnosis, and management protocols, along with the controversies and debates surrounding POIS.

The original version of the chapter has been revised. A correction to this chapter can be found at https://doi.org/10.1007/978-3-032-12423-4_16

O. A. Raheem (✉)
Department of Urology, Integrated Surgical Institute, Cleveland Clinic, Abu Dhabi, United Arab Emirates
e-mail: raheemo@ccad.ae

M. Alkassis
Department of Urology, University of Illinois Chicago, Chicago, IL, USA

A. Rashed
Urology Department, October 6th University, Cairo, Egypt

R. Shah et al. (eds.), *Diagnosis and Treatment of Male Sexual Dysfunction*,
https://doi.org/10.1007/978-3-032-12423-4_9

POIS Pathophysiology

Various theories have been developed on its etiology to better diagnose and treat POIS. The leading hypothesis is one of immunologic origin. After Waldinger and Schweitzer coined the term POIS, Waldinger et al. [1] further explored the condition and hypothesized that males with POIS have an autoimmune reaction to their own semen. Through this study, they were also able to establish diagnostic criteria. They recruited 45 Dutch Caucasian males suspected to have POIS based on symptoms including allergy and flu-like symptoms. Of this cohort, 33 consented to standardized evaluations and skin-prick tests with their own semen. Results showed that 88% had positive skin-prick tests. However, there was no associated increase in serum IgE levels. From this data, they concluded that the pathophysiology of POIS is rooted in a type 1 and type IV hypersensitivity to semen. Waldinger et al. [2] followed their initial study with a treatment trial of autologous semen injections administered subcutaneously in two men with POIS. They administered these injections every 2 weeks for 1 year and then every 4 weeks for the next 2 years. These injections resulted in 60% and 90% resolution of symptoms at 31 and 15 months respectively, leading them to conclude that hyposensitization is an effective therapy for POIS, further supporting their initial hypothesis. Other authors have also replicated this work; Wrotynska-Barczynska et al. [3] in 2022 performed immunotherapy in a 34-year-old male with success.

A report of a Korean man with POIS receiving intralymphatic immunotherapy (ILIT) showed promising results, as reported by Kim et al. [4] in 2018. They confirmed a positive serum IgE through SDS-PAGE, Western blotting, and ELISA. Fifteen months after ILIT, the patient had complete amelioration of his sneezing and improvement in other POIS-related symptoms except urinary symptoms and sore throat. The authors found that the patient had a decreased serum IgG3 and concluded that POIS likely involves several innate and adaptive immune system mediators, including T-helper cell type 1, 2, and 17 immunity. Depreux et al. [5] published a case report of a 30-year-old male being evaluated for malaise post-ejaculation. The patient had a negative skin prick test and was referred to a neurologist to be evaluated for a neurobiochemical mediator perspective, and and they did not find any neurological alterations that may explain the patient's symptoms.

One paper by Jiang et al. [6] postulated that POIS is a result of a mu-opioid receptor disorder, as some people experience withdrawal symptoms like nausea, vomiting, and anxiety. The Jiang's study concluded that IgE-mediated semen allergy in the reported case may not be the potential mechanism of POIS, as no semen-specific IgE reaction to diluted autologous subcutaneous injection was detected in the serum of the affected patient or three healthy males. A case report by Dexter [7] in 2010 about a 27-year-old man with a benign coital headache suggests that POIS could be caused by a lack of progesterone. During the first trimester of his wife's pregnancy, he experienced a spontaneous resolution of postcoital headaches, which returned after the birth of their child. He was then prescribed oral norethisterone, which treated his headaches going forward. Another study discusses the possibility of POIS being a form of Dhat syndrome, a cultural condition most commonly found in the Indian subcontinent. Dhat syndrome is the belief that loss of semen results in loss of energy and vitality, as reported by Jadhav in 2004 [8].

Angus-Leppan [9] reported two cases of paroxysmal neurologic symptoms during orgasm in a male and female. These two experiences may be considered their own syndromes outside of POIS, but they are helpful to include at this point in time, where very little data on POIS is available. The man experienced dizziness, sometimes accompanied by visual "aura-like" symptoms. He was prescribed diclofenac 50 mg 1 h before sex with good results. The woman experienced "bilateral leg weakness, tremor, oscillopsia, dizziness, and slurred speech." She was prescribed nifedipine 10 mg twice daily, which kept her symptoms at bay at her 3-year follow-up. Bolanos and Morgentaler [10] postulate that POIS could be caused by low testosterone, based on the successful treatment of a man with weakness, low energy, and anxiety post-ejaculation. Another case study by Takeshima et al. [11] supported the testosterone theory; the patient's symptom of fatigue was most improved after testosterone injections one to two times a month. Other published theories include an altered neuroendocrine response and autonomic nervous system dysregulation. Bignami et al. [12] suggest that people with POIS experience a "vegetative storm" after experiencing a surge of sympathetic activity and hormones. Several studies also describe a potential relationship between POIS and premature ejaculation, stating that some patients have these conditions comorbidly. The potential relationship between these conditions is ill-defined, as reported by Waldinger et al., part 1 and 2, in 2011 [1, 2].

There are very few clinical studies on the pathophysiology of POIS. Many medical providers experiment with treatments based on theoretical etiologies. These case reports contribute to the paucity of data and allow scientists to make inferences about the pathophysiology. While the data support the immunogenic etiology best, there are several sexual medicine experts who disagree with this current dogma. As a result, no two providers diagnose or treat POIS the same way. Perhaps it is best to consider POIS as having a multifaceted pathophysiology until more prospective studies are performed.

POIS Symptoms and Diagnostic Criteria

There are fewer than 100 cases of POIS in the literature, making standard symptom presentation difficult. That said, Waldinger et al. [13] created five diagnostic criteria:

1. A person must fall into one or more of the following symptom clusters:
   (a) General
      (i) Including extreme fatigue, exhaustion, palpitations, problems finding words, incoherent speech, dysarthria, concentration difficulties, quick irritation, inability to stand noise, photophobia, depressed mood
   (b) Flu-like
      (i) Including feeling feverish, extreme warmth, perspiration, shivery, ill with flu, feeling sick, feeling cold

   (c) Head
      (i) Including headache, foggy feeling in the head, heavy feeling in the head
   (d) Eyes
      (i) Including burning, red-injected eyes, blurred vision, watery, irritating, itching eyes, painful eyes
   (e) Nose
      (i) Including congested nose, watery, runny nose, sneezing
   (f) Throat
      (i) Including dirty taste in mouth, dry mouth, sore throat, tickling cough, hoarse voice
   (g) Muscle
      (i) Including muscle tension in the back or neck, muscle weakness, pain, heavy legs, and stiffness
2. All symptoms occur immediately (within seconds to minutes), or within a few hours after ejaculation that is initiated by coitus, and/or masturbation, and/or spontaneously (e.g., during sleep)
3. Symptoms occur always or nearly always (>90% of ejaculation events)
4. Most of these symptoms last for about 2–7 days
5. The symptoms disappear spontaneously

The diagnostic workup of a person who may have POIS should be approached from a multifactorial perspective. A review by Abdessater [14] laid out a workup outline which includes:

- Medical history: including allergies (seasonal and medication), sexually transmitted infections, and any history of prostatitis or other conditions that may mimic POIS.
- Neuropsychiatric: conduct an evaluation to assess for possible neurological or psychiatric disorders that may contribute to or mimic POIS symptoms.
- Sexual function: record a detailed sexual function interview, focusing on orgasm and ejaculatory disorders and relationship with their partner(s).
- Physical examination: perform a thorough physical examination, including a digital rectal examination (if indicated) following midstream urine collection for analysis and culture (if indicated).
- Labs (if indicated): including full blood count, serum electrolytes, creatinine, liver function tests, and hormones (follicle-stimulating hormone, luteinizing hormone, testosterone, etc.).
- Imaging (if indicated): consider brain MRI to rule out intracranial lesions or hemorrhages, such as arteriovenous malformation, which could lead to headaches after ejaculation.
- Specialized tests (if indicated): consider specialized tests such as perineal electromyography (EMG), neurovegetative tests, and cystoscopy to rule out uncommon urological conditions.
- Skin-prick test (if indicated): perform a protocolized intracutaneous skin-prick test with extremely diluted semen of the patient to assess for skin reactions. Most appropriate for patients who have atopic symptoms.

Diagnostic coding of POIS has evolved from not being a billable diagnosis in doctors' offices to falling under general male sexual dysfunction. The ICD-10 in 2024 includes:

- ICD-10-CM Diagnosis Code F52.3: Orgasmic disorder
- ICD-10-CM Diagnosis Code F52.31: Female orgasmic disorder
- ICD-10-CM Diagnosis Code F52.32: Male orgasmic disorder

POIS Therapeutic Management

POIS is treated through a multimodal approach. At this time, there is no cure for POIS, so it is approached from a symptom management standpoint. No single treatment has been shown to be effective for everyone with POIS. Based on the available literature, the following treatments have been explored:

Pharmacological Management

- Antihistamines and omalizumab
  - Because the leading hypothesis is immunologic, the most frequent therapy given is an antihistamine. There was one case report of successful use of omalizumab based on the immunogenic theory [15].
- Pain relievers (e.g., NSAIDs, acetaminophen)
  - Common clinical pathways focus more on symptomatic relief. Oftentimes, clinicians offer NSAIDs and acetaminophen for the headaches, myalgias, and muscle weakness seen in POIS patients [16].
- Alpha-1 antagonists (e.g., silodosin)
  - Silodosin was used in a study to produce anejaculation in 14 patients with POIS and was effective in 57% [17].
- Antidepressants and benzodiazepines
  - Researchers have proposed psychological etiologies for POIS and, whether there is one or not, most people experience psychological consequences because POIS significantly impairs quality of life [18].
- hCG
  - Based on the low testosterone theory [10].

Surgical Management

- Bilateral epididymectomy and bilateral vasoligation
  - Resulted in the successful resolution of one male's POIS symptoms. The authors hypothesized that symptoms were caused by repeated contact with sperm or epididymal fluid and circulating T-cells in the seminal tract [16].

Controversies Within POIS

Is It Truly "Immunogenic"?

Arguably, the most controversial component of POIS is the etiology. It is challenging to make generalizations about this condition with the paucity of available data. Many of the available data on POIS are replicated procedures or reviews of Waldinger et al.'s work [1, 2, 13]. The wide variation in symptoms (not confined to allergy and flu-like) opposes the type I and type IV hypersensitivity theory. Additionally, posts on online platforms and recent, currently unpublished survey results reveal that people experience an even wider array of symptoms than imagined or described by Waldinger et al. [1, 2, 13]. These posts also reveal that several different treatments have been tried, including but not limited to garlic, fenugreek, antibiotics, niacin, corticosteroids, caffeine, etc. I present these subjective findings to demonstrate that POIS presentation and treatment effectiveness vary tremendously, which has made it difficult for researchers to conclude that the etiology is limited to allergy and autoimmunity.

Re-Evaluation of Diagnostic Criteria

Due to underdiagnosis and underreporting, POIS diagnostic criteria have not changed since they were initially determined in 2002. Studies have reported new and wide variations in symptoms, numerous treatment options, and different lengths and severity of symptoms. One study observing the practice patterns of providers worldwide showed that medical providers are not following a standardized diagnostic or treatment protocol. They are approaching POIS from a multifactorial perspective, using their best clinical judgment, which is the best they can do given the currently available data. Hence, researchers have advocated for re-evaluating diagnostic criteria to better encompass the spectrum and chronicity of symptoms.

Post-Orgasmic Illness Syndrome in Females

Some experts do not categorize POIS in females as the same condition. In 2016, Waldinger reported the first case of POIS in a female [19]. However, the original report cannot be found online. All of the available data are based on males. However, the current diagnostic criteria are not gender-specific. Using that as the argument, females can have POIS. Differences in presentation between genders have not been thoroughly explored.

Advances and the Future of POIS

The largest limitation to continued research is related to the rarity and low recognizability of POIS. However, POIS research is on the rise. Scientists across the world are collaborating to better understand this condition. From reassessing the diagnostic criteria to collecting further data on varied presentations and possible treatment options, researchers are hopeful about the future of POIS.

Acknowledgments The author of this chapter would like to give special thanks to Dr. Olivia Paulsen and Ifeoma Ikedionwu for their dedicated efforts in the assistance with this chapter.

References

1. Waldinger MD, Meinardi MMHM, Zwinderman AH, Schweitzer DH. Postorgasmic illness syndrome (POIS) in 45 Dutch caucasian males: clinical characteristics and evidence for an immunogenic pathogenesis (part 1). J Sex Med. 2011;8(4):1164–70.
2. Waldinger MD, Meinardi MMHM, Schweitzer DH. Hyposensitization therapy with autologous semen in two Dutch caucasian males: beneficial effects in postorgasmic illness syndrome (POIS; part 2). J Sex Med. 2011;8(4):1171–6.
3. Wrotynska-Barczynska J, Swat E, Berger A, Pawelczyk L, Jedrzejczak P. Intensified hyposensitization is an effective treatment of postorgasmic illness syndrome (POIS). Sex Med. 2022;10(2):100474.
4. Kim TB, Shim YS, Lee SM, Son ES, Shim JW, Lee SP. Intralymphatic immunotherapy with autologous semen in a Korean man with post-orgasmic illness syndrome. Sex Med. 2018;6(2):174–9.
5. Depreux N, Basagaña M, Pascal M. Negative allergy study in a case of postorgasmic illness syndrome (POIS). Rev Int Androl. 2018;16(1):42–4.
6. Jiang N, Xi G, Li H, Yin J. Postorgasmic illness syndrome (POIS) in a Chinese man: no proof for IgE-mediated allergy to semen. J Sex Med. 2015;12(3):840–5.
7. Dexter S. Benign coital headache relieved by partner's pregnancies with implications for future treatment. BMJ Case Rep. 2010;2010:bcr10.2009.2359.
8. Jadhav S. Dhāt syndrome: a re-evaluation. Psychiatry. 2004;3(8):14–6.
9. Angus-Leppan H, Caulfield A. Orgasmic migraine aura: report of two cases. Cephalalgia. 2019;39(1):153–6.
10. Bolanos J, Morgentaler A. Successful treatment of post-orgasmic illness syndrome with human chorionic gonadotropin. Urol Case Rep. 2019;29:101078.
11. Takeshima T, Kuroda S, Yumura Y. Case of post-orgasmic illness syndrome associated with hypogonadism. IJU Case Rep. 2020;3(5):189–91.
12. Bignami B, Honore T, Turmel N, Haddad R, Weglinski L, Le Breton F, Amarenco G. Post-orgasmic illness syndrome. Prog Urol. 2017;27(7):446–8.
13. Waldinger MD, Schweitzer DH. Postorgasmic illness syndrome: two cases. J Sex Marital Ther. 2002;28(3):251–5.
14. Abdessater M, Elias S, Mikhael E, Alhammadi A, Beley S. Post orgasmic illness syndrome: what do we know till now? Basic Clin Androl. 2019;29:13.
15. McLean-Tooke A, Klinken E. Post-orgasmic illness syndrome successfully treated with omalizumab: a case report. J Sex Marital Ther. 2024;50:342–5.
16. Natale C, Gabrielson A, Tue Nguyen HM, Dick B, Hellstrom WJG. Analysis of the symptomatology, disease course, and treatment of postorgasmic illness syndrome in a large sample. J Sex Med. 2020;17(11):2229–35.

17. Nguyen HMT, Bala A, Gabrielson AT, Hellstrom WJG. Post-orgasmic illness syndrome: a review. Sex Med Rev. 2018;6(1):11–5.
18. Reisman Y. Clinical experience with post-orgasmic illness syndrome (POIS) patients-characteristics and possible treatment modality. Int J Impot Res. 2021;33(5):556–62.
19. Waldinger MD. Post orgasmic illness syndrome (POIS). Transl Androl Urol. 2016;5(4):602–6.

Chapter 10
Anhedonia and Orgasmic Dysfunction

Omer A. Raheem

Introduction and Definitions of Anhedonia

Anhedonia is a clinical condition characterized by the diminished ability to experience pleasure or interest in activities that were once enjoyable or fulfilling. It is considered a hallmark symptom of several psychiatric disorders, most notably depression, but can also be observed in other conditions such as schizophrenia, bipolar disorder, and substance use disorder [1]. While anhedonia is typically associated with a loss of pleasure in various life domains, including social interactions, hobbies, and food, one particular area where it manifests prominently is in sexual functioning. This phenomenon is often referred to as orgasmic anhedonia, a condition in which individuals experience a lack of pleasure or satisfaction during orgasm, which can significantly impact quality of life and interpersonal relationships.

The term "anhedonia" is derived from the Greek words "an" meaning "without," and "hēdonē," meaning "pleasure." Originally conceptualized as a symptom of depressive disorders, anhedonia has increasingly been understood as a multifaceted construct with both neurobiological and psychological dimensions [2]. The central aspect of anhedonia, particularly in the context of orgasmic dysfunction, is the inability to derive pleasure from sexual experiences despite the presence of physical arousal and orgasm.

O. A. Raheem (✉)
Department of Urology, Integrated Surgical Institute, Cleveland Clinic,
Abu Dhabi, United Arab Emirates

R. Shah et al. (eds.), *Diagnosis and Treatment of Male Sexual Dysfunction*,
https://doi.org/10.1007/978-3-032-12423-4_10

Historical Perspective of Anhedonia

The concept of anhedonia has its roots in the early clinical observations of depression. The term was first introduced by the French psychiatrist Paul-Émile Léon Viala in 1883 to describe a lack of pleasure in daily activities [3]. Sigmund Freud later contributed to the understanding of anhedonia, recognizing it as a symptom of melancholia, which he described as a loss of interest or pleasure in the world due to an overwhelming sense of guilt or self-reproach [4].

In the twentieth century, the understanding of anhedonia expanded as advances in psychology, psychiatry, and neurobiology provided a more detailed picture of its mechanisms. During the mid-twentieth century, researchers began exploring the physiological underpinnings of anhedonia, especially in relation to the dopaminergic pathways that mediate the brain's reward system [5]. These insights led to the classification of anhedonia as a core symptom of depression in diagnostic manuals, such as the *Diagnostic and Statistical Manual of Mental Disorders (DSM-III)*, which formalized the term's role in psychiatric conditions [1].

The specific intersection of anhedonia and orgasmic dysfunction has been less frequently explored in historical literature, though early psychoanalytic models, particularly those of Freud and others, alluded to sexual dissatisfaction as a possible manifestation of broader psychological distress [4].

Pathophysiology of Anhedonia

The pathophysiology of anhedonia, including orgasmic anhedonia, is complex and involves the interaction of neurobiological, psychological, and environmental factors. At the neurobiological level, anhedonia is thought to be primarily linked to dysfunction in the brain's reward system, particularly the dopaminergic pathways. The mesolimbic dopamine system, which includes structures such as the nucleus accumbens, ventral tegmental area, and prefrontal cortex, plays a crucial role in processing reward signals and the experience of pleasure [2].

In orgasmic anhedonia, there is often a disruption in the way that sexual stimuli are processed in the brain. Specifically, dysfunction in the reward system can result in a failure to experience pleasure despite physical arousal and orgasm. This can occur even when there are no apparent physical causes for sexual dysfunction, highlighting the psychological and neurobiological underpinnings of the disorder [6].

Psychologically, anhedonia is often linked to depressive states, where negative emotions and cognitive distortions such as low self-worth, hopelessness, and emotional numbness prevent the individual from engaging in or enjoying pleasurable activities, including sex [7]. Furthermore, psychological factors such as stress, trauma, and relationship dynamics can exacerbate orgasmic anhedonia by influencing sexual motivation and arousal. In some cases, individuals with anhedonia may experience an emotional disconnect from their sexual experiences, which further contributes to sexual dissatisfaction [8].

From an etiological perspective, anhedonia may be influenced by a variety of factors. Genetic predisposition, neurotransmitter imbalances, hormonal disturbances, and chronic medical conditions such as diabetes or neurological disorders can all contribute to the development of anhedonia In terms of environmental factors, childhood trauma, early life stress, and maladaptive coping mechanisms can also increase the risk of developing anhedonia [8].

Clinical Presentation and Comprehensive Medical Evaluation

The clinical presentation of anhedonia varies depending on the individual and the underlying condition. In the case of orgasmic anhedonia, the primary symptom is a lack of pleasure or satisfaction during orgasm, despite the physical ability to achieve orgasm. The symptoms may occur alongside other sexual dysfunctions, such as erectile dysfunction in men or vaginal dryness in women, which can complicate diagnosis and treatment [9].

Comprehensive medical evaluation is necessary to understand the full scope of the individual's condition. A thorough assessment should include a detailed medical history, psychological evaluation, and physical examination. Clinicians should screen for comorbid conditions such as depression, anxiety, and substance use, as these can contribute to both anhedonia and sexual dysfunction. Laboratory tests may be warranted to rule out endocrine disorders (e.g., hypothyroidism, testosterone deficiency) or other medical conditions that may contribute to sexual dysfunction.

In addition to medical evaluations, psychological assessments are crucial for identifying potential underlying psychological factors, such as trauma, relationship issues, or maladaptive coping strategies, that may be influencing the individual's experience of orgasmic anhedonia.

Physical and Psychological Consequences

The physical and psychological consequences of anhedonia, particularly orgasmic anhedonia, can be profound. Physically, individuals with orgasmic anhedonia may experience a diminished desire to engage in sexual activity, which can lead to a decrease in overall sexual functioning and intimacy. The inability to experience sexual pleasure can also contribute to frustration, anxiety, and reduced self-esteem, which may further perpetuate the cycle of sexual dysfunction.

Psychologically, anhedonia is often associated with feelings of isolation, sadness, and hopelessness. Individuals may withdraw from social and sexual interactions, leading to a sense of disconnection from partners and a reduction in overall life satisfaction. In some cases, sexual dysfunction can exacerbate feelings of depression and anxiety, creating a vicious cycle that is difficult to break without intervention [7].

In addition to the personal emotional consequences, orgasmic anhedonia can have a significant impact on interpersonal relationships. Partners of individuals with orgasmic anhedonia may experience frustration, confusion, and feelings of rejection, which can strain relationships and contribute to further psychological distress.

Treatment Considerations: Pharmacological and Therapeutic Interventions

The treatment of orgasmic anhedonia typically involves a combination of pharmacological and psychotherapeutic interventions. The first line of treatment often includes addressing any underlying psychiatric conditions, particularly depression, which is frequently associated with anhedonia. Antidepressant medications, particularly selective serotonin reuptake inhibitors (SSRIs), may be prescribed to alleviate depressive symptoms and restore the individual's ability to experience pleasure [10]. However, it is important to note that SSRIs themselves can sometimes contribute to sexual dysfunction, including orgasmic anhedonia, and alternative medications or dose adjustments may be necessary [11].

Dopamine agonists, such as pramipexole or bupropion, may also be used to enhance dopamine activity in the brain's reward system and improve the experience of pleasure. These medications have shown some promise in treating anhedonia and sexual dysfunction [12]. However, their use should be carefully monitored due to potential side effects.

Therapeutically, cognitive-behavioral therapy (CBT) is often employed to address the psychological factors contributing to anhedonia and sexual dysfunction. CBT can help individuals identify and challenge negative thought patterns, reduce anxiety, and develop healthier coping strategies for managing sexual difficulties [7]. In cases where trauma or relationship issues are present, specialized therapies such as trauma-focused CBT or sex therapy may be beneficial.

For individuals who experience orgasmic anhedonia as a result of trauma or relational issues, couples therapy and sexual counseling can help address communication problems and foster emotional intimacy. Mindfulness-based interventions, which focus on present-moment awareness and acceptance, have also been found to be effective in improving sexual satisfaction and overall well-being [13].

Conclusion

Orgasmic anhedonia, as a subset of the broader condition of anhedonia, presents a complex and multifaceted challenge in both clinical diagnosis and treatment. The interplay of neurobiological, psychological, and environmental factors creates a dynamic that requires a personalized approach to care. Addressing the underlying causes of anhedonia, whether through pharmacological or therapeutic means, is essential in helping individuals regain the ability to experience pleasure, not only in sexual contexts but in other areas of life. Given the profound impact of orgasmic anhedonia on mental health and relationships, comprehensive treatment strategies that incorporate both medical and psychological interventions are crucial for improving outcomes.

References

1. American Psychiatric Association. Diagnostic and statistical manual of mental disorders. 3rd ed. American Psychiatric Association; 1980.
2. Nestler EJ, Gould E, Manji H, Buncan M, Duman RS, Greshenfeld HK, Hen R, Koester S, Lederhendler I, Meaney M, Robbins T, Winsky L, Zalcman S. Neurobiology of depression. Neuron. 2002;34(1):13–25.
3. Viala P. Sur l'anhedonie [On Anhedonia]. Arch Psychol. 1883;4:251–67.
4. Freud S. Three essays on the theory of sexuality. Basic Books; 1905.
5. Wise RA. Dopamine, learning and motivation. Nat Rev Neurosci. 2004;5(6):483–94.
6. Pfaus JG. Neurobiology of sexual behavior and pleasure. J Sex Med. 2009;6(6):1533–53.
7. Hofmann SG, Sawyer AT, Fang A, Asnaani A. Cognitive behavioral therapy for depression and anhedonia. J Affect Disord. 2013;151(2):1–8.
8. Bress JN, Foti D, Kotov R, Klein DN, Hajcak G. Reward sensitivity and the electroencephalographic feedback negativity in adolescence: a prospective prediction of depression. J Abnorm Psychol. 2013;122(1):133–42.
9. Bancroft J. Human sexuality and its problems. 3rd ed. Churchill Livingstone/Elsevier; 2009.
10. Baldwin DS, Foong T, Croft HA. Antidepressants and sexual dysfunction: mechanisms and management. Psychopharmacology. 2014;231(16):3137–52.
11. Montejo AL, Llorca G, Izquierdo JA, Rico-Villademoros F. Sexual dysfunction in patients with depression treated with SSRIs: a prospective, multicenter, and descriptive clinical study of 1022 patients. J Clin Psychiatry. 2001;62(4):252–7.
12. Fitzgerald PB, Laird AR, Maller J, Daskalakis ZJ. Dopamine agonists in the treatment of anhedonia. J Clin Psychiatry. 2012;73(12):1678–83.
13. Dunne S, Dawson DL, Armstrong AR. Mindfulness, sexual difficulties, and sexual satisfaction. J Sex Med. 2012;9(7):1869–78.

Chapter 11
Epidemiology, Pathophysiology, and Diagnostic Approach of Priapism

Christopher Chee Kong Ho, Chu Ann Chai, and Ahmed El-Sakka

Epidemiology

Definition, Incidence, and Prevalence

Priapism is a urological emergency defined as a persistent and prolonged painful erection without sexual stimulation. It has varying incidence rates across different populations. In the United States, the incidence of priapism is estimated to range between 0.73 and 5.4 cases per 100,000 men per year [1]. This wide range is based on data from emergency departments across the country, highlighting that while priapism is relatively uncommon, it does represent a significant clinical concern, particularly in acute settings.

In Finland, the incidence of priapism is slightly lower, with reports ranging from 0.3 to 1.1 cases per 100,000 person-years. This study also observed a seasonal variation in priapism cases, with a higher occurrence noted during the warmer months [2]. Interestingly, the frequency of priapism is observed 30% more frequently during the summer months [3]. The reason behind this seasonal distribution remains unclear but may be related to factors such as increased recreational drug use or dehydration during the summer.

A study conducted in the Netherlands focused on the age-specific incidence of priapism, particularly in men aged 40 years and older. The findings indicated an

C. C. K. Ho (✉)
Department of Surgery, Taylor's University, Kuala Lumpur, Malaysia

C. A. Chai
Division of Urology, Department of Surgery, Faculty of Medicine, University of Malaya, Kuala Lumpur, Malaysia

A. El-Sakka
Faculty of Medicine, Suez Canal University, Ismailia, Egypt

R. Shah et al. (eds.), *Diagnosis and Treatment of Male Sexual Dysfunction*,
https://doi.org/10.1007/978-3-032-12423-4_11

incidence rate of 2.9 per 100,000 person-years in this age group [4]. This suggests that while priapism can occur at any age, there may be an increased susceptibility in older men, possibly due to underlying vascular or hematologic conditions.

Intracavernous injection therapy for erectile dysfunction (ED) is a known risk factor for priapism, with incidence rates ranging from 1.3% to 5.3% among patients receiving this treatment. Other studies have reported that there were no significant differences in the presence of priapism between office and self-injection programs [5, 6]. The explanation for a higher rate of priapism and penile fibrosis in self-injection programs could be attributed to increased duration of treatment, a higher number of injections per month and total number of injections, and a higher amount of vasoactive agent per month and total amount of this agent [4, 6]. Younger men and those with neurogenic or psychogenic erectile dysfunction are particularly at risk, as their underlying conditions may predispose them to the development of priapism following injection therapy [7].

Approximately 13% of patients presenting with priapism to emergency departments are admitted for further surgical intervention, underscoring the potential severity of this condition. While rare, cases of clitoral priapism have also been reported among female patients, highlighting the condition's potential to affect individuals beyond the male population [3].

Priapism is relatively rare in the pediatric population, with sickle cell disease (SCD) being the most common underlying cause. A comprehensive international multicenter survey conducted by Adeyoju et al. involved 130 patients with SCD, ranging in age from 4 to 66 years, with an average age of 25 years. The study found that 35% of these patients had experienced episodes of prolonged penile erection, with 72% of cases being recurrent or stuttering in nature. The average age at which the first episode occurred was 15 years [8].

Etiology: Risk Factors and Causes

The cause of priapism can be either primary, secondary, or idiopathic (Table 11.1).

Pathophysiology

Physiology of Normal Erection

Penile erection involves mainly four components—the central nervous system (CNS), the peripheral nervous system, the penile arteries, and the cavernosal trabecular smooth muscle [9]. For a normal erection to occur, the nervous and vascular systems need to work synergistically. Parasympathetic stimulation causes relaxation of trabecular smooth muscle, resulting in an increased compliance of the

Table 11.1 Various etiological factors that may cause priapism

Pharmacological agents	Neurological causes	Hematological conditions	Infective, toxic, and allergic	Neoplastic diseases	Traumatic and surgical
Prostaglandin	Multiple sclerosis	Sickle cell disease	Prostatitis	Lymphoma	Penile trauma
Papaverine	Herniated disc	Leukemia	Urethritis	Penile cancer	Spinal cord injury
Theophylline	Spinal tumor	Polycythemia	Syphilis	Prostate cancer	Perineal trauma
Cannabis	Spinal anesthesia	Coagulopathies	Mumps	Paraneoplastic	Pelvic trauma
Verapamil	Spinal tumor with compression				
Nitroglycerin	Ruptured cerebral aneurysm				
Haloperidol					

cavernosal sinusoids, and the arterial walls relax, causing a dilatation of the arterioles and arteries. This smooth muscle dilatation results in arterial engorgement. Expanding sinusoids are filled passively with blood, resulting in compression of the subtunical venous plexuses between the tunica albuginea and the peripheral sinusoids. This relaxation also affects the veins in the trabecular network, thereby reducing venous outflow [9]. Smooth muscle relaxation during erection depends on Ca^{2+} efflux. This relaxation of smooth muscle cells is mediated mainly by nitric oxide, which activates the enzyme guanylate cyclase, which in turn increases formation of the second messenger, cGMP. Elevated levels of peripheral cGMP result in the efflux of Ca^{2+} ions from the cavernosa smooth muscle cells. This phenomenon induces muscle relaxation, facilitates blood flow into the corpora cavernosa, and thereby helps to obtain and maintain penile erection [10]. Under physiological conditions, the process of penile detumescence, mediated by efferent sympathetic pathways, follows the tumescence phase. Adrenergic sympathetic nerves release norepinephrine, which acts on adrenoceptors in penile smooth muscle. These results in reduced arterial inflow, diminished lacunar space volume, and accelerated corporeal venous outflow. The flaccid state of the penis is maintained by contraction of penile smooth muscle cells mediated by the intracellular accumulation of Ca^{2+} ions, which is mainly affected by noradrenergic stimulation of a1-adrenergic receptors [10].

Low Flow (Ischemic) Priapism

The pathogenesis of ischemic conditions in the penile tissue is primarily due to the obstruction of venous outflow, which leads to increased intracorporal pressure, resulting in a compartment syndrome situation with minimal arterial inflow, tissue ischemia, hypoxia, and cavernosal acidosis, ultimately resulting in cellular damage [11]. Histological studies reveal that the extent of tissue damage is time-dependent. In the initial 12 hours, interstitial edema and tissue thickening are predominant, whereas after 24 hours, muscle necrosis and fibroblast proliferation become evident [12]. These processes contribute to endothelial damage and fibrosis of the corpus cavernosum, culminating in impaired erectile function. The vascular endothelium, which plays a crucial role in regulating smooth muscle tone and penile erection through nitric oxide (NO) production, is also affected [13]. Disruptions in NO pathways can alter smooth muscle contraction, as evidenced by animal studies showing exaggerated erectile responses and altered RhoA/Rho kinase activity in genetically modified mice [14].

High-Flow (Non-Ischemic) Priapism

High-flow priapism is a rare urological condition characterized by unregulated, continuous arterial inflow into the lacunar spaces of the penis, typically due to the formation of an arterial-lacunar fistula. This abnormality most often occurs following blunt or penetrating trauma that lacerates the cavernosal artery [15], leading to increased arterial flow that bypasses the helicine arteries. Unlike low-flow priapism, where the veno-occlusive mechanism is activated to trap blood within the penis, high-flow priapism does not activate this mechanism, which results in the condition being less painful and not ischemic [16].

The onset of high-flow priapism can be delayed, occurring up to 72 hours after the initial trauma. The penis in these cases is not fully rigid, and pulsations might be visible. This form of priapism is not associated with the risk of ischemia or subsequent fibrosis due to the arterial nature of the blood trapped in the penis. Goldstein's group in Boston described the underlying mechanism as an arterial-lacunar fistula where the blood bypasses the helicine arteries, leading directly into the lacunar spaces [17]. The increased flow within these spaces generates shear stress, which results in the release of nitric oxide, activation of the cGMP pathway, and subsequent smooth muscle relaxation and dilation of the trabeculae [18].

The pathophysiology of high-flow priapism includes a potential delay in the onset due to incomplete necrosis of the arterial wall post-trauma or the presence of clot formation at the injury site. Over time, the clot undergoes lysis, leading to the manifestation of high-flow priapism. Additionally, rare cases like Fabry's disease can present with high-flow priapism due to unregulated high arterial inflow [19]. Unlike ischemic priapism, which is an emergency due to the risk of tissue damage, high-flow priapism does not pose an immediate threat to penile tissue integrity, making it a less severe but still significant urological condition. Non-ischemic priapism can also occur idiopathically, particularly in the presence of congenital arterial malformations [20].

Stuttering/Recurrent/Intermittent Priapism

Stuttering or recurrent priapism, also known as intermittent priapism, is a condition characterized by repeated, prolonged, and often painful erections that occur without sexual arousal. This form of priapism is most commonly associated with hyperviscosity syndromes, particularly sickle cell disease (SCD), which remains the leading cause of priapism in children. In boys with SCD, the incidence of priapism is notably high, ranging from 18% to 27%. This condition is not exclusive to sickle cell disease and can also be seen in other hemoglobinopathies, though it is relatively rare outside of these contexts [21].

The pathophysiology of stuttering priapism involves repeated episodes of penile erection due to the abnormal aggregation of sickled red blood cells within the penile vasculature. These cells obstruct the normal outflow of blood, leading to a state of hyperviscosity and subsequent ischemia. The condition often manifests during sleep, with erections persisting upon waking. These episodes are usually not painful initially but can become increasingly uncomfortable and painful if the erection is prolonged, often taking about an hour for pain to set in [22].

Recurrent episodes of priapism can have severe consequences for penile health. The repeated ischemic events can lead to fibrosis in the corpora cavernosa. This fibrosis significantly increases the risk of ED later in life due to the structural damage and loss of normal penile tissue elasticity [22].

Beyond sickle cell disease, other hematologic disorders such as unstable hemoglobin variants (e.g., Hb Olmsted), thrombophilias, erythropoietin therapy, leukemia, and myeloma have also been linked to stuttering priapism. These conditions similarly contribute to abnormal blood flow dynamics, increasing the risk of recurrent priapism [23]. Despite its significant impact on quality of life and potential for long-term complications, the underlying mechanisms of stuttering priapism remain poorly understood, and it is often challenging to manage effectively. Treatment typically involves addressing the underlying hematologic disorder and using strategies to prevent or manage acute episodes to minimize long-term damage to the penile tissue.

The dysregulation of phosphodiesterase type 5 (PDE5) also plays a crucial role in the pathophysiology of non-hematological (idiopathic) stuttering priapism. Recurrent ischemic episodes lead to the downregulation of endothelial nitric oxide (NO) and PDE5 activity, resulting in reduced basal levels of NO and cyclic guanosine monophosphate (cGMP), which compromises PDE5 function [24]. This creates a lower threshold for smooth muscle relaxation in the penile tissue. During episodes of sexual stimulation, the surge of NO and cGMP overwhelms the diminished PDE5 activity, causing excessive and prolonged tissue relaxation, manifesting as priapism [25]. Champion et al. demonstrated this mechanism in studies using endothelial nitric oxide synthase knockout mice, where reduced PDE5 expression was associated with priapism, and restoring PDE5 expression corrected the condition [13]. PDE5 inhibitors like sildenafil help manage this effect by increasing basal cGMP levels and progressively reestablishing PDE5 expression and activity [26]. Long-term use of these inhibitors has been shown to alleviate recurrent episodes of priapism without negatively affecting normal erectile function [27].

Diagnostic Approach

History

The diagnostic approach to priapism relies heavily on a thorough and focused history-taking, as this can provide critical insights into the underlying cause and guide effective management. The history should encompass both sexual and medical aspects, with particular attention to medications, trauma, and predisposing comorbidities [28].

One of the key distinctions in priapism diagnosis is between low-flow (veno-occlusive) and high-flow (arterial) priapism, which can often be inferred based on the presence or absence of pain and the duration. Low-flow priapism is typically painful and associated with significant patient discomfort and anxiety, leading to prompt medical attention. In contrast, high-flow priapism is usually painless, resulting in less immediate concern from the patient, who may not seek treatment until days or even weeks after the initial injury.

The history of the priapic episode itself is crucial in determining the most appropriate treatment strategy. Key elements to explore include the following:

1. *Baseline Erectile Function*: Understanding the patient's normal erectile function can help differentiate between priapism and other potential causes of prolonged erections.
2. *Duration of Erection*: The length of time the erection has persisted is important, as prolonged episodes, especially beyond 4 hours, can lead to irreversible tissue damage.
3. *Degree of Pain*: The presence and intensity of pain can help distinguish between low-flow and high-flow priapism.
4. *Previous History of Priapism*: Any prior episodes and their management can offer insights into the recurrence risk and guide future treatment approaches.
5. *Drug Use*: Identifying any drugs or medications that might have triggered the priapism is essential. Certain medications, particularly those used to treat ED, as well as recreational drugs, are known to induce priapism (Table 11.2).

Table 11.2 Drugs/medication associated with priapism

Class	Drug/medication
Vasoactive erectile agents	Alprostadil, papaverine, prostaglandin E1
Oral phosphodiesterase type 5 inhibitors	Sildenafil, tadalafil, avanafil, and vardenafil
Hormonal agents	Testosterone, gonadotropin-releasing hormone
Antidepressants/antipsychotics	Chlorpromazine, clozapine, olanzapine, phenothiazines, risperidone
Attention deficit hyperactivity disorder	Atomoxetine
Alpha-adrenergic blockers	Silodosin, tamsulosin, and doxazosin
Antihypertensives	Propranolol, hydralazine, guanethidine
Anticoagulants	Warfarin, heparin
Recreational drugs	Marijuana, cocaine

6. *History of Trauma*: A history of pelvic, genital, or perineal trauma, especially a perineal straddle injury, should be noted, as these are common causes of high-flow priapism.
7. *Hematologic History*: Personal or family history of sickle cell disease or other hematologic abnormalities should be assessed, as these conditions are strongly associated with recurrent or stuttering priapism [29].
8. *Malignancy History*: A history of malignancies, particularly those affecting the genitourinary system, can also be a contributing factor.

Physical Examination

A careful and comprehensive physical examination that focuses on the genitalia, perineum, and abdomen is essential to identify the type and underlying cause of the condition.

Genital Examination

- *Corpora Cavernosa*: In cases of ischemic priapism, the corpora cavernosa will be fully rigid and tender due to prolonged blood entrapment. This rigidity and pain are hallmark features of ischemic priapism, indicating reduced blood flow and potential tissue ischemia. Conversely, in non-ischemic priapism, the corpora cavernosa exhibit only partial tumescence and are typically not painful. This difference helps distinguish between the two types of priapism and informs the urgency of treatment.

Perineal and Abdominal Examination

- *Perineum and pelvis*: The perineal and pelvic examination should assess for any signs of trauma, which is commonly associated with non-ischemic priapism, especially if there is a history of blunt injury to the area. Straddle injuries or perineal trauma may suggest arterial-cavernosal fistulas leading to high-flow priapism.

- *Abdomen*: The abdominal examination should focus on identifying any masses or signs of malignancy, particularly in cases where priapism may be secondary to pelvic or genitourinary cancers. These malignancies can lead to obstruction or compression of venous drainage, contributing to the development of priapism [30].

Laboratory Investigation

Blood Gas Analysis

Blood gas analysis of aspirated blood from the corpora cavernosa is crucial to differentiate between ischemic and non-ischemic priapism. In ischemic priapism, the blood is dark, hypoxic, and acidic, reflecting poor oxygenation and stasis. This condition is in contrast to non-ischemic priapism, where the blood remains well-oxygenated and bright red and has blood gas values similar to arterial blood, reflecting a non-ischemic state (Table 11.3). Blood gas analysis is a reliable way to diagnose ischemic priapism and guides the urgency of treatment.

Platelet Count and Coagulation Profile

Evaluating the coagulation status is important, as priapism can be linked to clotting disorders. Thrombophilias, or hypercoagulable states, may be associated with priapism, particularly in patients with a history of leukemia or myeloproliferative disorders.

Table 11.3 Key findings in different types of priapism

Key features	Ischemic	Non-ischaemic	Stuttering
Clinical features	Painful Rigid corpora	Painless Not fully rigid	It can be painful/painless Multiple recurrent episode
Laboratory (corporal blood gas)	Dark color pH < 7.25 PCO2 > 60 mmHg PO2 < 30 mmHg	Bright red pH > 7.25 PCO2 < 60 mmHg PO2 > 90 mmHg	Dark color pH < 7.25 PCO2 > 60 mmHg PO2 < 30 mmHg
Imaging	Reduced/absent Cavernous artery blood flow High-resistance flow of cavernous artery	Peak systolic velocity > 50 cm/s End diastolic velocity:0	Low peripheral resistance waveform Elevated variable cavernosal artery velocity

1. *Hemoglobin Electrophoresis*: This test is particularly useful when there is suspicion of hemoglobinopathies, such as sickle cell disease or other unstable hemoglobin variants, which are common causes of recurrent priapism [31].
2. *Toxicology Screening*: In cases where drug-induced priapism is suspected, urine toxicology screening can be beneficial to identify potential precipitating substances, particularly recreational drugs or medications used for erectile dysfunction.
3. *Genomic Testing*: Although not routinely recommended, genome-wide association studies have identified certain genetic polymorphisms, such as those in *LINC02537* and *NAALADL2*, that are associated with priapism in some populations [29].

Imaging Studies

In the acute setting, imaging is usually secondary to clinical assessment and blood gas analysis. However, in complex cases, imaging can be invaluable in guiding treatment. In prolonged or refractory ischemic priapism, MRI and PDUS provide insights into corporal viability and potential vascular anomalies, guiding both prognosis and intervention strategies.

Penile Color Doppler Ultrasound

Penile Doppler ultrasound (PDUS) is recommended after clinical diagnosis as an adjunct to cavernosal blood gas analysis. It can assist in differentiating between ischemic and non-ischemic priapism by assessing blood flow in the penile arteries [32].

- *Ischemic Priapism*: PDUS will show an absence or marked reduction of blood flow in the cavernosal arteries. This is indicative of low-flow priapism, where the blood is trapped within the corpora cavernosa and cannot exit. In successful interventions, the return of cavernosal artery flow can be detected by, indicating detumescence.
- *Non-Ischemic Priapism*: In high-flow priapism, PDUS shows increased systolic velocities (>50 cm/sec). It can also identify anatomical abnormalities, such as a cavernous artery fistula or pseudoaneurysm, typically found in the perineal portion of the corpora cavernosa after trauma [33]. The presence of a fistula, often resulting from trauma, may appear as a blush on the ultrasound, with a sensitivity of 100% and specificity of 73%.

Timing is crucial when performing PDUS. If done after corporal blood aspiration in ischemic priapism, reactive hyperemia may result in misleading findings that mimic non-ischemic priapism; hence, the recommendation is to perform the PDUS prior to aspiration [34].

Penile MRI

Magnetic resonance imaging (MRI) of the penis, particularly with T2-weighted gadolinium enhancement, is another valuable tool in the evaluation of ischemic priapism, especially in cases with delayed presentation (>48 hours) or refractory priapism. MRI can assess the viability of smooth muscle within the corpora cavernosa, which is critical for predicting future erectile function [34].

- *Smooth Muscle Viability*: In ischemic priapism, prolonged ischemia can lead to irreversible damage to the corpora cavernosa, resulting in erectile dysfunction. MRI has shown 100% sensitivity in detecting non-viable smooth muscle, a predictor of long-term erectile dysfunction. Patients with viable smooth muscle on MRI have a greater likelihood of maintaining erectile function after treatment [34].

Conclusion

Priapism represents a significant urological emergency with distinct pathophysiological mechanisms and clinical presentations, requiring timely diagnosis and intervention to prevent long-term complications, particularly ED. The condition's epidemiology varies widely across populations, with notable differences in incidence and etiology, with high prevalence among patients with sickle cell disease. The pathophysiology is complex, involving venous outflow obstruction, hypoxia, and acidosis in ischemic cases, and unregulated arterial inflow in non-ischemic cases. Diagnostic approaches must be thorough, integrating detailed patient history, physical examination, laboratory investigations, and advanced imaging techniques like color Doppler ultrasound and MRI. Understanding the underlying mechanisms and tailored therapeutic strategies is crucial in managing priapism effectively. Future research should focus on refining treatment algorithms to address the time-dependent nature of tissue damage and explore novel interventions that could mitigate long-term sequelae, enhancing patient outcomes in both acute and recurrent cases.

References

1. Roghmann F, Becker A, Sammon JD, Ouerghi M, Sun M, Sukumar S, Djahangirian O, Zorn KC, Ghani KR, Gandaglia G, et al. Incidence of priapism in emergency departments in the United States. J Urol. 2013;190(4):1275–80.
2. Kulmala RV, Lehtonen TA, Tammela TL. Priapism, its incidence and seasonal distribution in Finland. Scand J Urol Nephrol. 1995;29(1):93–6.
3. Medina CA. Clitoral priapism: a rare condition presenting as a cause of vulvar pain. Obstet Gynecol. 2002;100(5 Pt 2):1089–91.

4. Eland IA, van der Lei J, Stricker BH, Sturkenboom MJ. Incidence of priapism in the general population. Urology. 2001;57(5):970–2.
5. El-Sakka AI. Intracavernosal prostaglandin E1 self vs office injection therapy in patients with erectile dysfunction. Int J Impot Res. 2006;18(2):180–5.
6. El-Sakka AI. What is the current role of intracavernosal injection in management of erectile dysfunction? Int J Impot Res. 2016;28(3):88–95.
7. Linet OI, Neff LL. Intracavernous prostaglandin E1 in erectile dysfunction. Clin Investig. 1994;72(2):139–49.
8. Adeyoju AB, Olujohungbe AB, Morris J, Yardumian A, Bareford D, Akenova A, Akinyanju O, Cinkotai K, O'Reilly PH. Priapism in sickle-cell disease; incidence, risk factors and complications – an international multicentre study. BJU Int. 2002;90(9):898–902.
9. Dean RC, Lue TF. Physiology of penile erection and pathophysiology of erectile dysfunction. Urol Clin North Am. 2005;32(4):379–95. v
10. Morelli A, Filippi S, Vignozzi L, Mancina R, Maggi M. Physiology of erectile function: an update on intracellular molecular processes. EAU-EBU Update Ser. 2006;4(3):96–108.
11. Saenz de Tejada I, Kim NN, Daley JT, Royai R, Hypolite J, Broderick GA, Garcia-Diaz F, Levin R. Acidosis impairs rabbit trabecular smooth muscle contractility. J Urol. 1997;157(2):722–6.
12. Spycher MA, Hauri D. The ultrastructure of the erectile tissue in priapism. J Urol. 1986;135(1):142–7.
13. Champion HC, Bivalacqua TJ, Takimoto E, Kass DA, Burnett AL. Phosphodiesterase-5A dysregulation in penile erectile tissue is a mechanism of priapism. Proc Natl Acad Sci USA. 2005;102(5):1661–6.
14. Bivalacqua TJ, Ross AE, Strong TD, Gebska MA, Musicki B, Champion HC, Burnett AL. Attenuated RhoA/rho-kinase signaling in penis of transgenic sickle cell mice. Urology. 2010;76(2):510.e517–2.
15. Witt MA, Goldstein I, Saenz de Tejada I, Greenfield A, Krane RJ. Traumatic laceration of intracavernosal arteries: the pathophysiology of nonischemic, high flow, arterial priapism. J Urol. 1990;143(1):129–32.
16. Melman A, Serels S. Priapism. Int J Impot Res. 2000;12(Suppl 4):S133–9.
17. Ericson C, Baird B, Broderick GA. Management of Priapism: 2021 update. Urol Clin North Am. 2021;48(4):565–76.
18. Bastuba MD, Saenz de Tejada I, Dinlenc CZ, Sarazen A, Krane RJ, Goldstein I. Arterial priapism: diagnosis, treatment and long-term followup. J Urol. 1994;151(5):1231–7.
19. Foda MM, Mahmood K, Rasuli P, Dunlap H, Kiruluta G, Schillinger JF. High-flow priapism associated with Fabry's disease in a child: a case report and review of the literature. Urology. 1996;48(6):949–52.
20. Zouari M, Krichen E, Ben Saad N, Kraiem N, Rhaiem W, Mhiri R. Idiopathic high-flow priapism. Arch Iran Med. 2023;26(10):604–5.
21. Miller ST, Rao SP, Dunn EK, Glassberg KI. Priapism in children with sickle cell disease. J Urol. 1995;154(2 Pt 2):844–7.
22. Idris IM, Abba A, Galadanci JA, Aji SA, Jibrilla AU, Rodeghier M, Kassim A, Burnett AL, DeBaun MR. Incidence and predictors of priapism events in sickle cell anemia: a diary-based analysis. Blood Adv. 2022;6(20):5676–83.
23. Quigley M, Fawcett DP. Thrombophilia and priapism. BJU Int. 1999;83(1):155.
24. Lin CS. Phosphodiesterase type 5 regulation in the penile corpora cavernosa. J Sex Med. 2009;6(Suppl 3):203–9.
25. Burnett AL. Molecular pharmacotherapeutic targeting of PDE5 for preservation of penile health. J Androl. 2008;29(1):3–14.
26. Kovac JR, Mak SK, Garcia MM, Lue TF. A pathophysiology-based approach to the management of early priapism. Asian J Androl. 2013;15(1):20–6.
27. Burnett AL, Bivalacqua TJ, Champion HC, Musicki B. Feasibility of the use of phosphodiesterase type 5 inhibitors in a pharmacologic prevention program for recurrent priapism. J Sex Med. 2006;3(6):1077–84.

28. Montague DK, Jarow J, Broderick GA, Dmochowski RR, Heaton JP, Lue TF, Nehra A, Sharlip ID, Members of the Erectile Dysfunction Guideline Update P, Americal Urological A. American urological association guideline on the management of priapism. J Urol. 2003;170(4 Pt 1):1318–24.
29. Cintho Ozahata M, Page GP, Guo Y, Ferreira JE, Dinardo CL, Carneiro-Proietti ABF, Loureiro P, Mota RA, Rodrigues DOW, Belisario AR, et al. Clinical and genetic predictors of priapism in sickle cell disease: results from the recipient epidemiology and donor evaluation study III Brazil cohort study. J Sex Med. 2019;16(12):1988–99.
30. James Johnson M, Hallerstrom M, Alnajjar HM, Frederick Johnson T, Skrodzka M, Chiriaco G, Muneer A, Ralph DJ. Which patients with ischaemic priapism require further investigation for malignancy? Int J Impot Res. 2020;32(2):195–200.
31. Nolan VG, Wyszynski DF, Farrer LA, Steinberg MH. Hemolysis-associated priapism in sickle cell disease. Blood. 2005;106(9):3264–7.
32. von Stempel C, Zacharakis E, Allen C, Ramachandran N, Walkden M, Minhas S, Muneer A, Ralph D, Freeman A, Kirkham A. Mean velocity and peak systolic velocity can help determine ischaemic and non-ischaemic priapism. Clin Radiol. 2017;72(7):611.e9–611.e16.
33. Hakim LS, Kulaksizoglu H, Mulligan R, Greenfield A, Goldstein I. Evolving concepts in the diagnosis and treatment of arterial high flow priapism. J Urol. 1996;155(2):541–8.
34. Ralph DJ, Borley NC, Allen C, Kirkham A, Freeman A, Minhas S, Muneer A. The use of high-resolution magnetic resonance imaging in the management of patients presenting with priapism. BJU Int. 2010;106(11):1714–8.

Chapter 12
Advances in the Treatment of Priapism

Edoardo Pozzi, Fabio Castiglione, and Rupin Shah

Introduction

The management and treatment of priapism present a complex array of challenges that have evolved alongside some important advances in the last two decades [1]. Despite advances in understanding this condition, managing acute episodes and preventing long-term consequences remain a clinical challenge in everyday practice [1–3]. Moreover, the rarity of the disease, along with its unpredictable course, adds an extra layer of complexity to its management. As such, this chapter aims to provide a detailed outline of contemporary discoveries and recommendations in priapism treatment, reflecting the dynamic interplay between emerging scientific knowledge and modern clinical practice challenges.

E. Pozzi (✉)
Desai Sethi Urology Institute, Miller School of Medicine, University of Miami, Miami, FL, USA

Vita-Salute San Raffaele University, Milan, Italy

Division of Experimental Oncology/Unit of Urology, URI, IRCCS Ospedale San Raffaele, Milan, Italy
e-mail: pozzi.edoardo@hsr.it

F. Castiglione
King's College London Hospital, London, UK

R. Shah
Department of Urology, Lilavati Hospital & Research Centre, Mumbai, India

R. Shah et al. (eds.), *Diagnosis and Treatment of Male Sexual Dysfunction*, https://doi.org/10.1007/978-3-032-12423-4_12

Current Recommendations for Priapism Treatment

Ischemic Priapism

According to guidelines from the *European Association of Urology (EAU)* and the *American Urological Association (AUA)*, early management of ischemic priapism should begin within 4 to 6 hours from its onset [2, 3]. This involves a stepwise approach starting with decompressing the corpora cavernosa through penile aspiration and washout with saline solution (until bright blood is obtained) [2, 3]. If priapism persists despite aspiration, the next step is the intracavernosal injection of a sympathomimetic drug [2, 3]. *It is important not to inject a vasoconstrictor if the penis is partially detumesced, since in this situation the penile venous outflow has partially opened, and the sympathomimetic will enter the circulation, causing hypertension and tachycardia.* The first-line therapy is phenylephrine, with injections (aliquots of 200 µg) given every 3–5 minutes until detumescence is achieved [2, 3]. Surgery should only be considered when blood aspiration and intracavernosal injection of sympathomimetic drugs have failed, with distal shunt surgical procedures performed first and tunneling considered as the last solution [2, 3]. However, in cases of priapism secondary to intracavernosal injections of vasoactive agents, the initial step should be the intracavernosal injection of a sympathomimetic drug, replacing the initial standard step of blood aspiration, provided the presentation is within 4 hours [2, 3]. Likewise, in cases where the aforementioned steps fail, surgical shunts are the mainstay of treatment. In some instances, penile prosthesis implantation may be preferred over proximal shunting particularly in delayed (more than 48 hours) or refractory ischemic priapism [2, 3]. In cases in which a shunt has been performed, implantation of a penile prosthesis should be delayed to minimize the risk of infection and erosion of the implant [2, 3]. The decision on which type of implant to insert is dependent on patient suitability, surgeon's experience, and the availability and cost of the equipment [2, 3]. If a malleable penile prosthesis is implanted, it can later be exchanged for an inflatable penile implant if the patient desires. Patients must be fully counseled regarding the risks and benefits of implant insertion in cases of delayed presentation of refractory priapism [2, 3].

Stuttering Priapism

Stuttering priapism, the least prevalent subtype, is initially a self-resolving condition, with episodes usually lasting less than 3 to 4 hours [2–4]. However, there is a substantial chance that it can evolve into ischemic priapism [4, 5]. The causes of stuttering priapism are similar to those of ischemic priapism, even though in the majority of cases no evident cause is identifiable [2]. The primary goal in managing stuttering priapism is to prevent future episodes, apart from resolving the spontaneous attacks themselves [2, 3, 6–8]. The treatment of stuttering priapism for each acute episode is similar to that of ischemic priapism [2, 3, 6–8], and patients can be trained for intracavernosal self-injections of sympathomimetic drugs to be used at home when an acute episode occurs [2, 3]. For the prevention of future episodes in patients with frequent relapses, hormonal blockade with gonadotropin-releasing hormone agonists or antagonists, and/or antiandrogens may be considered [2, 3, 6–8]. Lastly, daily low-dose phosphodiesterase type 5 (PDE5) inhibitor treatment has been shown to prevent recurrent priapism while preserving normal erectile function in a small series of patients [2, 3].

Non-Ischemic Priapism

Non-ischemic priapism, which is less common than its ischemic counterpart, does not necessitate immediate surgical intervention [2, 4, 5]. The presence of oxygenated blood flow within the corpora and the absence of severe penile pain allow for initial conservative management [5]. From the outset, it is crucial to confirm an accurate diagnosis using color Doppler ultrasonography [2, 3]. In cases in which the etiology cannot be identified or relapses are frequent, a diagnostic angiography can be combined with super-selective embolization. Among cases treated with fistula embolization, erectile dysfunction (ED) rates have been reported as low as 5% when using temporary agents (blood clot and gel foam) and up to 39% with permanent agents (i.e., micro coils) [2, 3, 9, 10]. However, a recent study reported that ED rates were higher with temporary agents compared to permanent ones [10]. As such, even if the literature is contradictory regarding the ED rates, the choice of embolic agent is critical and should be tailored to each patient. Lastly, in some instances of long-standing non-ischemic priapism, patients can develop fibrosis within the distal corpora [2, 3, 9, 10]. Patients exhibiting distal flaccidity and fibrosis within the distal corpora should undergo a penile magnetic resonance imaging (MRI) scan, which is the optimal imaging modality in these scenarios to assess the extent and severity of fibrosis, providing information for treatment planning, guiding interventional procedures, and monitoring treatment outcomes [2, 3, 9–11].

Alternative Medications for Ischemic Priapism

The treatment of ischemic priapism, even though effective and standardized, has some limitations [2, 3]. Firstly, the evidence supporting the efficacy of higher doses of phenylephrine is not substantial, and the protocol is not standardized [1]. Although many studies have been published, the optimal dosage for the best clinical outcome still needs to be established. Meanwhile, other medications and treatment regimens have been studied, with many being under-discussed and needing to be investigated in prospective clinical trials.

Etilephrine

Etilephrine, an adrenergic agonist that stimulates both alpha- and beta-adrenergic receptors, has been suggested to be an efficacious treatment for priapism in men with sickle cell disease [3, 12, 13]. While mainly used for this condition, it has also demonstrated efficacy in treating priapism resulting from iatrogenic causes [13]. As the second-line sympathomimetic agent after phenylephrine, etilephrine is typically administered via intracavernosal injection, using a concentration of 2.5 mg in 1–2 mL of normal saline solution [13, 14].

Methylene Blue

Methylene blue may help counteract the smooth muscle relaxation that underlies priapism [2, 15, 16]. Small retrospective case studies have reported success in using this agent to terminate pharmacologically induced priapism of short duration [2, 15, 16]. The typical dosing is 50–100 mg injected directly into the corpora, left for 5 minutes, aspirated out, and followed by 5 more minutes of penile compression [2, 15, 16]. Side effects may include transient penile burning or blue discoloration [15, 16].

Adrenaline

Adrenaline, which acts as both an alpha- and beta-adrenergic agonist, has proven useful for ischemic priapism resulting from intracavernosal injection of vasoactive drugs [2, 17, 18]. By injecting 2 mL of 1/100,000 concentration (20 mcg) of adrenaline up to 5 times every 20 minutes directly into the corpus cavernosum, detumescence can often be achieved [2, 17, 18]. One case series found over 50% success after a single injection, with the overall efficacy reaching 95% with repeated injections [2]. As an alternative method (proposed by the co-author of this chapter—RS), one can directly draw 0.05 mL to 0.10 mL (equivalent to 50 mcg to 100 mcg) of adrenaline from the ampoule (which contains 1 mL of 1 mg adrenaline) into an insulin syringe and inject it into one of the corpora cavernosa. The dose may be repeated after 15 minutes if there is no detumescence. This method appears to be more convenient, as it eliminates the need to prepare a diluted adrenaline solution.

Oral Terbutaline

For prolonged erections lasting beyond 2.5 hours after intracavernosal injection, oral terbutaline has been studied [2, 19–21]. As a beta-2 agonist with some beta-1 and alpha effects, it is thought to aid in reversing the unwanted smooth muscle relaxation [2, 19–21]. However, terbutaline requires caution in patients with coronary disease, fluid overload, edema, or hypokalemia due to its mechanisms of action [2, 19–21]. An alternative beta-2 agonist, salbutamol, achieved detumescence in 34% of cases in one prospective study, though more data are still needed before definitively recommending it for ischemic priapism [2, 19–21].

Heparin and Anti-coagulation Drugs

Retrospective data from Ramstein et al. examined the use of antithrombotic medications—either subcutaneous heparin or oral aspirin 325 mg—in patients who underwent corporeal aspiration with or without phenylephrine injection for priapism [1, 22]. Those given antithrombotic therapy displayed significantly fewer recurrences after initial detumescence and higher rates of successful shunting [1, 22]. However, this data comes from a small cohort of only 18 patients, using varying doses and types of anticoagulants whose timing was not ideally measured [1, 22]. Further prospective, randomized trials are still required before recommending anticoagulation as treatment or a preventative adjunct for ischemic priapism [1].

Surgical Techniques for Ischemic Priapism

To date there is a lack of rigorous and precise data regarding the surgical management of priapism, with studies completed only on small cohorts [3, 23]. As such, clear recommendations regarding a specific shunting procedure cannot be made, but distal shunts are recognized as the primary surgical option carrying lower rates of postprocedural ED due to their less invasiveness as compared to other procedures [2, 3, 24–26].

Percutaneous Distal (Corpora-Glanular) Shunts

Winter's Procedure

This surgical procedure involves the use of a Tru-cut biopsy needle to create a fistulous passage between the glans and each of the corpora cavernosa [2, 27], thus allowing detumescence through the corpus spongiosum. The disadvantage of this technique lies in its limited efficacy due to the narrow diameter of the needle used, typically between 14 and 18 gauge [2, 27].

Ebbehoj's Technique

This surgical technique utilizes an 11-blade scalpel to make multiple percutaneous incisions through the glans into the distal tips of each of the corpora cavernosa [2, 28, 29].

T-Shunt

The T-shunt is a percutaneous surgical alternative that is commonly used in clinical practice. It consists of inserting a 10-size scalpel blade through the glans into the distal tip of the corpus cavernosum. Once the corpus is perforated, the blade is turned 90 degrees and withdrawn [2, 28, 29]. This procedure can either be performed on one side or on both sides if necessary. Hegar's dilators can also be used in order to promote and facilitate drainage of blood [2, 28, 29].

Al-Ghorab's Procedure

This surgical technique involves the removal of an elliptical segment from the distal end of each corpus cavernosum so as to create a large opening between the corpora and the glans [2, 30]. A 3-cm transversal incision is made on the dorsum of the glans penis, about 1 cm distal to the coronal sulcus, positioned over the rigid corpora, which can be felt through the glans. The incision is deepened until the corporal tips are exposed. The two corpora are incised, and some tunica is trimmed to create an adequate elliptical opening. The corpora are milked to drain the stagnated blood and establish free flow. The glans is closed with a superficial, watertight, continuous suture that leaves the fistula between the corpora and the glans tissue open [2, 30]. Patency of the fistula is demonstrated by squeezing the penis from base to tip which will cause the glans to swell up as blood flows from the corpora into the glans. Then, as the blood flows out of the glans through the spongiosum, they deflate. However, the penis will quickly re-erect and require the same milking action to detumesce again. Hence, it is important to instruct the patient to keep on performing this squeezing during his waking hours to keep the penis flaccid and allow recovery.

Burnett's Technique

This modifies the Al-Ghorab shunt by inserting a 7/8 Hegar dilator retrograde into the corpora cavernosa [2, 31–33]. This is useful if the blood has clotted in the corpora. After the clot is fragmented, it can be manually expressed from the base of the penis to the glans. After detumescence, the glans is closed as in Al-Ghorab's technique [2, 31–33]. However, complications like wound infection, penile skin necrosis, and urethrocutaneous fistulas have been documented [2, 31–33].

Open Proximal (Corpora-Spongiosal) Shunts

This more invasive approach creates a connection between the corpus cavernosum and corpus spongiosum via a trans-scrotal or perineal incision [1, 34]. Complications like urethrocavernous fistula, urethral stricture, or cavernositis may occur [1, 34]. The perineal route targeting the spongiosal bulb carries lower urethral injury risk [1, 34]. However, proximal shunts are generally more invasive with higher rates of ED [1, 34].

Peno-Scrotal Decompression

A novel proximal decompression technique has emerged with high success rates aimed at preserving the glans integrity [1, 35, 36]. It involves opening the proximal corpus cavernosum combined with proximal decompression, offering an alternative to traditional methods described above [1, 35, 36]. The procedure begins with a standard peno-scrotal incision and dissection, similar to those used in penile prosthesis implantation. A urethral catheter is inserted, and a specialized retractor system is then used to expose the corpora cavernosa [35]. A transverse incision is made, and dissection continues until the tunica albuginea of one corporal body is exposed. Traction sutures are placed on the corpora, followed by a 2-cm incision to allow drainage of ischemic blood [35]. Corporal decompression is accomplished by employing a pediatric suction tip to extract deoxygenated blood from both the ipsilateral and contralateral corpora via cross-septal egress [35]. If unilateral decompression successfully resolves the priapism, indicated by a return of bright red blood, the corpora are irrigated with saline, and the incision is closed [35]. However, in severe cases where unilateral dilation is insufficient, bilateral corporal dilation is performed in the same manner [35].

Penile Prosthesis Implantation

Failure to achieve detumescence following the aforementioned treatment approaches will inevitably lead to irreversible smooth muscle necrosis and ED [2, 3]. An erection persisting for 24 to 48 hours inexorably results in permanent smooth muscle damage and subsequent fibrosis [2, 3]. The high rates of impotence, corporal fibrosis, and loss of penile length and girth that occur after a prolonged priapism suggest the need for an alternative approach. Hence, it was proposed that these patients with treatment-refractory priapism may benefit from immediate penile prosthesis implantation [2, 3, 37]. Such an approach would allow for a relatively easy implantation before fibrosis sets in and will maintain the penile length and girth. The use of a malleable prosthesis has been recommended in these cases since it does not have multiple components and hence is associated with a lower infection risk [2, 3, 36–41]. After 3 weeks of a priapism, the insertion of a penile prosthesis becomes more challenging due to progressive cavernous fibrosis [2, 3, 36–41]. Alnajjar et al. highlighted some considerations to avoid complications during an early implantation [1}. Downsizing a malleable device by 1–2 cm will reduce the risk of distal erosion and extrusion, particularly if the patient has recently undergone a distal shunt [1, 38]. Moreover, they also recommended a 2-week interval between the shunt and malleable prosthesis insertion to allow the fistula to heal properly [1, 38]. After 6 months, the malleable prosthesis can be replaced with a three-piece inflatable prosthesis, allowing for cylinder upsizing [1, 38]. If an early penile implant is not done in a case of prolonged priapism, then severe fibrosis with shortening will develop. This condition can be minimized by daily use of a vacuum erection device, which will result in visible increase in length and girth. However, even then, the fibrosis will be extensive, and corporal dilatation will be very difficult needing special cavernotomes and a highly experienced surgeon. In severely fibrotic and challenging cases, penile prosthesis implantation simultaneous with total corporal reconstruction may be the only option [1, 38]. Nevertheless, complication rates are significantly higher due to severe fibrosis, and therefore, patient counseling and managing expectations become crucial. Consequently, patients should be assessed on a case-by-case basis and counseled on the risks and benefits of early versus delayed penile prosthesis insertion [1, 38]. Currently, there is no absolute evidence regarding the ideal device or timing of implantation [1, 38]. However, several reports do detail the advantages and disadvantages of malleable versus inflatable prostheses and of acute versus delayed implantation [2, 3, 36–41]. The current guidelines support the concept of early penile prosthesis placement in men with untreated acute ischemic priapism lasting over 36 hours or in men who have not benefited from a shunting procedure [3]. After many years of translational research, it has been established that time-dependent irreversible changes are inevitable in refractory cases; therefore, early penile prosthesis placement has become the standard of care in specialist centers [1, 37, 38, 41].

Although this belief holds true, cases of spontaneous recovery even after prolonged times of ischemia have been reported [1]. In this regard, the use of penile magnetic resonance imaging (MRI) can have a potential role [42]. It has been demonstrated that penile MRI during an episode of priapism can accurately assess smooth muscle viability and areas of early fibrosis [42]. As a matter of speculation, penile MRI could potentially predict and assess candidates for early vs. late penile prosthesis implantation. It may help identify areas of the corpora cavernosa that are not perfused or show patchy perfusion, suggesting fibrosis or smooth muscle necrosis, and may detect segmental cavernosal thrombosis.

Alternative Medications for Stuttering Priapism

As mentioned before in this chapter, stuttering priapism represents the least frequent subtype, typically presenting as a self-limiting condition [5]. However, there is a significant risk of cases progressing to full ischemic priapism [2–5]. It is also important to underline that the underlying etiologies are frequently shared with the ischemic forms [2–5]. The goal for stuttering priapism management is preventing recurrence rather than resolving spontaneously acute episodes [2–5].

Dutasteride and Phosphodiesterase 5 Inhibitors A recent small study identified daily dutasteride therapy as a promising treatment option to reduce the frequency and severity of painful episodes without significant side effects. In another small case series, daily low-dose phosphodiesterase 5 inhibitor (PDE5i) treatment prevented priapism recurrence while preserving normal erectile function [43]. A recent cohort study evaluated the efficacy of various treatments in patients with sickle cell-related stuttering priapism [14]. This study demonstrated that hydroxyurea and automated exchange transfusion were the most effective options, but hormone manipulation and alpha-agonist (e.g., etilephrine) therapies were beneficial in both idiopathic and sickle cell-related cases [14].

Procedures for Non-Ischemic Priapism

Persistent semi-erection due to non-ischemic priapism is often attributed to an increased arterial blood flow to the penile corpora, which may be idiopathic or follow an injury to the penis or the perineal area resulting in a traumatic fistula [2, 3, 10]. This type of priapism is less prevalent than its ischemic counterpart and does not typically necessitate immediate surgical treatment [2, 3, 10]. The presence of oxygen-rich blood in the corpora and the absence of intense penile pain allow for an initial conservative approach to management [2, 3, 10]. Accurate diagnosis is crucial from the start, and this is typically verified through arterial blood gas analysis, Doppler ultrasound imaging, and angiography [2, 3, 10].

Angiography and Vessel Embolization For those with prolonged and relapsing non-ischemic priapism, there is a risk of developing fibrosis in the distal corpora, making early intervention with targeted embolization imperative to prevent such complications [2, 4]. Selective arterial embolization can be performed using temporary substances, such as autologous blood clots and gel foam, or permanent substances, such as micro coils, ethylene-vinyl alcohol copolymer (PVA), and N-butyl-cyanoacrylate (NBCA) [2].

The complications of selective arterial embolization include penile gangrene, cavernositis, gluteal ischemia, and perineal abscesses [9]. As stated before in this chapter, the rates of post-embolization ED vary according to the type of substances used (temporary or permanent), ranging from 5% to 39% [10].

Artificial Intelligence: Powered Tools for Priapism

Despite significant progress in understanding the pathophysiology of this condition, clinicians continue to struggle to tackle the acute episode while preserving long-term erectile function along with preventing future occurrences [44]. Despite significant progress in understanding the pathophysiology of this condition, clinicians continue to struggle to tackle the acute episode while preserving long-term erectile function along with preventing future occurrences [44]. Conversely, having sickle cell disease as the etiology of priapism emerged as a protective factor against the need for shunting [44]. Lastly, by using machine learning models, including a forest algorithm, the authors accurately predicted the requirement for shunting in 87.2% men [44]. Although it is the only study conducted using AI in the context of priapism to date, this work represents a significant step forward in the application of AI within the field of priapism and offers insights into how technology can support clinical decision-making in such complex cases [44].

Conclusion and Future Directions

While treating this rare urological condition remains an ongoing challenge, our comprehension and approach have progressed significantly thanks to years of clinical and fundamental scientific research. Advancements in pharmacology have greatly improved the management of stuttering priapism and the prospects for resolution in cases of ischemic priapism when treated within the first few hours of onset. However, the management of non-ischemic priapism is primarily expectant, with super-selective embolization considered only in persistent cases. Arguably, the most crucial diagnostic step is distinguishing between ischemic and non-ischemic states, as this determination guides further interventions, including surgical shunts and early penile prosthesis implantation for refractory cases. AI models may have a specific and impactful role in such a challenge.

References

1. Alnajjar HM, Muneer A. Recent advances in understanding and treating priapism. Fac Rev. 2022;11:23. https://doi.org/10.12703/r/11-23.
2. Salonia A, Bettocchi C, Capogrosso P, Carvalho J, Corona G, Hatzichristodoulou G, Jones TH, Kadioglu A, Martinez-Salamanca JI, Minhas S, Serefoglu EC, Verze P, Boeri L, Cocci A, Dimitropoulos K, Falcone M, Gül M, Kalkanli A, Morgado LA, Milenkovic U, Russo G, Tharakan T. EAU guidelines on sexual and reproductive health. Arnhem: EAU Guidelines Office; 2023. ISBN 978-94-92671-19-6. Available at: https://uroweb.org/guidelines/sexual-and-reproductive-health n.d
3. Bivalacqua TJ, Allen BK, Brock GB, Broderick GA, Chou R, Kohler TS, et al. The diagnosis and management of recurrent Ischemic Priapism, priapism in sickle cell patients, and non-ischemic priapism: an AUA/SMSNA guideline. J Urol. 2022;208:43–52. https://doi.org/10.1097/JU.0000000000002767.
4. Morrison BF, Burnett AL. Stuttering priapism: insights into pathogenesis and management. Curr Urol Rep. 2012;13:268–76. https://doi.org/10.1007/s11934-012-0258-9.
5. Liguori G, Rizzo M, Boschian R, Cai T, Palmieri A, Bucci S, et al. The management of stuttering priapism. Minerva Urol E Nefrol Ital J Urol Nephrol. 2020;72:173–86. https://doi.org/10.23736/S0393-2249.19.03323-X.
6. Broderick GA, Kadioglu A, Bivalacqua TJ, Ghanem H, Nehra A, Shamloul R. Priapism: pathogenesis, epidemiology, and management. J Sex Med. 2010;7:476–500. https://doi.org/10.1111/j.1743-6109.2009.01625.x.
7. Zacharakis E, Garaffa G, Raheem AA, Christopher AN, Muneer A, Ralph DJ. Penile prosthesis insertion in patients with refractory ischaemic priapism: early vs delayed implantation. BJU Int. 2014;114:576–81. https://doi.org/10.1111/bju.12686.
8. Welliver RC, Fonseca AN, West BL, McVary KT, Köhler TS. Autoinflation leading to failure of two-piece ambicor implantable penile prosthesis: an outcome from a methodical treatment of recalcitrant stuttering priapism. Case Rep Urol. 2014;2014:529037. https://doi.org/10.1155/2014/529037.
9. Biebel MG, Gross MS, Munarriz R. Review of ischemic and non-ischemic priapism. Curr Urol Rep. 2022;23:143–53. https://doi.org/10.1007/s11934-022-01096-8.
10. Ingram AR, Stillings SA, Jenkins LC. An update on non-ischemic priapism. Sex Med Rev. 2020;8:140–9. https://doi.org/10.1016/j.sxmr.2019.03.004.
11. Junior AR, Schmid BP, Nasser F, Borges LL. The role of magnetic resonance imaging in the Management of High-Flow Priapism: an essential tool when everything Else fails. J Vasc Interv Radiol JVIR. 2022;33:470–3. https://doi.org/10.1016/j.jvir.2021.12.031.
12. Saffon Cuartas JP, Sandoval-Salinas C, Martínez JM, Corredor HA. Treatment of priapism secondary to drugs for erectile dysfunction. Adv Urol. 2019;2019:6214921. https://doi.org/10.1155/2019/6214921.
13. Serrate RG, Prats J, Regué R, Rius G. The usefulness of ethylephrine (Efortil-R) in the treatment of priapism and intraoperative penile erections. Int Urol Nephrol. 1992;24:389–92. https://doi.org/10.1007/BF02550631.
14. Gbadoé AD, Atakouma Y, Kusiaku K, Assimadi JK. Management of sickle cell priapism with etilefrine. Arch Dis Child. 2001;85:52–3. https://doi.org/10.1136/adc.85.1.52.
15. Hübler J, Szántó A, Könyves K. Methylene blue as a means of treatment for priapism caused by intracavernous injection to combat erectile dysfunction. Int Urol Nephrol. 2003;35:519–21. https://doi.org/10.1023/b:urol.0000025617.97048.ae.
16. Martínez Portillo F, Hoang-Boehm J, Weiss J, Alken P, Jünemann K. Methylene blue as a successful treatment alternative for pharmacologically induced priapism. Eur Urol. 2001;39:20–3. https://doi.org/10.1159/000052407.
17. Keskin D, Cal C, Delibaş M, Ozyurt C, Günaydin G, Nazli O, et al. Intracavernosal adrenalin injection in priapism. Int J Impot Res. 2000;12:312–4. https://doi.org/10.1038/sj.ijir.3900539.

18. van Driel MF, Mooibroek JJ, Mensink HJ. Treatment of priapism by injection of adrenaline into the corpora cavernosa penis. Scand J Urol Nephrol. 1991;25:251–4. https://doi.org/10.3109/00365599109024554.
19. Lowe FC, Jarow JP. Placebo-controlled study of oral terbutaline and pseudoephedrine in management of prostaglandin E1-induced prolonged erections. Urology. 1993;42:51–3.; discussion 53–4. https://doi.org/10.1016/0090-4295(93)90338-b.
20. Gupta A, Seth T, Gupta A. Successful use of terbutaline in persistent priapism in a 12-year-old boy with chronic myeloid leukemia. Pediatr Hematol Oncol. 2009;26:70–3. https://doi.org/10.1080/08880010802435146.
21. Priyadarshi S. Oral terbutaline in the management of pharmacologically induced prolonged erection. Int J Impot Res. 2004;16:424–6. https://doi.org/10.1038/sj.ijir.3901180.
22. Ramstein JJ, Lee A, Cohen AJ, Mmonu NA, Rios N, Enriquez A, et al. Clinical outcomes of Periprocedural antithrombotic therapy in ischemic priapism management. J Sex Med. 2020;17:2260–6. https://doi.org/10.1016/j.jsxm.2020.07.013.
23. Fantus RJ, Brannigan RE, Davis AM. Diagnosis and Management of Priapism. JAMA. 2023;330:559–60. https://doi.org/10.1001/jama.2023.13377.
24. Zacharakis E, Raheem AA, Freeman A, Skolarikos A, Garaffa G, Christopher AN, et al. The efficacy of the T-shunt procedure and intracavernous tunneling (snake maneuver) for refractory ischemic priapism. J Urol. 2014;191:164–8. https://doi.org/10.1016/j.juro.2013.07.034.
25. Brant WO, Garcia MM, Bella AJ, Chi T, Lue TF. T-shaped shunt and intracavernous tunneling for prolonged ischemic priapism. J Urol. 2009;181:1699–705. https://doi.org/10.1016/j.juro.2008.12.021.
26. Burnett AL, Pierorazio PM. Corporal "snake" maneuver: corporoglanular shunt surgical modification for ischemic priapism. J Sex Med. 2009;6:1171–6. https://doi.org/10.1111/j.1743-6109.2008.01176.x.
27. Winter CC. Cure of idiopathic priapism: new procedure for creating fistula between glans penis and corpora cavernosa. Urology. 1976;8:389–91. https://doi.org/10.1016/0090-4295(76)90498-2.
28. Ebbehoj J. A new operation for priapism. Scand J Plast Reconstr Surg. 1974;8:241–2. https://doi.org/10.3109/02844317409084400.
29. Lund K, Ebbehøj J. Results of glando-cavernous anastomosis in 18 cases of priapism. Scand J Plast Reconstr Surg. 1980;14:269–72. https://doi.org/10.3109/02844318009106720.
30. Bella A, Wang R, Shamloul R, Zappavigna C, Ahmed M, Sadeghi-Nejad Hossein. 1859 3-piece inflatable penile prosthesis insertion post t-shunt for priapism with dilation/corporal snake maneuver and comparison to post al-ghorab shunt ipp outcomes. J Urol. 2012;187:e751–2. https://doi.org/10.1016/j.juro.2012.02.1971.
31. Burnett AL, Bivalacqua TJ. Priapism: new concepts in medical and surgical management. Urol Clin North Am. 2011;38:185–94. https://doi.org/10.1016/j.ucl.2011.02.005.
32. Althof SE, Rosen RC, Perelman MA, Rubio-Aurioles E. Standard operating procedures for taking a sexual history. J Sex Med. 2013;10:26–35. https://doi.org/10.1111/j.1743-6109.2012.02823.x.
33. Burnett AL. Surgical management of ischemic priapism. J Sex Med. 2012;9:114–20. https://doi.org/10.1111/j.1743-6109.2011.02446.x.
34. Segal RL, Readal N, Pierorazio PM, Burnett AL, Bivalacqua TJ. Corporal Burnett "Snake" surgical maneuver for the treatment of ischemic priapism: long-term followup. J Urol. 2013;189:1025–9. https://doi.org/10.1016/j.juro.2012.08.245.
35. Fuchs JS, Shakir N, McKibben MJ, Mathur S, Teeple S, Scott JM, et al. Penoscrotal decompression-promising new treatment paradigm for refractory ischemic priapism. J Sex Med. 2018;15:797–802. https://doi.org/10.1016/j.jsxm.2018.02.010.
36. Baumgarten AS, VanDyke ME, Yi YA, Keith CG, Fuchs JS, Ortiz NM, et al. Favourable multi-institutional experience with penoscrotal decompression for prolonged ischaemic priapism. BJU Int. 2020;126:441–6. https://doi.org/10.1111/bju.15127.

37. Muneer A, Ralph DJ. Immediate placement of a penile prosthesis as first-line treatment for the management of Ischaemic Priapism. Eur Urol Focus. 2019;5:529–30. https://doi.org/10.1016/j.euf.2019.01.009.
38. Zacharakis E, De Luca F, Raheem AA, Garaffa G, Christopher N, Muneer A, et al. Early insertion of a malleable penile prosthesis in ischaemic priapism allows later upsizing of the cylinders. Scand J Urol. 2015;49:468–71. https://doi.org/10.3109/21681805.2015.1059359.
39. Sansalone S, Garaffa G, Djinovic R, Antonini G, Vespasiani G, Ieria FP, et al. Simultaneous total corporal reconstruction and implantation of a penile prosthesis in patients with erectile dysfunction and severe fibrosis of the corpora cavernosa. J Sex Med. 2012;9:1937–44. https://doi.org/10.1111/j.1743-6109.2012.02748.x.
40. Martínez-Salamanca JI, Mueller A, Moncada I, Carballido J, Mulhall JP. Penile prosthesis surgery in patients with corporal fibrosis: a state of the art review. J Sex Med. 2011;8:1880–9. https://doi.org/10.1111/j.1743-6109.2011.02281.x.
41. Mishra K, Loeb A, Bukavina L, Baumgarten A, Beilan J, Mendez M, et al. Management of Priapism: a contemporary review. Sex Med Rev. 2020;8:131–9. https://doi.org/10.1016/j.sxmr.2019.01.001.
42. Ralph DJ, Borley NC, Allen C, Kirkham A, Freeman A, Minhas S, et al. The use of high-resolution magnetic resonance imaging in the management of patients presenting with priapism. BJU Int. 2010;106:1714–8. https://doi.org/10.1111/j.1464-410X.2010.09368.x.
43. Burnett AL, Bivalacqua TJ, Champion HC, Musicki B. Feasibility of the use of phosphodiesterase type 5 inhibitors in a pharmacologic prevention program for recurrent priapism. J Sex Med. 2006;3:1077–84. https://doi.org/10.1111/j.1743-6109.2006.00333.x.
44. Masterson TA, Parmar M, Tradewell MB, Nackeeran S, Rainer Q, Blachman-Braun R, et al. Using artificial intelligence to predict surgical shunts in men with ischemic priapism. J Urol. 2020;204:1033–8. https://doi.org/10.1097/JU.0000000000001183.

Chapter 13
Management of Testosterone Deficiency Syndrome

Hyun Jun Park, V. S. Karthikeyan, and Eric Chung

Introduction to Testosterone Deficiency Syndrome

Testosterone levels gradually decrease in men after middle age. If the testosterone level falls below a certain level, related symptoms appear. Testosterone deficiency syndrome (TDS) is defined as the presence of typical symptoms along with low serum testosterone levels in aging men. This clinical and biochemical syndrome associated with aging is also referred to as late-onset hypogonadism (LOH) [1, 2] or adult-onset testosterone deficiency syndrome because it is not a congenital testosterone deficiency (Table 13.1).

According to the guidelines for TDS published in various academic societies, symptoms associated with sexual function are the most important for diagnosing TDS. However, the cutoff values of testosterone levels for laboratory diagnosis differ slightly according to each guideline (Table 13.2). The International Society for the Study of the Aging Male and the International Society for Sexual Medicine use a serum total testosterone level of <350 ng/dL as the standard, while the Endocrine Society and the American Urological Association follow the cutoff value of a serum total testosterone level of <300 ng/dL [3].

In patients with TDS, the treatment goal is to restore the decreased serum testosterone level to a physiological level [4]. Currently available formulations include

H. J. Park (✉)
Department of Urology, Pusan National University Hospital, Pusan National University School of Medicine, Busan, Korea (Republic of)

V. S. Karthikeyan
Apollo Hospitals, Chennai, India

E. Chung
Department of Urology, Princess Alexandra Hospital, University of Queensland, Brisbane, QLD, Australia

AndroUrology Centre, Brisbane, QLD, Australia

R. Shah et al. (eds.), *Diagnosis and Treatment of Male Sexual Dysfunction*,
https://doi.org/10.1007/978-3-032-12423-4_13

Table 13.1 Evolution of guidelines for diagnosis and treatment of TDS

	Title	Year of release and update
Expert opinion	Clinical practice guidelines for screening and monitoring male patients receiving testosterone supplementation therapy	1996
ISSAM	Investigation, treatment, and monitoring of late-onset hypogonadism in males. Official recommendations of ISSAM	2002, 2005, 2008, 2015
Endocrine Society	Testosterone therapy in men with hypogonadism	2006, 2010, 2018
ISSM	Diagnosis and treatment of testosterone deficiency: Recommendations from the fourth international consultation for sexual medicine (ICSM)	2015, 2019
AUA	Evaluation and management of testosterone deficiency	2018
EAA	EAA guidelines on investigation, treatment, and monitoring of functional hypogonadism in males	2020
Society for Endocrinology (UK)	Society for Endocrinology guidelines for testosterone replacement therapy in male hypogonadism	2022
BSSM	BSSM Guidelines on Male Testosterone Deficiency	2023
EAU	EAU Guidelines on Sexual and Reproductive Health—Chapter: Male Hypogonadism	2024
KSMHA	Male Hypogonadism: The Korean Society of Men's Health and Aging Position Statement	2025

ISSAM International Society for the Study of the Aging Male, *ISSM* International Society for Sexual Medicine, *ICSM* International Consultation for Sexual Medicine, *AUA* American Urological Association, *EAA* European Academy of Andrology, *BSSM* British Society for Sexual Medicine, *EAU* European Urological Association, *KSMHA* Korean Society of Men's Health and Aging

oral, buccal, transdermal, and intramuscular injections, which vary in route of administration, dose, formulations, and safety profiles [1, 5, 6]. When starting treatment, short-acting formulations, which can be easily stopped if side effects occur, are preferred [1], but in general, each formulation is selected through consultation between the patient and the physician.

The prevalence of TDS varies widely based on the population studied and the diagnostic criteria used [7]. Epidemiological studies suggest that approximately 2.1%–5.6% of men under 60 years old experience TDS, with this figure rising to about 20% in men over 60 and up to 50% in men over 80 years old [6, 8, 9].

The etiology of TDS can be broadly classified into primary, secondary, and mixed hypogonadism. Primary hypogonadism, also known as testicular failure, is characterized by an inability of the testes to produce sufficient testosterone. This condition can result from genetic conditions such as Klinefelter syndrome, as well as acquired conditions like mumps orchitis, testicular trauma, or chemotherapy. Secondary hypogonadism is due to dysfunctions in the hypothalamus or pituitary gland, which regulate testosterone production. Conditions such as pituitary tumors, hypothalamic diseases, or systemic illnesses like obesity and diabetes can disrupt

Table 13.2 Cutoff values of testosterone for laboratory diagnosis

National or international guidelines	TT cutoff (ng/mL)
AUA	3.0
EAU	3.5
ES	3.0
ISSM	3.5
ISSAM	3.5
BSSM	3.5
KSMHA	2.6

T testosterone, *TT* total testosterone, *AUA* American Urological Association, *EAU* European Association of Urology, *ES* Endocrine Society, *ISSM* International Society of Sexual Medicine, *ISSAM* International Society for the Study of the Aging Male, *BSSM* British Society for Sexual Medicine, *KSMHA* Korean Society for Men's Health and Aging

this regulatory axis. Mixed hypogonadism, involving both testicular and hypothalamic-pituitary dysfunctions, is common, particularly in the context of aging and chronic diseases.

Several risk factors are associated with an increased likelihood of developing TDS. Age is the most significant risk factor, with testosterone levels naturally declining by about 1%–2% per year after the age of 30 [10]. Obesity is another crucial risk factor; adipose tissue can convert testosterone to estrogen, leading to reduced testosterone levels. Metabolic syndrome, characterized by insulin resistance, hypertension, dyslipidemia, and abdominal obesity, is also strongly associated with TDS. Moreover, chronic illnesses such as type 2 diabetes, chronic obstructive pulmonary disease, and HIV/AIDS can contribute to the development of TDS. Lifestyle factors, including excessive alcohol consumption, smoking, and lack of physical activity, further exacerbate the risk [11].

Genetic predispositions play a role in the risk of developing TDS. Mutations or polymorphisms in genes involved in the hypothalamic-pituitary-gonadal axis, androgen receptor function, and testosterone metabolism can influence susceptibility to TDS [12]. Additionally, environmental factors such as exposure to endocrine-disrupting chemicals, including bisphenol A (BPA) and phthalates, have been implicated in disrupting testosterone production and action [13].

Clinical Manifestations and Diagnosis

The diagnosis of TDS is controversial. TDS is diagnosed based on symptoms (and signs) and laboratory values. The symptoms of TDS can mimic other chronic medical conditions.

Symptoms of TDS

The symptoms of TDS could be specific or non-specific. Symptoms such as erectile dysfunction, reduced nocturnal erections, and male infertility, especially due to sperm abnormalities, can be specific to TDS. Non-specific symptoms may be difficult to attribute to TDS alone; this is due to the wide range of functions of testosterone in the human body. These non-specific symptoms include generalized tiredness, fatigue, malaise, weakness, reduced energy levels, increased body fat deposition, and reduced level of cognition. This also includes reduced strength, endurance, and muscle mass, bone mineral density, and reduced sleep. Symptoms such as depression, feeling lonely, irritated, and unable to concentrate also are some of the non-specific symptoms of TDS [14–16].

Differential Diagnosis

The differential diagnosis for TDS includes anemia of chronic disease, chronic medical illnesses, depression, nutritional deficiency, obesity, and metabolic syndrome.

Clinical and Laboratory Assessments

Physical Examination

- Clinical physical examination is an important adjunct in the diagnosis of TDS. A normal clinical examination may not be able to rule out TDS; however, in the presence of specific signs, it adds great value toward making a diagnosis of TDS in the presence of suggestive symptoms.
- General examination includes body habitus, androgenization, and also other markers of chronic lifestyle diseases.
- An obese body habitus, tending toward central/abdominal obesity, is a definite clue toward TDS.
- Androgenization is more useful in younger adults presenting especially with low sperm counts, specifically for gynecomastia and reduced body hair.
- Testicular volume is an important predictor, with volume <10 ml being considered a strong predictor. Some information to be considered before deciding the testicular volume as pathological includes a history of chronic illness, previous testicular trauma, torsion, chemotherapy, or surgery. Other findings to look for are asymmetry of the testes, a palpable mass in the testes, varicocele, and scrotal skin thickness [6, 16].

Table 13.3 Key points for laboratory diagnosis

Testosterone levels	Total testosterone levels: <2.6–3.5 ng/ml (see Table 13.2) 1. Measurement: CMAJ. 2. Measurements: ISSM, BSSM, ES, EAU.	
Factors affecting testosterone levels	Sleep, glucose and food intake, stress, daily activities, acute illness, androgens, chronic medical illness, and depression	
SHBG alterations—Key conditions	Reduced: Obesity, steroid use, diabetes mellitus, hypothyroidism, nephrotic syndrome	Increased: Age, hyperthyroidism, HIV, cirrhosis, estrogen use, anticonvulsants

ES Endocrine Society, *ISSM* International Society for Sexual Medicine, *BSSM* British Society for Sexual Medicine, *EAU* European Association of Urology, *CMAJ* Canadian Medical Association Journal

Hormone Level Testing

TDS may not be diagnosed only based on low testosterone levels. A single low testosterone level should not be the only basis for diagnosing TDS. Whilst TDS can be suspected on history and physical examination, proving testosterone deficiency needs meticulous testing for the same. Due to diurnal variation, especially in younger adults (<45 years), it is best estimated in morning samples (7–11 AM), and a fasting sample is preferred, though not mandatory. The test has to be repeated after 1–2 weeks in case of a low value [14]. The normal values for total testosterone range from 300 to 1000 ng/dl. The absolute cutoff value for labeling TDS is controversial; however, it is considered 300–350 ng/dl based on various guidelines, and treatment is beneficial in men with levels <230 ng/dl. Liquid chromatography mass spectrometry appears to be a reproducible method for total testosterone estimation [15, 16].

The circulating testosterone levels can be affected by stress, sleep, general illness, and also levels of sex hormone binding globulin. In case of obesity or other specific diseases such as thyroid dysfunction and liver diseases, it would be required to evaluate free testosterone or calculated bioavailable testosterone values. The usage of estimated free or calculated bioavailable testosterone levels is controversial. However, when it is difficult to standardize free testosterone measurements (equilibrium dialysis is the best method), calculated bioavailable testosterone values appear to be reliable [6] (Table 13.3).

The other hormones that are important in the evaluation of TDS include estradiol (to quantify peripheral aromatization and guide therapy) and pituitary gonadotropins (LH and, if required, FSH) levels to identify the cause. In case of severe testosterone deficiency (persistent low total testosterone <100–150 ng/dl), prolactin estimation (and cranial MRI) might be useful [6, 14, 17].

Treatment

Various formulations of testosterone are available for the treatment of TDS. The primary principle in TDS treatment is to initiate therapy only when patients have TDS symptoms and decreased blood testosterone levels have been confirmed [1, 18]. The ideal hormone therapy should maintain serum testosterone levels as close to physiological levels as possible. Current formulations include subcutaneous implants, intramuscular injections, oral tablets, transdermal patches, and gels, each with distinct pharmacokinetic profiles. Determining the superior formulation is challenging, but starting with short-acting formulations to assess efficacy and side effects before transitioning to long-acting formulations is recommended [1, 3, 19]. The characteristics, advantages, and disadvantages of testosterone therapies used in TDS treatment are discussed below.

Injectable Formulations

Testosterone enanthate injections involve administering 250 mg intramuscularly every 2–3 weeks. A major drawback is the rapid rise to supraphysiological levels post-injection, followed by a drop below the physiological level. Testosterone undecanoate is a slow-release formulation that provides a stable level in the mid-range with effects lasting up to three months. Each vial contains 4 ml of 250 mg/ml testosterone undecanoate in a benzyl benzoate/castor oil solution, administered as 1000 mg deep intramuscularly every 10–14 weeks.

Gel Formulations

Transdermal patches are no longer produced due to inconvenience and side effects, but gels remain available. These gels often include alcohol to enhance absorption and bioavailability. They should be applied to clean, dry, intact skin of the shoulder and upper arms, on the abdomen, or divided between the inner thighs. Rotating application sites daily between the abdomen and thighs is recommended to minimize local reactions. Avoid application to the scrotum or genitals. The dosage varies from 40 mg to 100 mg of testosterone per day depending on the formulation and the monitored rise in testosterone. Testosterone gel is available in single packs containing 25 mg or 50 mg of testosterone and also in multi-dose metered bottles. The gel should be gently rubbed in and allowed to dry before covering with loose clothing. Hands must be washed with soap and water after application, and bathing should be avoided for at least two hours post-application to ensure optimal absorption.

Recently, a nasal gel formulation has become available. The recommended starting dose is twice daily, one spray per nostril per administration, delivering 5.5 mg per spray, for a total of 22 mg daily. For twice-daily dosing, it should be administered with at least six hours between doses, preferably at the same time each day. Patients should be instructed to fully depress the pump to ensure proper dosage. For three-times-daily dosing, it should be administered with 6–8 hour intervals, preferably at consistent times daily.

Oral formulations of testosterone are also available and are discussed in Table 13.4.

Advantages and Disadvantages of Each Formulation

Testosterone enanthate injections require visits every 2–3 weeks and pose a thrombosis risk due to the rapid post-injection peak, necessitating caution in elderly patients or those with cardiovascular diseases. Testosterone undecanoate injections are convenient with quarterly dosing, making them suitable for patients requiring long-term testosterone therapy, but are expensive and cause injection site pain. Gel formulations offer the advantage of maintaining near-physiological levels and allow for immediate discontinuation in case of side effects. However, gels require waiting for absorption post-application and pose a transmission risk through skin contact. Nasal gels avoid transmission risks and maintain physiological testosterone levels

Table 13.4 Features, advantages, and disadvantages of each formulation

Ingredient	Dosing methods	Advantages	Disadvantages
Testosterone enanthate 250 mg	Intramuscular injections every 2–3 weeks	Short-acting formulation allows immediate discontinuation in the event of side effects	Large fluctuations in blood testosterone levels
Testosterone undecanoate 1000 mg	Intramuscular injections every 10–14 weeks	Blood testosterone levels remain constant	Long-lasting and difficult-to-deal-with side effects. Cost
Oral testosterone undecanoate	Dose varies with the product. The recommended starting dose of Jatenzo® is 237 mg taken orally twice daily, once in the morning and once in the evening. Take with food, and then titrate up or down	Convenience of oral administration. Improved adherence. Steady hormone levels	Cost, daily dosing. Variable absorption
Transdermal testosterone gel	Apply daily to the shoulders and upper arms, inner thighs, or abdomen	Blood testosterone levels remain constant	Transmission through skin-to-skin contact. Cost, daily dosing
Nasal testosterone gel	Twice daily. Self-administered using a nasal applicator	Blood testosterone levels remain constant. No skin transmission concerns	Foreign body sensation in the nasal cavity Cost, daily dosing

with minimal impact on the hypothalamic-pituitary-gonadal axis, thereby preserving spermatogenesis and presenting a lower polycythemia risk compared to injectables [20].

A recent study tracking 640 patients over 10 years found that the one-year treatment continuation rate was approximately 75.9%, with discontinuation reasons including inconvenience, cost, side effects, and insufficient efficacy. Among the formulations, undecanoate had the highest treatment adherence rate [21].

In conclusion, the choice of testosterone therapy should begin with short-acting injections or gels to assess patient response and side effects [1]. Once efficacy and tolerability are confirmed, switching to long-acting injectables may be considered for maintaining physiological testosterone levels over the long term. The advantages and disadvantages of each treatment are briefly summarized in Table 13.4.

Effectiveness of TRT

TRT has been shown to effectively ameliorate many symptoms of TDS. Clinical studies have demonstrated that TRT can significantly improve sexual function, including libido and erectile function. A meta-analysis of randomized controlled trials indicated that TRT resulted in a substantial improvement in sexual desire and satisfaction [6].

In addition to sexual health, TRT positively impacts mood and cognitive function. Men undergoing TRT have reported improvements in mood, reductions in depressive symptoms, and an enhanced overall sense of well-being. Cognitive benefits, such as improved memory and spatial ability, have also been observed, although more research is needed to confirm these effects [22].

TRT has a notable impact on body composition. It is associated with increased lean body mass, decreased fat mass, and improved muscle strength. These changes are particularly beneficial for older men, who often experience sarcopenia and increased adiposity. Furthermore, TRT has been linked to improved bone mineral density, thereby reducing the risk of osteoporosis and fractures in aging men [23]. The effects of TRT and how they are measured are summarized in Table 13.5.

Side Effects of TRT

While TRT can be highly beneficial, it is not without potential side effects. One of the most significant concerns is the risk of cardiovascular events. Some studies suggest that TRT may increase the risk of heart attacks, strokes, and other cardiovascular issues, particularly in older men with preexisting heart conditions. However, other studies have shown no significant increase in cardiovascular risk, indicating that further research is needed to clarify these findings [24, 25].

Table 13.5 Benefits of testosterone therapy and outcome measures

Benefits of testosterone therapy	Estimated time to effects	Outcome measures
Improved sexual desire and erectile function	3–6 weeks	IIEF, AMS, HADS, GEQ, PDQ, DISF/DISF-SR
Improved energy, mood, and vitality	3–6 weeks	AMS, HADS, GEQ, SF-12, fatigue (MFI), PHQ-9, BDI-II, BAI
Increased lean body mass	12–16 weeks	DXA
Reduced waist circumference	12–16 weeks	Waist circumference
Reduced total body fat mass	12–16 weeks	DXA
Increased bone mineral density	6 months	DXA
Increased insulin sensitivity	Few days	HOMA
Reduced blood glucose	3–12 months	Glycated hemoglobin (HbA1c), fasting plasma glucose
Increased muscle strength	12–16 weeks	Maximum weight lift, bench, and leg press exercises

IIEF International index of erectile function, *AMS* aging male symptom questionnaire, *HADS* hospital anxiety and depression scale, *GEQ* global efficacy question, *PDQ* psychosexual daily questionnaire, *DISF/DISF-SR* derogatis interview for sexual function, *SF-12* short-form-12, *MFI* multidimensional fatigue inventory, *PHQ-9* patient health questionnaire-9, *BDI-II* Beck depression inventory, *BAI* Beck anxiety inventory, *DXA* dual energy X-ray absorptiometry, *HOMA* homeostasis model assessment index of insulin resistance

In the multicenter, randomized, double-blind, placebo-controlled, noninferiority TRAVERSE trial, 5246 men aged 45–80 with preexisting or high risk of cardiovascular disease, who reported symptoms of hypogonadism and had two fasting testosterone levels below 300 ng/dL, were enrolled. A primary cardiovascular endpoint event occurred in 182 patients (7.0%) in the testosterone group and in 190 patients (7.3%) in the placebo group (hazard ratio, 0.96; 95% confidence interval, 0.78–1.17; $P < 0.001$ for noninferiority). The results showed that in men with hypogonadism and preexisting or high risk of cardiovascular disease, testosterone-replacement therapy was noninferior to placebo regarding the incidence of major adverse cardiac events [25].

Another concern is the potential for TRT to exacerbate prostate diseases. Historically, it was believed that testosterone stimulates the growth of prostate tissue, thereby increasing the risk of benign prostatic hyperplasia (BPH) and prostate cancer. However, more recent evidence suggests that the relationship between TRT and prostate cancer is more complex and not necessarily causal. Large randomized controlled trials and meta-analyses have not demonstrated a significant increase in prostate cancer incidence among men receiving TRT, although vigilance is warranted [25]. Current guidelines from the American Urological Association (2018) and the Endocrine Society (2018) recommend that men on TRT undergo regular monitoring of prostate-specific antigen (PSA) levels and digital rectal examinations to detect any clinically significant changes early. Thus, while TRT does not appear to increase prostate cancer risk in appropriately selected patients, ongoing surveillance remains essential [1, 6, 25].

Polycythemia, defined as an abnormal increase in red blood cell mass, is another well-recognized side effect of TRT. The Endocrine Society and AUA guidelines recommend that therapy should be withheld or adjusted if hematocrit exceeds 54%, as this level significantly increases blood viscosity and the risk of thromboembolic events [6, 20]. Baseline hematocrit should be measured before initiation of TRT, repeated at 3–6 months, and thereafter annually. If hematocrit rises above 50%, closer monitoring and dose adjustment should be considered. In patients exceeding 54%, TRT should be discontinued until hematocrit normalizes, and alternative strategies such as dose reduction, switching to a different formulation, or therapeutic phlebotomy may be required [6, 20].

Other side effects include sleep apnea, skin reactions at the site of testosterone application, and changes in cholesterol levels. TRT can also impact fertility by suppressing spermatogenesis, which is particularly relevant for men desiring to father children [26].

Precautions and Monitoring

To ensure the safe and effective use of TRT, appropriate patient selection and monitoring are crucial. Prior to initiating TRT, a thorough evaluation should be conducted, including a detailed medical history, physical examination, and baseline laboratory tests to confirm hypogonadism and rule out contraindications.

During treatment, regular follow-up visits are necessary to monitor the patient's response to therapy and to detect any adverse effects. This includes periodic assessment of testosterone levels, hematocrit, lipid profiles, liver function, and PSA levels. Additionally, patients should be educated about the potential side effects and instructed to report any unusual symptoms promptly.

The Ideal Goal of TRT: Maintaining Testosterone Levels or Managing Symptoms?

Typically, the goal of TRT is to restore blood testosterone to normal levels. When used to treat men with hypogonadism, it may also result in other benefits, including (i) improved sexual desire and erectile function, (ii) improved energy, mood, and vitality, (iii) increased lean body mass, (iv) reduced waist circumference, (v) reduced total body fat mass, (vi) increased bone mineral density, (vii) increased insulin sensitivity, (viii) reduced blood glucose and hemoglobin A1c, and (ix) increased muscle strength, as shown in the table below [1]. Improvement in libido generally occurs within 6 weeks of treatment, whereas other benefits usually take up to 12 months [27]. Thus, the effects of TRT are very diverse. Several clinical trials have been conducted, and the effects of TRT have already been well established in published papers [28]. The questions that most practitioners prescribing TRT have are regarding the realistic therapeutic endpoints that must be set for TRT. According to the currently published guidelines, it is recommended that the concentration of testosterone be restored to the mid-normal range (International Society for Sexual Medicine) [29] or to the middle tertile of the normal reference range (American Urological Association) [1]. These recommendations, however, do not provide appropriate answers to the practitioners in real-world settings. In addition, many published studies on TRT have used different outcome measures depending on the research themes, as shown in Table 13.5. Another problem that confuses practitioners is that serum testosterone levels and symptoms are not mechanically correlated. In some cases, the testosterone level is restored to normal without any improvement in symptoms after a sufficient period of time, whereas in other cases, testosterone levels are still low with the improvement in symptoms. Although very difficult, it is necessary to set the ideal TRT goal for practitioners who start TRT in these situations. However, it is recommended that treatment goals be established to achieve an appropriate level of testosterone (e.g., 3–5 ng/mL) rather than subjective symptom improvement. This is because the duration of treatment required for the improvement in subjective symptoms varies according to each symptom. In addition, there are different test methods that can objectively evaluate each symptom. Therefore, it is difficult to assess all the symptoms related to testosterone deficiency in real practice settings. It is important to identify the symptoms that are most obvious and uncomfortable for the patients before treatment. After treatment, it is recommended that the focus be directed toward assessing whether the serum testosterone level has reached the normal range and whether symptoms have improved. If the symptoms are sexual libido or erectile dysfunction, patients are more likely to appreciate the effects of treatment on them. However, symptoms such as changes in body composition, bone mineral density, lean body mass, and muscle strength are difficult for the patient to appreciate immediately and require an assessment of the treatment effects and feedback on the test results. This increases the patient's satisfaction with treatment and induces self-awareness for improvement in symptoms. If there is an improvement in the subjective symptoms after treatment without any change in serum testosterone levels, these might be placebo effects. It is therefore advisable to discontinue TRT as recommended in the guidelines [1, 29]. In summary, the ideal goal of TRT is to focus on the recovery of serum testosterone levels. Regarding the improvement of subjective symptoms, it is recommended that patients are encouraged to be self-aware or provide feedback by appropriate tests.

Conclusion

Testosterone deficiency syndrome (TDS), also known as late-onset hypogonadism (LOH), represents a growing health concern in the aging male population. It is defined by a progressive decline in serum testosterone levels that manifests clinically as symptoms such as decreased libido, fatigue, loss of muscle mass, and impaired well-being. Accurate diagnosis requires both the recognition of characteristic symptoms and biochemical confirmation of low testosterone levels.

Testosterone replacement therapy (TRT) remains the cornerstone of management and has demonstrated significant benefits across multiple domains, including sexual function, mood, cognition, body composition, and bone health. At the same time, therapy must be individualized, as potential risks—such as cardiovascular events, prostate-related changes, and polycythemia—necessitate careful patient selection, structured monitoring, and adherence to guideline-based recommendations.

Recent evidence, particularly the TRAVERSE trial published in 2023, has provided important reassurance regarding cardiovascular safety, showing that TRT was noninferior to placebo in men with hypogonadism and preexisting or high cardiovascular risk. These findings underscore that, when appropriately indicated and closely monitored, TRT can be used safely even in patients with elevated baseline cardiovascular risk.

In conclusion, the management of TDS requires a balanced approach that integrates clinical judgment, individualized therapy, and ongoing surveillance. Patient education and regular follow-up are essential to achieving safe and effective outcomes. Continued research will further clarify the long-term benefits and risks of TRT and refine our strategies for optimizing the care of men with TDS.

References

1. Mulhall JP, Trost LW, Brannigan RE, Kurtz EG, Redmon JB, Chiles KA, et al. Evaluation and management of testosterone deficiency: AUA guideline. J Urol. 2018;200(2):423–32.
2. Khera M, Adaikan G, Buvat J, Carrier S, El-Meliegy A, Hatzimouratidis K, et al. Diagnosis and treatment of testosterone deficiency: recommendations from the fourth international consultation for sexual medicine (ICSM 2015). J Sex Med. 2016;13(12):1787–804.
3. Park HJ, Ahn ST, Moon DG. Evolution of guidelines for testosterone replacement therapy. J Clin Med. 2019;8(3)
4. Moon DG, Park HJ. The ideal goal of testosterone replacement therapy: maintaining testosterone levels or managing symptoms? J Clin Med. 2019;8(3)
5. Isidori AM, Buvat J, Corona G, Goldstein I, Jannini EA, Lenzi A, et al. A critical analysis of the role of testosterone in erectile function: from pathophysiology to treatment-a systematic review. Eur Urol. 2014;65(1):99–112.
6. Bhasin S, Brito JP, Cunningham GR, Hayes FJ, Hodis HN, Matsumoto AM, et al. Testosterone therapy in men with hypogonadism: an Endocrine Society Clinical Practice Guideline. J Clin Endocrinol Metab. 2018;103(5):1715–44.
7. Wu FC, Tajar A, Beynon JM, Pye SR, Silman AJ, Finn JD, et al. Identification of late-onset hypogonadism in middle-aged and elderly men. N Engl J Med. 2010;363(2):123–35.
8. McLachlan RI, Allan CA. Defining the prevalence and incidence of androgen deficiency in aging men: where are the goal posts? J Clin Endocrinol Metab. 2004;89(12):5916–9.
9. Feldman HA, Longcope C, Derby CA, Johannes CB, Araujo AB, Coviello AD, et al. Age trends in the level of serum testosterone and other hormones in middle-aged men: longitudinal results from the Massachusetts male aging study. J Clin Endocrinol Metab. 2002;87(2):589–98.

10. Harman SM, Metter EJ, Tobin JD, Pearson J, Blackman MR, Baltimore Longitudinal Study of A. Longitudinal effects of aging on serum total and free testosterone levels in healthy men. Baltimore Longitudinal Study of Aging. J Clin Endocrinol Metab. 2001;86(2):724–31.
11. Grossmann M, Matsumoto AM. A perspective on middle-aged and older men with functional hypogonadism: focus on holistic management. J Clin Endocrinol Metab. 2017;102(3):1067–75.
12. Zitzmann M. The role of the CAG repeat androgen receptor polymorphism in andrology. Front Horm Res. 2009;37:52–61.
13. Giwercman A, Rylander L, Lundberg GY. Influence of endocrine disruptors on human male fertility. Reprod Biomed Online. 2007;15(6):633–42.
14. Mulhall JP, Trost LW, Brannigan RE, et al. Evaluation and Management of Testosterone Deficiency: AUA guideline. J Urol. 2018;200(2):423–32.
15. Kwong JCC, Krakowsky Y, Grober E. Testosterone deficiency: a review and comparison of current guidelines. J Sex Med. 2019;16(6):812–20.
16. McBride JA, Carson CC, Coward RM. Diagnosis and management of testosterone deficiency. Asian J Androl. 2015;17(2):177–86.
17. Salter CA, Mulhall JP. Guideline of guidelines: testosterone therapy for testosterone deficiency. BJU Int. 2019;124(5):722–9.
18. Minhas S, Bettocchi C, Boeri L, Capogrosso P, Carvalho J, Cilesiz NC, et al. European Association of Urology guidelines on male sexual and reproductive health: 2021 update on male infertility. Eur Urol. 2021;80(5):603–20.
19. Lee DS, Park HJ. Efficacy and safety of testosterone therapy based on guideline recommendations; re: clinical practice guideline by the American College of Physicians. World J Mens Health. 2020;38(4):397–401.
20. Rivero MJ, Ory J, Diaz P, Thirumavalavan N, Han S, Reis IM, et al. Comparison of hematocrit change in testosterone-deficient men treated with intranasal testosterone gel vs intramuscular testosterone Cypionate: a randomized clinical trial. J Urol. 2023;210(1):162–70.
21. Kang B, Noh M, Park HJ. Compliance with testosterone replacement therapy in patients with testosterone deficiency syndrome: a 10-year observational study in Korea. World J Mens Health. 2022;40(4):686–92.
22. Corona G, Guaraldi F, Rastrelli G, Sforza A, Maggi M. Testosterone deficiency and risk of cognitive disorders in aging males. World J Mens Health. 2021;39(1):9–18.
23. Shin MJ, Jeon YK, Kim IJ. Testosterone and sarcopenia. World J Mens Health. 2018;36(3):192–8.
24. Morgentaler A, Miner MM, Caliber M, Guay AT, Khera M, Traish AM. Testosterone therapy and cardiovascular risk: advances and controversies. Mayo Clin Proc. 2015;90(2):224–51.
25. Lincoff AM, Bhasin S, Flevaris P, Mitchell LM, Basaria S, Boden WE, et al. Cardiovascular safety of testosterone-replacement therapy. N Engl J Med. 2023;389(2):107–17.
26. Kim SD, Cho KS. Obstructive sleep apnea and testosterone deficiency. World J Mens Health. 2019;37(1):12–8.
27. Saad F, Aversa A, Isidori AM, Zafalon L, Zitzmann M, Gooren L. Onset of effects of testosterone treatment and time span until maximum effects are achieved. Eur J Endocrinol. 2011;165(5):675–85.
28. Elliott J, Kelly SE, Millar AC, Peterson J, Chen L, Johnston A, et al. Testosterone therapy in hypogonadal men: a systematic review and network meta-analysis. BMJ Open. 2017;7(11):e015284.
29. Dean JD, McMahon CG, Guay AT, Morgentaler A, Althof SE, Becher EF, et al. The international society for sexual medicine's process of care for the assessment and management of testosterone deficiency in adult men. J Sex Med. 2015;12(8):1660–86.

Chapter 14
Sexual Pain in Men

Marwan Alkassis and Omer A. Raheem

Introduction

"Sexual pain" in men is a very vague entity. In fact, it could indicate discomfort or pain in the genital area independent of sexual activity, or it could designate pain during physical activity marked by painful erection and painful ejaculation. Sexual pain is a multifactorial condition with significant physical and psychosocial consequences. It may present as penile, scrotal, ejaculatory, or erectile pain and can arise from diverse etiologies.

Conditions Associated with Sexual Pain in Men

Vasectomy Vasectomy is a sterilization technique consisting in ligating both vas deferens. This surgical procedure can lead to post-vasectomy pain syndrome, which is a chronic complication characterized by an intermittent or constant testicular pain persisting for more than 3 months [4]. This pain can be unilateral or bilateral and is associated with painful ejaculation and pain on physical activity, like sexual intercourse. The prevalence of PVPS varies, with up to 33% of men reporting some level of chronic scrotal discomfort, while approximately 1% to 6% experience clinically significant pain that may impair quality of life. Preventive strategies include optimizing surgical techniques—such as using open-ended or fascial interposition

M. Alkassis
Department of Urology, University of Illinois Chicago, Chicago, IL, USA

O. A. Raheem (✉)
Department of Urology, Integrated Surgical Institute, Cleveland Clinic, Abu Dhabi, United Arab Emirates
e-mail: raheemo@ccad.ae

R. Shah et al. (eds.), *Diagnosis and Treatment of Male Sexual Dysfunction*,
https://doi.org/10.1007/978-3-032-12423-4_14

methods—minimally invasive approaches like the no-scalpel technique, and providing thorough preoperative counselling to manage patient expectations and identify those at higher risk. Additionally, effective postoperative care, including rest, scrotal support, and anti-inflammatory medications, along with early intervention for acute complications, may reduce the likelihood of developing PVPS [4].

Inguinal Hernia The definition of sexual pain related to inguinal hernia remains unclear. In fact, authors used multiple definitions to describe this entity. While some define it as erectile or ejaculatory pain [53], others describe it as pain in the groin, scrotum, penile shaft, glans, and the suprapubic area during sexual activity [11, 20, 57].

Pudendal Nerve Entrapment Pudendal nerve entrapment or pudendal neuralgia is responsible for multiple sexual symptoms such as persistent genital arousal, erectile dysfunction, premature ejaculation, ejaculatory pain, as well as pain including the glans penis, the scrotum, and the perineum [3, 45]. Patients describe a burning, tingling, or stabbing pain that progresses throughout the day, which can also appear after ejaculation or may worsen during intercourse [31].

Peyronie's Disease Peyronie's disease is a progressive fibrotic disorder affecting the tunica albuginea of the penis and is characterized by an acute and a chronic phase. The acute phase corresponds to the inflammatory phase and the plaque formation and involves penile pain during erection and intercourse [16]. During the chronic phase, the inflammation attenuates and the plaque becomes palpable. Contrary to popular belief, the rigid albuginea plaque in the chronic phase may lead to penile pain with rigid erection.

Chronic Prostatitis/Chronic Pelvic Pain Syndrome Chronic prostatitis/chronic pelvic pain syndrome (CP/CPPS) corresponds to the National Institutes of Health (NIH) type III prostatitis [27]. It is characterized by abdominal, pelvic, and genital pain in the absence of a bacterial infection [58]. Besides anatomical pain, ejaculatory pain is a common feature of CP/CPPS and could affect 24 to 50% of males with this syndrome [9, 47].

Ejaculatory Duct Obstruction Ejaculatory duct obstruction corresponds to the partial or complete obstruction of one or both ejaculatory ducts [52]. Based on the type and location of the obstruction, patients can experience multiple symptoms such as oligoasthenospermia, hematospermia, infertility, and painful ejaculation [22].

Infection and Inflammation of the Uro-genital Tract Infection of the prostate, testis, epididymis, and urethra by common or sexually transmitted germs is responsible lower urinary tract symptoms and ejaculatory pain [42]. Prostatitis can lead to ejaculatory pain and pain during anal intercourse in men who have sex with pain, while orchitis, epididymitis, and orchi-epididymitis are responsible for contact pain.

Some sexually transmitted diseases like genital herpes and chancroid caused by *H. ducreyi* lead to painful skin lesions preventing sexual intercourse [14].

Genital Skin Lesions Lichen sclerosus is a chronic dermatologic condition characterized inflammation and white, sclerotic plaques affecting the prepuce and glans penis [40]. This condition leads to meatal structure resulting in lower urinary tract symptoms as well as genital scarring and severe phimosis leading to painful erection and intercourse [12].

Diagnosis of Sexual Pain in Men

Evaluation of sexual pain in men can be challenging because an underlying cause is not always present. A thorough history and physical exam are needed to guide the clinician toward the possible etiology as they provide information regarding the pain characteristics as well as the associated symptoms and comorbidities.

A history of vasectomy and a scrotal pain appearing afterward indicates a probable post-vasectomy pain syndrome, encountered in 15% of men after vasectomy [4]. An inguinal hernia on physical exam or a history of hernia repair might indicate the reason for the sexual pain that might present as erectile or ejaculatory pain or pain in the groin or perineal area [53]. However, these diagnoses remain diagnoses of exclusion, and more serious and evident causes should be ruled out first.

Chronic pelvic pain syndrome is another diagnosis of exclusion, as it implies a pain in the pelvic is lasting for a minimum of three months in the absence of malignancy, infection, neurologic disease, and any anatomical or functional pelvic disorder.

Urine culture can help ruling out or confirming a urinary tract infection, and in case of a suspected sexually transmitted disease, special cultures, Nucleic Acid Amplification Test (NAAT), and polymerase chain reaction can help in identifying the offending agent.

Penile inspection can identify characteristic sexually transmitted disease. Genital herpes appear as vesicles with yellowish content, grouped "in clusters" on an erythematous base that will rupture and form ulcers. Chancroid presents as erythematous papules that will transform into pustules that will rupture leading to ulcers with pyonecrotic exudate [14].

Peyronie's disease assessment should focus on the presence of actual pain as this might indicate an acute phase [56]. Physical exam should focus on assessing the penile length and the localization of the plaque if the patient is seen during the chronic phase. A penile duplex ultrasound can help in assessing the degree of the curvature, the identification of the penile plaque, and the vascular flow rate.

Pudendal disease entrapment can lead to multiple sexual dysfunction in men and women [3]. The pain associated with pudendal neuralgia is described as burning, tingling, or stabbing appearing in the scrotum, the glans, and the perineum. This pain characteristic might guide the clinician toward a neurologic cause. Pudendal neuralgia is diagnosed based on the Nantes criteria: (1) pain in the anatomical territory of the pudendal nerve, (2) worsened by sitting, (3) the patient is not woken at night by the pain, (4) no objective sensory loss on clinical examination, and (5) positive anesthetic pudendal nerve block [29]. It is worthy to note that a normal imaging, not explaining the patient's symptoms, is required to proceed with the pudendal neuralgia diagnosis.

Ejaculatory duct obstruction is usually diagnosed during infertility workup and semen analysis abnormalities; however, patients may report hematospermia and ejaculatory pain [22]. Ejaculatory duct obstruction can be acquired or congenital. In case of congenital obstruction, the clinician should evaluate for the cystic fibrosis gene mutation because cystic fibrosis is present in 50% of the patient with idiopathic obstruction of the ejaculatory duct [23]. Diagnosis of ejaculatory duct obstruction is based on the trans-rectal ultrasound showing a seminal vesicle width greater than 1.5 cm or ejaculatory duct diameter greater than 2.3 mm. Trans-rectal ultrasound can also show a cyst or calcification along the duct, which helps in confirming the diagnosis [35, 52]. Complementary procedures such as seminal vesicle aspiration, seminal vesiculography, and chromotubation can help in confirming the diagnosis.

Treatment of Sexual Pain in Men

Post-vasectomy pain syndrome remains a rare, yet a challenging complication of vasectomy, and the literature tackling the treatment of this syndrome is rare. Post-vasectomy pain syndrome should initially be treated as idiopathic testicular pain with non-steroidal anti-inflammatory drugs over a period of 2–4 weeks. In the absence of relief, patients should be treated with tricyclic antidepressant (amitriptyline) or anticonvulsant (gabapentin or pregabalin). These drugs have proven to be effective on idiopathic and neurologic testicular pain; however, patients with post-vasectomy pain syndrome do not show much improvement [49]. If medical therapy fails, Tan et Levine proposed to re-assess the exact location of the pain [55]. If the pain is localized at the transected vas, a vasectomy reversal should be attempted, followed by microdenervation of the spermatic cord and orchiectomy if the pain persists. In case of a diffuse pain along the cord or testicle, patients who improve more than 90% after cord block should proceed with microdenervation of the spermatic cord followed by orchiectomy if no improvement. Patients who do not improve with cord block should remain on medical therapy and associated pelvic floor physical therapy, radiofrequency, or acupuncture, leaving the microdenervation of the cord and orchiectomy as last resorts.

Vasectomy reversal, whether by vasovasostomy or vasoepididymostomy, has been evaluated in multiple series. Myers et al. showed that 84% of men operated with vasectomy reversal were satisfied or pain free following the procedure, knowing that three of these patients required a second vasectomy reversal [38]. Lee et al. reported a satisfaction rate in all the 22 operated patients after a mean follow-up of

3.22 years [30]. Polackwich et al. reported the longest follow-up (8.4 years) with a rate of satisfaction of 80.6%, showing that the benefit of vasectomy reversal on post-vasectomy pain syndrome remains after many years [44].

Laparoscopic or open hernia repair are associated with an improvement in sexual pain. Some authors suggest that minimally invasive surgery has an advantage over open surgery in reducing sexual pain [6, 20, 57]; however, others did not find a difference between both techniques [54]. Hernia repair can be a double-edged blade as it could lead to de-novo sexual pain especially with the open technique, and patients should be informed about this risk during the preoperative discussions [11, 53].

Pudendal nerve entrapment could lead to debilitating sexual symptoms including genital pain. Pharmacologic treatments should be tried first and consist primarily in tricyclic antidepressants and antiepileptic agents [26]. Pudendal nerve infiltration remains a good option for the short term as it provides symptoms improvement up to 82% after the procedure, declining to 62% at 3 months and 12% at 1 year [59]. Surgical decompression of the pudendal nerve remains the last resort. Laparoscopic pudendal nerve release consists in releasing the pudendal nerve below the sacrospinous ligament or at the entry of the Alcock's canal [10]. This technique has proven to be effective in reducing sexual symptoms as well as sexual pain in men and women [3, 10].

Peyronie's disease treatment depends on the sexual function limitation, the degree of bother, and the phase of disease. It includes observation, oral agents, topical therapies, shock wave therapy, mechanical therapy, intralesional injections, and surgery [64]. Observation is a good option in patients with minimal bother; however, they should be monitored regularly as symptom progression varies between 42% and 48% [19, 37]. While the AUA has recommended against the use of tamoxifen, vitamin E, omega-3-fatty acids, procarbazine, and vitamin E/L combination [39], some experts continue to use oral therapy. In fact, the association of pentoxifylline, L-citrulline, and tadalafil daily in case of associated erectile dysfunction seems to yield good results [60]. Topical treatments such as verapamil alone, verapamil associated with electromotive drug administration to help in tissue penetration, and a combination of nicardipine, superoxide dismutase, and emu oil have been studied as therapeutic options for Peyronie's disease. However, the AUA do not recommend these treatments due to the lack of supportive data [39]. Shock wave treatment has yielded satisfactory results regarding the pain and the size of the plaque [18, 28], but it is not recommended for the treatment of penile curvature [39]. Mechanical therapy consists in vacuum therapy or penile traction therapy and may be used as monotherapy or in association with other treatment modalities [64]. Mechanical therapy has proved to improve penile curvature and stretched penile length [36, 62, 63]. There is no consensus on the duration of the applied traction; however, mechanical therapy seems to be an interesting therapeutic modality that needs further investigation. Injecting drugs directly into the plaque provide some benefits, and agents used include verapamil, interferon alfa 2b, and Collagenase Clostridium histolyticum [46]. Verapamil may be indicated for penile pain, while interferon alfa 2b has proven to be effective for penile pain and restoring penile length [21, 24, 39]. Collagenase

Clostridium histolyticum injection is a promising therapeutic option, especially in decreasing penile curvature. However, care must be taken to the side effects consisting mainly of penile ecchymosis and swelling [64]. Surgical treatment is considered in severe penile curvature and indentation deformity making sexual intercourse difficult, and it should be considered during the chronic phase of the disease [13]. Surgical techniques consist of penile plication or corporoplasty, plaque incision or partial excision with grafting, and penile prosthesis placement with straightening maneuvers; each one has its own indications and risks [64].

Chronic prostatitis/Chronic pelvic pain syndrome can be challenging to treat. Phenotypically directed multimodal therapy has provided some improvement in understanding and management of pelvic pain syndrome [48]. Pelvic floor physiotherapy and physical activity help reduce pelvic pain and improve quality of life, as patients with chronic pelvic pain syndrome have often pelvic floor muscle dysfunction [43]. Early identification and management of associated psychological comorbidities such as depression and anxiety plays a crucial role in the management of pelvic pain syndrome, and psychological interventions may reduce pain and its associated healthcare burden [7]. Simple analgesics like paracetamol and nonsteroidal anti-inflammatory drugs may be used; however, data regarding their specific use in chronic pelvic pain syndrome is missing. While neuromodulators like tricyclic antidepressants and anticonvulsants may be more useful, care should be taken because of their frequent side effects [32, 61]. α-Blockers, such as terazosin, alfuzosin, doxazosin, tamsulosin, and silodosin have shown to reduce pelvic pain and voiding symptoms [2]. 5-α-Reductase inhibitors are recommended for chronic pelvic pain syndrome [2]. A trial of antibiotics (quinolones for six weeks or tetracycline for 12 weeks) may improve pelvic pain symptoms; however, persistence of symptoms after six weeks should warrant change of treatment, and caution in avoiding unnecessary antibiotic use should be taken to prevent bacterial resistance.

Ejaculatory Duct Obstruction Transurethral resection of the ejaculatory ducts (TURED) is the mainstay treatment for ejaculatory duct obstruction. Care should be taken to avoid the bladder neck and the external urinary sphincter, as well as coagulation should be limited to avoid secondary stenosis [5]. Ejaculatory duct desobstruction does not just improve fertility, but it helps in reducing sexual symptoms. Some reports showed that TURED improved testicular pain in patients with ejaculatory duct obstruction [34]. Another therapeutic surgical modalities include incision using the cold-knife [17], or a combination of hook electrode and endoscissors [33]. These treatments showed an improvement in semen analysis, hematospermia, and painful ejaculation.

Infection and inflammation of the uro-genital tract which includes bacterial prostatitis, epididymitis, orchitis, and orchi-epididymitis are treated with antibiotics depending and the urine culture results and the susceptibility profile. Duration of the treatment depends on the antibacterial agent used and the frequency of infection. For example, acute bacterial prostatitis are treated with fluoroquinolones for at least 14 days, while azithromycin and doxycycline treatments should be extended to at least three to four weeks [50, 51]. Chancroid are treated with azithromycin 1 g orally in a single dose or ceftriaxone 250 mg IM in a single dose or ciprofloxacin 500 mg orally twice a day for 3 days [1]. Genital herpes are treated with acyclovir, valacyclovir, or famciclovir [8].

In *Genital skin lesions* like lichen sclerosus, treatment is crucial to preserve quality of life and to avoid urinary and sexual dysfunction [25]. Local treatments are considered first-line therapy and consist in topical corticosteroid or topical calcineurin inhibitors [25, 41]. Systemic treatments such as pulsed high-dose corticosteroid with low-dose methotrexate or systemic retinoid are indicated if widespread lichen sclerosus is present or if disease is resistant to topical treatment [15]. Complete circumcision is indicated if the patient remains symptomatic after a sufficient conservative treatment. Complete foreskin removal significantly decreases the recurrence of the disease [25].

I reviewed the uploaded chapter "*Sexual Pain in Men*" and drafted a *Concluding Section* that synthesizes the main points in a formal, textbook-appropriate style:

Conclusion

Sexual pain in men is a complex, multifactorial clinical entity that demands careful evaluation and a multidisciplinary approach. Although often underrecognized, it significantly impacts quality of life, psychological well-being, and intimate relationships. Etiologies range from urologic and dermatologic conditions to musculoskeletal, neurologic, and psychogenic factors, underscoring the importance of a comprehensive diagnostic framework.

Successful management requires individualized treatment strategies, guided by accurate diagnosis and attention to both physical and psychosocial contributors. Advances in minimally invasive therapies, pharmacologic interventions, and psychosexual counseling continue to expand the therapeutic landscape. At the same time, barriers such as stigma, underreporting, and limited provider familiarity hinder timely recognition and intervention.

Ultimately, optimizing outcomes for men with sexual pain rests on improving awareness among clinicians, fostering collaboration across specialties, and advancing research into pathophysiology and evidence-based treatment algorithms. By integrating clinical vigilance with empathetic patient-centered care, providers can better address this challenging and often overlooked domain of male sexual health.

References

1. Ahmed J, Rawre J, Dhawan N, Dudani P, Khanna N, Dhawan B. Genital ulcer disease: a review. J Family Med Prim Care. 2022;11(8):4255–62. https://doi.org/10.4103/jfmpc.jfmpc_2111_21.
2. Anothaisintawee T, Attia J, Nickel JC, Thammakraisorn S, Numthavaj P, McEvoy M, Thakkinstian A. Management of chronic prostatitis/chronic pelvic pain syndrome: a system-

atic review and network meta-analysis. JAMA. 2011;305(1):78–86. https://doi.org/10.1001/jama.2010.1913.
3. Aoun F, Alkassis M, Tayeh GA, Chebel JA, Semaan A, Sarkis J, Mansour R, Mjaess G, Albisinni S, Absil F, Bollens R, Roumeguère T. Sexual dysfunction due to pudendal neuralgia: a systematic review. Transl Androl Urol. 2021;10(6):2500–11. https://doi.org/10.21037/tau-21-13.
4. Auyeung AB, Almejally A, Alsaggar F, Doyle F. Incidence of post-vasectomy pain: systematic review and meta-analysis. Int J Environ Res Public Health. 2020;17(5):1788. https://doi.org/10.3390/ijerph17051788.
5. Avellino GJ, Lipshultz LI, Sigman M, Hwang K. Transurethral resection of the ejaculatory ducts: etiology of obstruction and surgical treatment options. Fertil Steril. 2019;111(3):427–43. https://doi.org/10.1016/j.fertnstert.2019.01.001.
6. Aykanat IC, Er S, Senel C, Comcali B, Aslan Y, Balci M, Yuksel BC, Tuncel A. Comparison of the impact of open and laparoscopic inguinal hernia operations on male sexual function and pain during sexual activity. Andrologia. 2022;54(1):e14254. https://doi.org/10.1111/and.14254.
7. Bajaj P, Bajaj P, Madsen H, Arendt-Nielsen L. Endometriosis is associated with central sensitization: a psychophysical controlled study. J Pain. 2003;4(7):372–80. https://doi.org/10.1016/s1526-5900(03)00720-x.
8. Batteiger TA, Rietmeijer CA. Herpes simplex virus: a practical guide to diagnosis, management, and patient counseling for the primary care clinician. Med Clin North Am. 2024;108(2):311–23. https://doi.org/10.1016/j.mcna.2023.08.016.
9. Blanker MH, Bosch JL, Groeneveld FP, Bohnen AM, Prins A, Thomas S, Hop WC. Erectile and ejaculatory dysfunction in a community-based sample of men 50 to 78 years old: prevalence, concern, and relation to sexual activity. Urology. 2001;57(4):763–8. https://doi.org/10.1016/s0090-4295(00)01091-8.
10. Bollens R, Mjaess G, Sarkis J, Chemaly AK, Nemr E, Daher K, Semaan A, Chebel JA, Absil F, Aoun F. Laparoscopic transperitoneal pudendal nerve and artery release for pudendal entrapment syndrome. Surg Endosc. 2021;35(11):6031–8. https://doi.org/10.1007/s00464-020-08092-4.
11. Calisir A, Ece I, Yilmaz H, Alptekin H, Colak B, Yormaz S, Gul M, Sahin M. Pain during sexual activity and ejaculation following hernia repair: a retrospective comparison of transabdominal preperitoneal versus Lichtenstein repair. Andrologia. 2021;53(2):e13947. https://doi.org/10.1111/and.13947.
12. Charlton OA, Smith SD. Balanitis xerotica obliterans: a review of diagnosis and management. Int J Dermatol. 2019;58(7):777–81. https://doi.org/10.1111/ijd.14236.
13. Chung E, Wang R, Ralph D, Levine L, Brock G. A worldwide survey on Peyronie's disease surgical practice patterns among surgeons. J Sex Med. 2018;15(4):568–75. https://doi.org/10.1016/j.jsxm.2018.01.025.
14. Cunha Ramos M, Nicola MRC, Bezerra NTC, Sardinha JCG, Sampaio de Souza Morais J, Schettini AP. Genital ulcers caused by sexually transmitted agents. An Bras Dermatol. 2022;97(5):551–65. https://doi.org/10.1016/j.abd.2022.01.004.
15. De Luca DA, Papara C, Vorobyev A, Staiger H, Bieber K, Thaçi D, Ludwig RJ. Lichen sclerosus: the 2023 update. Front Med (Lausanne). 2023;10:1106318. https://doi.org/10.3389/fmed.2023.1106318.
16. Di Maida F, Cito G, Lambertini L, Valastro F, Morelli G, Mari A, Carini M, Minervini A, Cocci A. The natural history of Peyronie's disease. World J Mens Health. 2021;39(3):399–405. https://doi.org/10.5534/wjmh.200065.
17. Fuse H, Nishio R, Murakami K, Okumura A. Transurethral incision for Hematospermia caused by ejaculatory duct obstruction. Arch Androl. 2003;49(6):433–8. https://doi.org/10.1080/01485010390219890.
18. Gao L, Qian S, Tang Z, Li J, Yuan J. A meta-analysis of extracorporeal shock wave therapy for Peyronie's disease. Int J Impot Res. 2016;28(5):161–6. https://doi.org/10.1038/ijir.2016.24.

19. Gelbard MK, Dorey F, James K. The natural history of Peyronie's disease. J Urol. 1990;144(6):1376–9. https://doi.org/10.1016/s0022-5347(17)39746-x.
20. Gutlic A, Rogmark P, Gutlic N, Petersson U, Montgomery A. Pain with sexual activity at 1 and 3 years: comparing total extraperitoneal with Lichtenstein inguinal hernia repair in a randomized setting (TEPLICH trial). Surgery. 2022;172(5):1463–70. https://doi.org/10.1016/j.surg.2022.07.013.
21. Hellstrom WJG, Kendirci M, Matern R, Cockerham Y, Myers L, Sikka SC, Venable D, Honig S, McCullough A, Hakim LS, Nehra A, Templeton LE, Pryor JL. Single-blind, multicenter, placebo controlled, parallel study to assess the safety and efficacy of intralesional interferon alpha-2B for minimally invasive treatment for Peyronie's disease. J Urol. 2006;176(1):394–8. https://doi.org/10.1016/S0022-5347(06)00517-9.
22. Ilie CP, Mischianu DL, Pemberton RJ. Painful ejaculation. BJU Int. 2007;99(6):1335–9. https://doi.org/10.1111/j.1464-410X.2007.06664.x.
23. Jarvi K, Zielenski J, Wilschanski M, Durie P, Buckspan M, Tullis E, Markiewicz D, Tsui L-C. Cystic fibrosis transmembrane conductance regulator and obstructive azoospermia. Lancet. 1995;345(8964):1578. https://doi.org/10.1016/S0140-6736(95)91131-6.
24. Kendirci M, Usta MF, Matern RV, Nowfar S, Sikka SC, Hellstrom WJG. The impact of intralesional interferon alpha-2b injection therapy on penile hemodynamics in men with Peyronie's disease. J Sex Med. 2005;2(5):709–15. https://doi.org/10.1111/j.1743-6109.2005.00110.x.
25. Kirtschig G, Becker K, Günthert A, Jasaitiene D, Cooper S, Chi C-C, Kreuter A, Rall KK, Aberer W, Riechardt S, Casabona F, Powell J, Brackenbury F, Erdmann R, Lazzeri M, Barbagli G, Wojnarowska F. Evidence-based (S3) guideline on (anogenital) lichen sclerosus. J Eur Acad Dermatol Venereol. 2015;29(10):e1–43. https://doi.org/10.1111/jdv.13136.
26. Knowles CH, Cohen RC. Chronic anal pain: a review of causes, diagnosis, and treatment. Cleve Clin J Med. 2022;89(6):336–43. https://doi.org/10.3949/ccjm.89a.21102.
27. Krieger JN, Nyberg L, Nickel JC. NIH consensus definition and classification of prostatitis. JAMA. 1999;282(3):236–7. https://doi.org/10.1001/jama.282.3.236.
28. Krieger JR, Rizk PJ, Kohn TP, Pastuszak A. Shockwave therapy in the treatment of Peyronie's disease. Sex Med Rev. 2019;7(3):499–507. https://doi.org/10.1016/j.sxmr.2019.02.001.
29. Labat J-J, Riant T, Robert R, Amarenco G, Lefaucheur J-P, Rigaud J. Diagnostic criteria for pudendal neuralgia by pudendal nerve entrapment (Nantes criteria). Neurourol Urodyn. 2008;27(4):306–10. https://doi.org/10.1002/nau.20505.
30. Lee JY, Chang JS, Lee SH, Ham WS, Cho HJ, Yoo TK, Lee KS, Kim TH, Moon HS, Choi HY, Lee SW. Efficacy of vasectomy reversal according to patency for the surgical treatment of postvasectomy pain syndrome. Int J Impot Res. 2012;24(5):202–5. https://doi.org/10.1038/ijir.2012.17.
31. Leslie SW, Antolak S, Feloney MP, Soon-Sutton TL (2023) Pudendal neuralgia. In: StatPearls. Treasure Island (FL): StatPearls Publishing.
32. Lunn MPT, Hughes RAC, Wiffen PJ. Duloxetine for treating painful neuropathy, chronic pain or fibromyalgia. Cochrane Database Syst Rev. 2014;2014(1):CD007115. https://doi.org/10.1002/14651858.CD007115.pub3.
33. Manohar T, Ganpule A, Desai M. Transrectal ultrasound- and fluoroscopic-assisted transurethral incision of ejaculatory ducts: a problem-solving approach to nonmalignant hematospermia due to ejaculatory duct obstruction. J Endourol. 2008;22(7):1531–5. https://doi.org/10.1089/end.2007.0415.
34. Medeiros Lacerda JI, Hasegawa E, Fraietta R, Bertolla RP, Cedenho AP, Ortiz V. Transurethral resection of the ejaculatory duct in a fertile man. Fertil Steril. 2008;89(5):1260.e13–5. https://doi.org/10.1016/j.fertnstert.2007.05.006.
35. Modgil V, Rai S, Ralph DJ, Muneer A. An update on the diagnosis and management of ejaculatory duct obstruction. Nat Rev Urol. 2016;13(1):13–20. https://doi.org/10.1038/nrurol.2015.276.
36. Moncada I, Krishnappa P, Romero J, Torremade J, Fraile A, Martinez-Salamanca JI, Porst H, Levine L. Penile traction therapy with the new device "Penimaster PRO" is effective

and safe in the stable phase of Peyronie's disease: a controlled multicentre study. BJU Int. 2019;123(4):694–702. https://doi.org/10.1111/bju.14602.
37. Mulhall JP, Schiff J, Guhring P. An analysis of the natural history of Peyronie's disease. J Urol. 2006;175(6):2115–8; discussion 2118. https://doi.org/10.1016/S0022-5347(06)00270-9.
38. Myers SA, Mershon CE, Fuchs EF. Vasectomy reversal for treatment of the post-vasectomy pain syndrome. J Urol. 1997;157(2):518–20.
39. Nehra A, Alterowitz R, Culkin DJ, Faraday MM, Hakim LS, Heidelbaugh JJ, Khera M, Kirkby E, McVary KT, Miner MM, Nelson CJ, Sadeghi-Nejad H, Seftel AD, Shindel AW, Burnett AL, American Urological Association Education and Research, Inc. Peyronie's disease: AUA guideline. J Urol. 2015;194(3):745–53. https://doi.org/10.1016/j.juro.2015.05.098.
40. Nguyen ATM, Holland AJA. Balanitis xerotica obliterans: an update for clinicians. Eur J Pediatr. 2020;179(1):9–16. https://doi.org/10.1007/s00431-019-03516-3.
41. Papini M, Russo A, Simonetti O, Borghi A, Corazza M, Piaserico S, Feliciani C, Calzavara-Pinton P, Mucous Membrane Disorders Research Group of SIDeMaST. Diagnosis and management of cutaneous and anogenital lichen sclerosus: recommendations from the Italian Society of Dermatology (SIDeMaST). Ital J Dermatol Venerol. 2021;156(5):519–33. https://doi.org/10.23736/S2784-8671.21.06764-X.
42. Parnham A, Serefoglu EC. Retrograde ejaculation, painful ejaculation and hematospermia. Transl Androl Urol. 2016;5(4):592–601. https://doi.org/10.21037/tau.2016.06.05.
43. Parsons BA, Baranowski AP, Berghmans B, Borovicka J, Cottrell AM, Dinis-Oliveira P, Elneil S, Hughes J, Messelink BEJ, de C Williams AC, Abreu-Mendes P, Zumstein V, Engeler DS. Management of chronic primary pelvic pain syndromes. BJU Int. 2022;129(5):572–81. https://doi.org/10.1111/bju.15609.
44. Polackwich AS, Tadros NN, Ostrowski KA, Kent J, Conlin MJ, Hedges JC, Fuchs EF. Vasectomy reversal for Postvasectomy pain syndrome: a study and literature review. Urology. 2015;86(2):269–72. https://doi.org/10.1016/j.urology.2015.04.013.
45. Robert R, Prat-Pradal D, Labat JJ, Bensignor M, Raoul S, Rebai R, Leborgne J. Anatomic basis of chronic perineal pain: role of the pudendal nerve. Surg Radiol Anat. 1998;20(2):93–8. https://doi.org/10.1007/BF01628908.
46. Russo GI, Milenkovic U, Hellstrom W, Levine LA, Ralph D, Albersen M. Clinical efficacy of injection and mechanical therapy for Peyronie's disease: a systematic review of the literature. Eur Urol. 2018;74(6):767–81. https://doi.org/10.1016/j.eururo.2018.07.005.
47. Shoskes DA, Landis JR, Wang Y, Nickel JC, Zeitlin SI, Nadler R, Chronic Prostatitis Collaborative Research Network Study Group. Impact of post-ejaculatory pain in men with category III chronic prostatitis/chronic pelvic pain syndrome. J Urol. 2004;172(2):542–7. https://doi.org/10.1097/01.ju.0000132798.48067.23.
48. Shoskes DA, Nickel JC, Kattan MW. Phenotypically directed multimodal therapy for chronic prostatitis/chronic pelvic pain syndrome: a prospective study using UPOINT. Urology. 2010;75(6):1249–53. https://doi.org/10.1016/j.urology.2010.01.021.
49. Sinclair AM, Miller B, Lee LK. Chronic orchialgia: consider gabapentin or nortriptyline before considering surgery. Int J Urol. 2007;14(7):622–5. https://doi.org/10.1111/j.1442-2042.2007.01745.x.
50. Skerk V, Krhen I, Schonwald S, Cajic V, Markovinovic L, Roglic S, Zekan S, Andracevic AT, Kruzic V. The role of unusual pathogens in prostatitis syndrome. Int J Antimicrob Agents. 2004;24(Suppl 1):S53–6. https://doi.org/10.1016/j.ijantimicag.2004.02.010.
51. Skerk V, Schönwald S, Krhen I, Banaszak A, Begovac J, Strugar J, Strapac Z, Vrsalovic R, Vukovic J, Tomas M. Comparative analysis of azithromycin and ciprofloxacin in the treatment of chronic prostatitis caused by Chlamydia trachomatis. Int J Antimicrob Agents. 2003;21(5):457–62. https://doi.org/10.1016/s0924-8579(03)00056-6.
52. Smith JF, Walsh TJ, Turek PJ. Ejaculatory duct obstruction. Urol Clin N Am. 2008;35(2):221–7. https://doi.org/10.1016/j.ucl.2008.01.011.
53. Ssentongo AE, Kwon EG, Zhou S, Ssentongo P, Soybel DI. Pain and dysfunction with sexual activity after inguinal hernia repair: systematic review and meta-analysis. J Am Coll Surg. 2020;230(2):237–250.e7. https://doi.org/10.1016/j.jamcollsurg.2019.10.010.

54. Supsamutchai C, Wattanapreechanon P, Saengsri S, Wilasrusmee C, Poprom N. Sexual dysfunction between laparoscopic and open inguinal hernia repair: a systematic review and meta-analysis. Langenbeck's Arch Surg. 2023;408(1):277. https://doi.org/10.1007/s00423-023-03006-z.
55. Tan WP, Levine LA. An overview of the management of post-vasectomy pain syndrome. Asian J Androl. 2016;18(3):332–7. https://doi.org/10.4103/1008-682X.175090.
56. Taylor FL, Levine LA. Peyronie's disease. Urol Clin North Am. 2007;34(4):517–34, vi. https://doi.org/10.1016/j.ucl.2007.08.017.
57. Tolver MA, Rosenberg J. Pain during sexual activity before and after laparoscopic inguinal hernia repair. Surg Endosc. 2015;29(12):3722–5. https://doi.org/10.1007/s00464-015-4143-8.
58. Tran CN, Shoskes DA. Sexual dysfunction in chronic prostatitis/chronic pelvic pain syndrome. World J Urol. 2013;31(4):741–6. https://doi.org/10.1007/s00345-013-1076-5.
59. Tricard T, Munier P, Story F, Lang H, Saussine C. The drug-resistant pudendal neuralgia management: a systematic review. Neurourol Urodyn. 2019;38(1):13–21. https://doi.org/10.1002/nau.23824.
60. Valente EGA, Vernet D, Ferrini MG, Qian A, Rajfer J, Gonzalez-Cadavid NF. L-arginine and phosphodiesterase (PDE) inhibitors counteract fibrosis in the Peyronie's fibrotic plaque and related fibroblast cultures. Nitric Oxide. 2003;9(4):229–44. https://doi.org/10.1016/j.niox.2003.12.002.
61. Wiffen PJ, Derry S, Moore RA, McQuay HJ. Carbamazepine for acute and chronic pain in adults. Cochrane Database Syst Rev. 2011;1:CD005451. https://doi.org/10.1002/14651858.CD005451.pub2.
62. Yafi FA, Pinsky MR, Stewart C, Sangkum P, Ates E, Trost LW, Sikka SC, Hellstrom WJG. The effect of duration of penile traction therapy in patients undergoing Intralesional injection therapy for Peyronie's disease. J Urol. 2015;194(3):754–8. https://doi.org/10.1016/j.juro.2015.03.092.
63. Ziegelmann M, Savage J, Toussi A, Alom M, Yang D, Kohler T, Trost L. Outcomes of a novel penile traction device in men with Peyronie's disease: a randomized, single-blind, controlled trial. J Urol. 2019;202(3):599–610. https://doi.org/10.1097/JU.0000000000000245.
64. Ziegelmann MJ, Bajic P, Levine LA. Peyronie's disease: contemporary evaluation and management. Int J Urol. 2020;27(6):504–16. https://doi.org/10.1111/iju.14230.

Chapter 15
Oncosexology and Oncofertility in Men

Christopher Ho Chee Kong

Introduction

Oncosexology is the field that studies the impact of cancer and its treatments on a patient's sexual health and sexuality, addressing issues like loss of libido, erectile dysfunction, and psychological impacts.

Oncofertility is the related field focused on preserving fertility in cancer patients by managing the effects of cancer treatments on reproductive health and exploring options for fertility preservation before or during treatment.

The Association Between Cancer and Male Sexual Dysfunction

Kidney Cancer and Male Sexual Dysfunction

In a study by Anastasiadis et al. on patients with kidney cancer after treatment (operation, radiation, or chemotherapy), most patients were found to have remained sexually active in non-distressed relationships, but 51% of men reported depressive symptoms, and sexual functioning may be worse than in comparable chronically ill populations [1].

In another study by Christiansen et al. who evaluated patients who underwent nephrectomy or nephroureterectomy, 54.7% of sexually active males were shown to have some degree of ED after surgery [2].

C. H. C. Kong (✉)
Department of Urology, Taylor's University, Kuala Lumpur, Malaysia

R. Shah et al. (eds.), *Diagnosis and Treatment of Male Sexual Dysfunction*, https://doi.org/10.1007/978-3-032-12423-4_15

Advanced kidney cancer treated with molecular targeted therapy (MTT); antiangiogenic therapies (sunitinib, sorafenib, and bevacizumab); and mTOR inhibitors (temsirolimus and everolimus) can lead to a decline of erectile function scores and sexual activity after treatment and negatively affect male sexual function [3, 4].

This can be attributed to the adverse effects of targeted therapy of mRCC, such as fatigue, pain, anorexia, asthenia, or hypothyroidism. In a study by Tsimafeyeu et al. involving patients with mRCC, mild erectile dysfunction (ED) was observed in 19 out of 25 treatment-naïve males, while severe ED was reported in 8 out of 25 after the first month of first-line targeted therapy [5].

Prostate Cancer (PCa) and Sexual Dysfunction

Treatment for localized prostate cancer involves surgery. Recovery of erectile function was found to be 68% of preoperatively potent men treated with bilateral and 47% treated with unilateral nerve-sparing open retropubic prostatectomy (ORP) surgery [6]. For laparoscopic radical prostatectomy (LRP), 66% had preserved erections and could engage in spontaneous intercourse. For robotic-assisted laparoscopic radical prostatectomy (RALP), 78% of patients were potent with or without the use of oral medications after one year [7]. Besides ED, patients after radical prostatectomy undergo sexual changes, which include loss of penile length, reduced sexual desire, and orgasmic dysfunction, including painful orgasm and climacturia [8–10].

ED can occur after radiotherapy (RT). This could be attributed to penile neurovascular and cavernosal damage. ED usually occurs after six months post radiation therapy as compared to radical prostatectomy, where it is an immediate side effect. Besides ED, sexual desire, sexual satisfaction, orgasmic function, and general satisfaction also occur after RT [11].

There are other treatments that have fewer sexual dysfunction side effects: For focal therapy (FT), it has been observed that sexual function returned to baseline within 9–12 months [12]. For high-intensity focused ultrasound (HIFU), erectile function was preserved in 78% of patients [13]. Androgen deprivation therapy (ADT) for patients with metastatic prostate cancer can also cause sexual dysfunction, including loss of libido and ED [14, 15].

Penile Cancer (PEC) and Sexual Dysfunction

Penile cancer is rare, and there are very few studies analyzing the impact of penile cancer on sexual dysfunction. All types of treatment for PEC can impact quality of life and sexual function. Partial or total penectomy can be associated with significant sexual dysfunction, probably due to the shame of the small penis size and the absence of the glans. Patients post partial or total penectomy have been reported to have significant reduction in erectile and orgasmic function and reduced global sexual score [16–18].

Testicular Cancer (TC) and Sexual Dysfunction

TC treatment can cause changes in body image, and this can have a negative impact on sexuality, fertility, mental health, and quality of life. Anxiety and depression seemed to be associated with impaired masculinity, sexual function, and quality of life. Changes in body image after orchiectomy can impact self-confidence and sexuality, and to mitigate this, a testicular prosthesis implant can be offered at the time of surgery [19–21]. Significantly reduced or absent orgasm and ejaculatory dysfunction can persist for up to two years after treatment [22].

Bladder Cancer and Sexual Dysfunction

Gut et al. showed that the incidence of ED increased in patients under the age of 45 years after TURBT (15.8% before vs. 52.6% after), and they concluded that psychological and emotional burdens are the main causes of sexual dysfunction in these cases [23].

Patients who received intravesical BCG might present with pelvic pain and may experience a negative impact on sexual activity after the initial treatment. ED after BCG treatment is generally transient and reversible [24–26].

Radical cystectomy (RC) is associated with ED due to surgical trauma to the neurovascular bundle. Nerve-sparing RC can often provide preservation or recovery of erectile function, and 36% of RC patients recovered sexual intercourse at 3 years and 57% at 5 years. This recovery depends on the preoperative erectile function and age of the patient. Function can be improved after sexual rehabilitation with intracavernous injection therapy or oral phosphodiesterase inhibitors after surgery [27, 28].

The type of urinary diversion can also affect sexual activity. Patients with ileal conduit diversion may have a greater impact on sexual function compared to those who underwent orthotopic diversion, likely due to depression or anxiety associated with changes in body image [29].

Trimodality therapy (TMT), which consists of maximal TURBT followed by radical RT with concurrent chemotherapy, impairs male sexual function less compared to RC. A total of 39% of men reported no erections in the past 4 weeks, 54% were capable of orgasm and 50% of ejaculation, while only 8% were dissatisfied with their sex lives [30].

The Association Between Cancer and Fertility in Men

Testicular Cancer and Fertility

Factors involved:

1. The destruction of the testicular parenchyma due to pressure effects. In the case of tumors that cause destruction of over 50% of the normal testis, a 50% reduced chance of normal spermatogenesis was found [31].
2. Neoangiogenesis causes alterations in local blood flow, which in turn elevates inner scrotal temperature; however, these concepts have not been supported by robust scientific evidence.
3. Testicular dysgenesis, which is associated with cancer, is seen with testicular hypotrophy, a history of cryptorchidism, and pre-existing infertility, which may coexist [32].
4. Testicular tumors may also secrete gonadotropins like beta-hCG, which can cause negative feedback and downregulation of the hypothalami-pituitary axis [33]. Also, elevated levels of beta-hCG and alpha fetoprotein seen in some tumors have been associated with reduced sperm count and increased estradiol and prolactin levels [34, 35].
5. Induction of autoimmune mechanisms, e.g., anti-sperm antibodies, which may interrupt blood-testicular barriers.
6. Treatment of testicular cancer.

   (a) Surgical.

      (i) Unilateral orchiectomy reduces sperm count as reported by Rives et al. and Fossa et al. [36, 37]. Hansen et al. reported that 40% of patients were azoospermic oroligospermic 3 weeks after a unilateral orchiectomy [38].
      (ii) Retroperitoneal lymphadenectomy (RPLND) may also cause damage to thoracolumbar orthosympathetic pathways, which will then give rise to retrograde ejaculation or anejaculation. Consequently, this may lead to "de facto" physiological infertility.

   (b) Radiotherapy.

      (i) Germinal epithelium has a high proliferative index, making it one of the most radiosensitive tissues. Therefore, even low doses of radiation can cause significant tissue damage. To add to this, spermatogonia (spermatogonial stem cells) due to their high growth index are more radiosensitive than mature tissue [39].
      (ii) Fertility recovery after irradiation is considered a slow process, depending on the amount of doses administered, and requires a time of 9–18 months for doses below 1 Gy, while higher doses can result in permanent azoospermia [40].

(c) Chemotherapy.

Chemotherapy also destroys germinal epithelium because it acts on rapidly replicating cells, both cancerous and healthy, therefore causing tissue damage leading to oligo-azoospermia. The effect of chemotherapy on fertility is directly proportional to the cumulative dose of the drugs [41, 42]. A single course of carboplatin is a minimally invasive chemotherapy that has proven to be effective and is now increasingly indicated in stage 1 seminomas after orchiectomy instead of retroperitoneal lumbo-aortic prophylactic radiotherapy. It has been reported that this treatment preserves spermatogenesis and testosterone levels [43].

Prostate Cancer and Fertility

During radical prostatectomy, the vas deferens is occluded, and this causes permanent obstructive azoospermia, thus preventing natural fertility. The significant rates of erectile dysfunction in cases without nerve-sparing techniques are leaded to infertility and indirectly.

Prostatic radiotherapy may also cause hypogonadism due to the proximity of the testes to the prostate. Daniel et al. reported that after external radiotherapy on the prostate area, total and free testosterone levels decreased by 27% and 31% respectively [44].

Hormone therapy alone, or in combination with radiotherapy, generally produces azoospermia or severe oligospermia [45].

Chemotherapy with taxanes, for the most advanced forms of cancer, produces oligo-azoospermia [46].

Bladder Cancer and Fertility

Radical cystoprostatectomy, where there is removal of the prostate and seminal vesicles and the closure of the vas deferens, with possible damage to the neurovascular bundles, can lead to obstructive azoospermia. Neoadjuvant chemotherapy may cause cytotoxic sperm effects [47, 48].

Penile Cancer and Fertility

Partial or total penile amputations are usually done for invasive penile tumors (T2 or more). This interrupts sexual intercourse for the couple, thus affecting their fertility.

Genital HPV infection, which is considered a causal factor of penile cancer, may cause infertility via seminal HPV infection [49].

Kidney Cancer and Fertility

Kidney cancer may cause fertility indirectly via sexual dysfunction, as discussed earlier on sexual dysfunction and cancers.

The Association Between Infertility and Male Sexual Dysfunction Among Cancer Survivors

In a study by Liu et al., the prevalence of sexual dysfunction in the infertile group was higher compared to the control [50]. The authors found that male infertility was associated with an increase in the prevalence of sexual dysfunction, with the areas most affected being erectile function, orgasm, and sexual desire. Therefore, physicians involved in reproductive health and human sexuality should be aware of this problem in order to evaluate and treat patients to improve their quality of life and seek to avoid problems that may arise during diagnosis and treatment for infertility. The authors also recommended investigating the sexual function, general health, and psychological status of men in infertile couples, especially young men with azoospermia, to improve reproductive health, general health and sexual health. Guidance and monitoring must start with the diagnosis of infertility and continue until the end of the treatment period, including the process of assisted reproduction. Psychotherapy monitoring has also been recommended to minimize the occurrence of sexual dysfunction and improve the patient's quality of life [51]. Therefore, in order to increase the success rate of assisted reproductive treatments, we can improve their sexual and emotional relationships by providing couples with sexual dysfunction counseling and proposing treatment strategies that may be useful.

Inability to have a child has a negative impact on an individual's feelings, with couples describing the period of diagnosis and treatment of infertility as one of the most stressful periods of their lives [52]. Reproduction is closely connected with self-image, self-respect, and sexuality. Sexual intercourse, which is supposed to be spontaneous and erotic, loses this value because the main aim now becomes conception. The ability for intimate sexuality will be affected, and such changes in turn will provoke certain sexual dysfunctions [53, 54].

Management of infertility usually entails controlling the frequency and timing of sexual intercourse. This means that the usual intimate experience becomes regulated and controlled; giving couples the feeling that the medical team is also symbolically present during their most personal act [55]. The emotional impact of the diagnosis and forced and dictated sexual relations as part of the treatment and management of the problem usually compounds the problem of sexual dysfunction [56]. Interestingly, sexual dysfunction can be triggered by or cause infertility [57].

In a study by Song et al., the authors found that men's sexual function is more impaired during their partner's fertile period, which can be attributed to sexual anxiety; the most common sexual dysfunction reported was erectile dysfunction (50.9%) [58]. However, in another study, premature ejaculation was found to be the most common sexual dysfunction, concurring with results from another publication [59, 60].

Researchers have associated greater ED severity with worse semen parameters [61]. The European Society of Sexual Medicine (ESSM) recommends that phosphodiesterase type 5 inhibitors (PDE5is) can be safely used to treat ED among infertile men. It also noted that male partners of infertile couples are at higher risk of premature ejaculation (PE). Retrograde ejaculation (RE) and anejaculation are causes of infertility and can be managed with electroejaculation (EEJ) or penile vibratory stimulation (PVS) or, alternatively, with oral treatments. Low sexual desire has been reported by one-third of men of infertile couples.

In cancer patients, infertility often occurs because of anticancer therapies that impair spermatogenesis. This involves damage of testosterone-producing Leydig cells or local nerves, along with germ cell damage, all of which can be induced by chemotherapy and radiotherapy, as well as influenced by cancer localization, stage, and psychological factors. While some men recover their fertility after remission, others suffer from decreased sperm count and azoospermia. Fertility-preserving modalities can preserve spermatogenesis following cancer therapy. Patients who can ejaculate and have sperm in their semen should cryopreserve it. However, for patients who have never ejaculated before puberty or in whom spermatogenesis has not been established, a testis biopsy is performed to collect and preserve sperm or germ cells [62].

In a study by Frederick et al., it was shown that there was a strong psychological association between fertility and sexuality in which more than half of the included male childhood cancer survivors spontaneously expressed concerns about their fertility when asked about their sexual function [63].

Other studies found a higher incidence of male sexual dysfunction in patients suffering from anxiety disorders, in particular post-traumatic stress disorder (PTSD) [64–67]. Cancer has lately been recognized as one possible stressor inducing PTSD, with a prevalence of PTSD between 7 and 75% among cancer patients [68]. [Dahl AA, Østby-Deglum M, Oldenburg J et al. (2016) Aspects of posttraumatic stress disorder in long-term testicular cancer survivors: cross-sectional and longitudinal findings. J Cancer Surviv 10:842–849].

Strategy for Improvement

Strategies for improving oncofertility (cancer and fertility care) and oncosexology (cancer and sexual health) include multidisciplinary collaboration, enhanced patient education and counseling, advancements in reproductive technologies like in vitro follicle maturation and cryopreservation, and the integration of psychosocial and emotional support throughout the treatment and survivorship journey. Developing national guidelines, improving communication between healthcare providers and patients, and creating networks for sharing best practices are also key [69–71].

For Oncofertility

- Technological Advancements.
- Focus on improving cryopreservation methods for eggs and reproductive tissues and enhancing in vitro follicle maturation to achieve better results in preserving fertility.
- Multidisciplinary Care.
- Foster strong coordination and collaboration between oncologists, reproductive specialists, nurses, and patient navigators to provide comprehensive care.
- Improved Patient Communication and Education.
- Develop clear, culturally sensitive materials and decision aids to help patients understand their options and make informed choices about fertility preservation.
- Psychosocial Integration.
- Incorporate the psychosocial needs and well-being of cancer survivors into their overall fertility treatment plan and provide appropriate counseling resources.
- Policy and Access.
- Advocate for insurance and government policies to cover oncofertility services, ensuring improved funding, infrastructure, and access to these essential services.

For Oncosexology

- Provider Training and Education.
- Equip healthcare professionals with the knowledge and confidence to discuss sexual health concerns, provide counseling, and offer timely interventions for patients affected by cancer and its treatments.
- Standardized Care Pathways.

- Develop and implement integrated strategies and national guidelines that incorporate the sexual health needs of cancer patients from the time of diagnosis through survivorship.
- Access to Specialized Care.
- Ensure that patients have access to oncosexology specialists, psychologists, and other professionals who can provide tailored support for sexual health and intimacy issues.
- Supportive Resources.
- Provide patients with information, counseling services, and support groups to help them navigate the emotional, physical, and relational impacts of cancer on their sexuality.
- Research and Monitoring.
- Establish longitudinal studies and national registries to monitor the long-term effects of cancer treatments on sexual health and to evaluate the effectiveness of interventions.
- Overall Strategies for Both Fields
- Interdisciplinary Networks.
- Create and utilize networks for sharing best practices and resources across different oncofertility and oncosexology programs internationally.
- Addressing Barriers.
- Identify and implement strategies to overcome personal perspectives and barriers faced by healthcare providers when delivering fertility and sexual health care.
- Longitudinal Patient Monitoring.
- Implement frameworks for long-term monitoring to assess the impact of interventions and the ongoing needs of cancer survivors.

Future Directions

Future directions in oncosexology include improving patient access to sexual health resources and integrating sexual health education into routine oncology care, while oncofertility will focus on advancing fertility preservation techniques like in vitro maturation (IVM) of eggs, developing artificial ovaries, expanding oocyte and ovarian tissue cryopreservation, and further improving assisted reproductive technologies (ART) for survivors [70, 72].

Future Directions in Oncofertility

- *Enhanced Fertility Preservation Methods.*
- Research and development will continue to refine techniques for preserving fertility before cancer treatment.
  - *Ovarian Tissue Cryopreservation*: Continued refinement of this technique, which involves freezing ovarian tissue for later reimplantation and potential restoration of fertility.

  - *In Vitro Maturation (IVM)*: Further development of IVM to mature immature oocytes (eggs) in the lab and create viable embryos.
  - *Artificial Ovaries*: Research into the creation of functional artificial ovaries could offer new possibilities for fertility restoration.

- *Advancements in Assisted Reproductive Technologies (ART).*
- Improving ART techniques like IVF and IUI for cancer survivors, making them more successful and accessible.
- *Global Accessibility.*
- Efforts to make oncofertility services and fertility preservation options available to a wider range of patients worldwide, including those in underserved areas
- *Oncosexology Integration.*
- More closely linking oncosexology with oncofertility care to ensure that patients receive comprehensive support for both their reproductive and sexual health needs throughout and after cancer treatment.
- Future Directions in Oncosexology
- *Improved Patient Access and Screening.*
- Expanding access to specialized sexual health resources for cancer patients and integrating systematic sexual health screenings into routine cancer care.
- *Enhanced Education and Support.*
- Developing more comprehensive sexual health education materials and support services for patients and healthcare providers.
- *Personalized Care.*
- Tailoring sexual health interventions and support to the specific needs and concerns of individual patients, considering their cancer type, treatment, and personal preferences.
- *Addressing Psychosocial Aspects.*
- A greater focus on the psychological and emotional impacts of cancer and its treatment on sexual well-being and developing integrated support systems.
- *Research on Long-Term Effects.*

- Conducting more research to understand the long-term effects of various cancer treatments on sexual health and to develop effective, long-lasting interventions.

Conclusions

With advancements in cancer therapy, long-term survival rates have greatly improved. Hence, the protection and preservation of fertility in patients with malignant tumors has received increasing attention worldwide. Greater awareness among physicians is required regarding oncosexology and oncofertility. The Oncofertility Consortium, established in 2017, plays a major role in collaborating and training the next generation of oncofertility collaborators to undertake a multidisciplinary, multinational approach, as well as to engage all stakeholders, in order to ensure continued rapid transfer of sound science to quality medical practice.

References

1. Anastasiadis AG, Davis AR, Sawczuk IS, Fleming M, Perelman MA, Burchardt M, et al. Quality of life aspects in kidney cancer patients: data from a national registry. Support Care Cancer. 2003;11:700–6.
2. Christiansen RS, Azawi N, Højgaard A, Lund L. Informing patients about the negative effect of nephrectomy on sexual function. Turk J Urol. 2020;46:18–25.
3. Bessede T, Massard C, Albouy B, Leborgne S, Gross-Goupil M, Droupy S, et al. Sexual life of male patients with advanced renal cancer treated with angiogenesis inhibitors. Ann Oncol. 2011;22:2320–4.
4. Marcon J, Trottmann M, Rodler S, Becker AJ, Stief CG, Bauer RM, et al. Impact of antiangiogenic treatment on the erectile function in patients with advanced renal cell carcinoma. Andrologia. 2021;53:e13881.
5. Tsimafeyeu I, Zukov R, Demidov L, Borisov P, Kuznetsov V, Leonenko V, Bondarenko A, Zakurdaeva K, Tishova Y. Erectile dysfunction in patients with metastatic renal cell carcinoma. Ann Oncol. 2019;30(suppl_5):v718–46.
6. Catalona WJ, Carvalhal GF, Mager DE, Smith DS. Potency, continence and complication rates in 1,870 consecutive radical retropubic prostatectomies. J Urol. 1999;162:433–8.
7. Patel VR, Thaly R, Shah K. Robotic radical prostatectomy: outcomes of 500 cases. BJU Int. 2007;99:1109–12.
8. Messaoudi R, Menard J, Ripert T, Parquet H, Staerman F. Erectile dysfunction and sexual health after radical prostatectomy: impact of sexual motivation. Int J Impot Res. 2011;23:81–6.
9. Frey A, Sønksen J, Jakobsen H, Fode M. Prevalence and predicting factors for commonly neglected sexual side effects to radical prostatectomies: results from a cross-sectional questionnaire-based study. J Sex Med. 2014;11:2318–26.
10. Capogrosso P, Ventimiglia E, Serino A, Stabile A, Boeri L, Gandaglia G, et al. Orgasmic dysfunction after robot-assisted versus open radical prostatectomy. Eur Urol. 2016;70:223–6.
11. Guzle Adas Y, Kekilli E, Altundag MB. The evaluation of sexual functions of prostate cancer patients receiving radiotherapy. J BUON. 2021;26:2106–10.
12. Nahar B, Bhat A, Reis IM, Soodana-Prakash N, Becerra MF, Lopategui D, et al. Prospective evaluation of focal high intensity focused ultrasound for localized prostate cancer. J Urol. 2020;204:483–9.
13. Rischmann P, Gelet A, Riche B, Villers A, Pasticier G, Bondil P, et al. Focal high intensity focused ultrasound of unilateral localized prostate cancer: A prospective multicentric Hemiablation study of 111 patients. Eur Urol. 2017;71:267–73.
14. Ahmadi H, Daneshmand S. Androgen deprivation therapy: evidence-based management of side effects. BJU Int. 2013;111:543–8.
15. Tucci M, Leone G, Buttigliero C, Zichi C, DI Stefano RF, Pignataro D, et al. Hormonal treatment and quality of life of prostate cancer patients: new evidence. Minerva Urol Nefrol. 2018;70:144–51.
16. Romero FR, Romero KR, Mattos MA, Garcia CR, Fernandes Rde C, Perez MD. Sexual function after partial penectomy for penile cancer. Urology. 2005;66:1292–5.
17. Monteiro LL, Skowronski R, Brimo F, Carvalho PDC, Neto, Vasconcelos RAL, Pacheco CRCV, et al. Erectile function after partial penectomy for penile cancer. Int Braz J Urol. 2021;47:515–22.
18. Opjordsmoen S, Waehre H, Aass N, Fossa SD. Sexuality in patients treated for penile cancer: patients' experience and doctors' judgement. Br J Urol. 1994;73:554–60.
19. Smith AB, Butow P, Olver I, Luckett T, Grimison P, Toner GC, et al. The prevalence, severity, and correlates of psychological distress and impaired health-related quality of life following treatment for testicular cancer: a survivorship study. J Cancer Surviv 2016;10:223–233.
20. Rincones O, Smith A', Naher S, Mercieca-Bebber R, Stockler M. An updated systematic review of quantitative studies assessing anxiety, depression, fear of cancer recurrence or psychological distress in testicular cancer survivors. Cancer Manag Res. 2021;13:3803–16.

21. Adshead J, Khoubehi B, Wood J, Rustin G. Testicular implants and patient satisfaction: a questionnaire-based study of men after orchidectomy for testicular cancer. BJU Int. 2001;88:559–62.
22. Nazareth I, Lewin J, King M. Sexual dysfunction after treatment for testicular cancer: a systematic review. J Psychosom Res. 2001;51:735–43.
23. Guo P, Wang Y, Xie YF, Lv TB. Erectile dysfunction in nonmuscle-invasive bladder cancer patients before and after transurethral resection (TUR) of bladder tumor in China. Asian J Androl. 2022;24:509–12.
24. Mack D, Frick J. Quality of life in patients undergoing bacille Calmette-Guérin therapy for superficial bladder cancer. Br J Urol. 1996;78:369–71.
25. van der Aa MN, Steyerberg EW, Sen EF, Zwarthoff EC, Kirkels WJ, van der Kwast TH, et al. Patients' perceived burden of cystoscopic and urinary surveillance of bladder cancer: a randomized comparison. BJU Int. 2008;101:1106–10.
26. Sighinolfi MC, Micali S, De Stefani S, Mofferdin A, Ferrari N, Giacometti M, et al. Bacille Calmette-Guérin intravesical instillation and erectile function: is there a concern? Andrologia. 2007;39:51–4.
27. Miyao N, Adachi H, Sato Y, Horita H, Takahashi A, Masumori N, et al. Recovery of sexual function after nerve-sparing radical prostatectomy or cystectomy. Int J Urol. 2001;8:158–64.
28. Titta M, Tavolini IM, Dal Moro F, Cisternino A, Bassi P. Sexual counseling improved erectile rehabilitation after non-nerve-sparing radical retropubic prostatectomy or cystectomy--results of a randomized prospective study. J Sex Med. 2006;3:267–73.
29. Bessa A, Martin R, Häggström C, Enting D, Amery S, Khan MS, et al. Unmet needs in sexual health in bladder cancer patients: a systematic review of the evidence. BMC Urol. 2020;20:64.
30. Zietman AL, Sacco D, Skowronski U, Gomery P, Kaufman DS, Clark JA, et al. Organ conservation in invasive bladder cancer by transurethral resection, chemotherapy and radiation: results of a urodynamic and quality of life study on long-term survivors. J Urol. 2003;170:1772–6.
31. Moody JA, Ahmed K, Horsfield C, et al. Fertility preservation in testicular cancer – predictors of spermatogenesis. BJU Int. 2018;122:236–42.
32. Sharpe RM, Skakkebaek NE. Testicular dysgenesis syndrome: mechanistic insights and potential new downstream effects. Fertil Steril. 2008;89:e33–8.
33. Carroll PR, Whitmore WF Jr, Herr HW, et al. Endocrine and exocrine profiles of men with testicular tumors before orchiectomy. J Urol. 1987;137:420–3.
34. Hansen PV, Trykker H, Andersen J, et al. Germ cell function and hormonal status in patients with testicular cancer. Cancer. 1989;64:956–61.
35. de Bruin D, de Jong IJ, Arts EG, et al. Semen quality in men with disseminated testicular cancer: relation with human chorionic gonadotropin beta-subunit and pituitary gonadal hormones. Fertil Steril. 2009;91:2481–6.
36. Rives N, Perdrix A, Hennebicq S, et al. The semen quality of 1158 men with testicular cancer at the time of cryopreservation: results of the French National CECOS Network. J Androl. 2012;33:1394–401.
37. Fosså SD, Aabyholm T, Vespestad S, et al. Semen quality after treatment for testicular cancer. Eur Urol. 1993;23:172–6.
38. Hansen PV, Trykker H, Helkjoer PE, et al. Testicular function in patients with testicular cancer treated with orchiectomy alone or orchiectomy plus cisplatin-based chemotherapy. J Natl Cancer Inst. 1989;81:1246–50.
39. De Felice F, Marchetti C, Marampon F, et al. Radiation effects on male fertility. Andrology. 2019;7:2–7.
40. Maltaris T, Koelbl H, Seufert R, et al. Gonadal damage and options for fertility preservation in female and male cancer survivors. Asian J Androl. 2006;8:515–33.
41. Puscheck E, Philip PA, Jeyendran RS. Male fertility preservation and cancer treatment. Cancer Treat Rev. 2004;30:173–80.
42. Brydøy M, Fosså SD, Klepp O, et al. Sperm counts and endocrinological markers of spermatogenesis in long-term survivors of testicular cancer. Br J Cancer. 2012;107:1833–9.

43. Gandini L, Sgrò P, Lombardo F, et al. Effect of chemo- or radiotherapy on sperm parameters of testicular cancer patients. Hum Reprod. 2006;21:2882–9.
44. Daniell HW, Clark JC, Pereira SE, et al. Hypogonadism following prostate-bed radiation therapy for prostate carcinoma. Cancer. 2001;91:1889–95.
45. Boyd BG, McCallum SW, Lewis RW, et al. Assessment of patient concern and adequacy of informed consent regarding infertility resulting from prostate cancer treatment. Urology. 2006;68:840–4.
46. Chatzidarellis E, Makrilia N, Giza L, et al. Effects of taxane-based chemotherapy on inhibin B and gonadotropins as biomarkers of spermatogenesis. Fertil Steril. 2010;94:558–63.
47. Wallace WH, Anderson RA, Irvine DS. Fertility preservation for young patients with cancer: who is at risk and what can be offered? Lancet Oncol. 2005;6:209–18.
48. van Buul PP, Goudzwaard JH. Bleomycin-induced structural chromosomal aberrations in spermatogonia and bone-marrow cells of mice. Mutat Res. 1980;69:319–24.
49. Lyu Z, Feng X, Li N, et al. Human papillomavirus in semen and the risk for male infertility: a systematic review and meta-analysis. BMC Infect Dis. 2017;17:714.
50. Liu Y, Wang Y, Pu Z, Wang Y, Zhang Y, Dong C, Zeng Y, Zhou S. Sexual dysfunction in infertile men: a systematic review and meta-analysis. Sex Med. 2022 Aug;10(4):100528.
51. Gao J, Zhang X, Su P, et al. Relationship between sexual dysfunction and psychological burden in men with infertility: a large observational study in China. J Sex Med. 2013;10:1935–42.
52. aniluk JC, Koert E, Breckon E. Sexuality and infertility. In: Binik YM, Hall KSK, editors. Principles and practice of sex therapy. 5th ed. New York: The Guilford Press; 2014. p. 419–36.
53. Daniluk JC, Koert E, Breckon E. Sexuality and infertility. In: Binik YM, Hall KSK, editors. Principles and practice of sex therapy. 5th ed. New York: The Guilford Press; 2014. p. 419–36.
54. Piva I, Lo Monte G, Graziano A, Marci R. A literature review on the relationship between infertility and sexual dysfunction: does fun end with baby making? Eur J Contracept Reprod Health Care. 2014;19(4):231–7.
55. Braverman AM. Psychosocial aspect of infertility: sexual dysfunction. Int Congr Ser. 2004;1266:270–6.
56. Globevnik Velikonja V. Psihološko svetovanje ob neplodnosti. In: Vrtačnik Bokal E, Jančar N, editors. Sodobne oblike zdravljenja neplodnosti/IV spominski sestanek akad. prof. dr. Lidije An- dolšek-Jeras. Ljubljana: Slovensko društvo za reproduktivno medicine; 2007. p. 102–7.
57. Starc A, Trampuš M, Pavan Jukić D, Rotim C, Jukić T, Polona MA. Infertility and sexual dysfunctions: a systematic literature review. Acta Clin Croat. 2019 Sep;58(3):508–15.
58. Song SH, Kim DS, Yoon TK, Hong JY, Shim SH. Sexual function and stress level of male partners of infertile couples during the fertile period. BJU Int. 2016;117(1):173–6.
59. Bakhtiari A, Basirat Z, Aghajani Mir M. Sexual dysfunction in men seeking infertility treatment: the prevalence and associa- tions. Caspian J Reprod Med. 2015;1(3):2–6.
60. Wischmann TH. Sexual disorders in infertile couples. J Sex Med. 2010;7(5):1868–76.
61. Capogrosso P, Jensen CFS, Rastrelli G, et al. Male Sexual Dysfunctions in the Infertile Couple–Recommendations From the European Society of Sexual Medicine (ESSM). J Sex Med. 2021;9:100377.
62. Yumura Y, Takeshima T, Komeya M, Kuroda S, Saito T, Karibe J. Fertility and sexual dysfunction in young male cancer survivors. Reprod Med Biol. 2022;21:e12481.
63. Frederick NN, Recklitis CJ, Blackmon JE, Bober S. Sexual dysfunction in young adult survivors of childhood cancer. Pediatr Blood Cancer. 2016;63:1622–8.
64. Velurajah R, Brunckhorst O, Waqar M, et al. Erectile dysfunction in patients with anxiety disorders: a systematic review. Int J Impot Res. 2021; https://doi.org/10.1038/s41443-020-00405-4.
65. Bird ER, Piccirillo M, Garcia N, et al. Relationship between posttraumatic stress disorder and sexual difficulties: a systematic review of veterans and military personnel. J Sex Med. 2021;18:1398–426.
66. Wang S-C, Chien W-C, Chung C-H, et al. Posttraumatic stress disorder and the risk of erectile dysfunction: a nationwide cohort study in Taiwan : PTSD and erectile dysfunction. Ann General Psychiatry. 2021;20:48.

67. Bulut EC, Ertaş K, Bulut D, et al. The effect of COVID- 19 epidemic on the sexual function of healthcare professionals. Andrologia. 2021;53:e13971.
68. Dahl AA, Østby-Deglum M, Oldenburg J, et al. Aspects of posttraumatic stress disorder in long-term testicular cancer survivors: cross-sectional and longitudinal findings. J Cancer Surviv. 2016;10:842–9.
69. Ghaemi M, Rokhzadi I, Dashtkoohi M, Doosti M, Rezaeinejad M, Shariat M, Hantoushzadeh S, Keikha F, Eshraghi N, Fakehi M. Knowledge, attitudes, and practices of healthcare providers among women oncofertility in Iran: a cross-sectional study. BMC Cancer. 2024;24(1):1044.
70. Gupta D, Singh S, Shukla S, Shrivastava S. Oncofertility: treatment options from bench to bedside. Cancer Pathog Ther. 2023;1(4):284–9. https://doi.org/10.1016/j.cpt.2023.05.001. PMID: 38327602; PMCID: PMC10846294
71. Su HI, Lacchetti C, Letourneau J, Partridge AH, Qamar R, Quinn GP, Reinecke J, Smith JF, Tesch M, Wallace WH, Wang ET, Loren AW. Fertility preservation in people with cancer: ASCO Guideline Update. J Clin Oncol. 2025;43(12):1488–515. https://doi.org/10.1200/JCO-24-02782. Epub 2025 Mar 19. Erratum in: J Clin Oncol. 2025 May 20;43(15):1847. https://doi.org/10.1200/JCO-25-00662. Erratum in: J Clin Oncol. 2025 Aug;43(22):2553. https://doi.org/10.1200/JCO-25-01373. PMID: 40106739
72. Waimey KE, Duncan FE, Su HI, Smith K, Wallach H, Jona K, Coutifaris C, Gracia CR, Shea LD, Brannigan RE, Chang RJ, Zelinski MB, Stouffer RL, Taylor RL, Woodruff TK. Future directions in Oncofertility and fertility preservation: a report from the 2011 Oncofertility consortium conference. J Adolesc Young Adult Oncol. 2013;2(1):25–30. https://doi.org/10.1089/jayao.2012.0035. PMID: 23610740; PMCID: PMC3604786

Correction to: Post-Orgasmic Illness Syndrome: Systematic Review of the Literature

Omer A. Raheem, Marwan Alkassis, and Ayman Rashed

Correction to:
Chapter 9 in: R. Shah et al. (eds.), *Diagnosis and Treatment of Male Sexual Dysfunction*, https://doi.org/10.1007/978-3-032-12423-4_9

The original version of the chapter "**Chapter 9** – Post-Orgasmic Illness Syndrome: Systematic Review of the Literature" was inadvertently published with incorrect author details. The updated author details are listed below:

Current author order:
Omer A. Raheem
Marwan Alkassis

Updated author order:
Omer A. Raheem
Marwan Alkassis
Ayman Rashed

Affiliation of new author:
Urology Department
October 6th University, Cairo, Egypt

The updated version of this chapter can be found at
https://doi.org/10.1007/978-3-032-12423-4_9

R. Shah et al. (eds.), *Diagnosis and Treatment of Male Sexual Dysfunction*,
https://doi.org/10.1007/978-3-032-12423-4_16

Index

R. Shah et al. (eds.), *Diagnosis and Treatment of Male Sexual Dysfunction*,
https://doi.org/10.1007/978-3-032-12423-4

MIX
Papier aus verantwortungsvollen Quellen
Paper from responsible sources
FSC® C105338

If you have any concerns about our products,
you can contact us on
ProductSafety@springernature.com

In case Publisher is established outside the EU,
the EU authorized representative is:
Springer Nature Customer Service Center GmbH
Europaplatz 3, 69115 Heidelberg, Germany

Printed by Libri Plureos GmbH
in Hamburg, Germany